ADVANCED TECHNIQUES IN BONE REGENERATION

Edited by **Alessandro Rozim Zorzi** and **João Batista de Miranda**

Advanced Techniques in Bone Regeneration
http://dx.doi.org/10.5772/61425
Edited by Alessandro Rozim Zorzi and João Batista de Miranda

Contributors

ZuFu Lu, Yogambha Ramaswamy, Khoon S Lim, Hala Zreiqat, Hossein Ghanbari, Roghayyeh Vakili-Ghartavol, Carlo Galli, Anna Tampieri, Simone Sprio, Monica Sandri, Michele Iafisco, Silvia Panseri, Monica Montesi, Andrea Ruffini, Alessio Adamiano, Alberto Ballardini, Anca Hermenean, Sorina Dinescu, Mariana Ionita, Marieta Costache, Tomoki Aoyama, Orlando Chaparro, Itali Linero, Hans-Dieter Volk, Katharina Schmidt-Bleek, Christian H. Bucher, Hong Lei, Georg N. Duda, Inga Marijanovic, Alan Ivkovic, Igor Matic, Maja Antunovic, Marina Panek, Giorgio Maria Calori, Samit Nandi, Mohammed Elbadawi, James Meredith, Lynne Hopkins, Sultan Olmez, Carlos Vinicius Buarque De Gusmao, Jose Alves, William Dias Belangero, Eduardo José Mariotoni Bronzatto, Helder Groenwold Campos, Bruna Olivotti Lahan Martins, Daniel Miranda Ferreira

Published by InTech

Janeza Trdine 9, 51000 Rijeka, Croatia

Publishing Process Manager Sandra Bakic

Technical Editor SPi Global

Cover InTech Design team

First published August, 2016

Printed in Croatia

Additional hard copies can be obtained from orders@intechopen.com

Advanced Techniques in Bone Regeneration, Edited by Alessandro Rozim Zorzi and João Batista de Miranda

p. cm.

Print ISBN 978-953-51-2538-9
Online ISBN 978-953-51-2539-6

For EU product safety concerns:
IN TECH d.o.o., Prolaz Marije Krucifikse Kozulić 3, 51000 Rijeka, Croatia,
info@intechopen.com or visit our website at intechopen.com.

Meet the editors

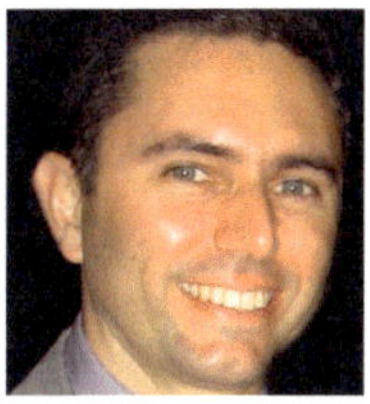

Dr. Alessandro Rozim Zorzi is an orthopedic surgeon at the State University of Campinas, Brazil, where he practices surgeries such as knee arthroscopy and total joint arthroplasties. He also develops didactic activities with medical students, orthopedic fellows, and postgraduates. He obtained MSc with a randomized clinical study on the use of bone grafting, and then later, he obtained PhD with an experimental study on regeneration of articular cartilage with the use of mesenchymal stem cells. He is the author of dozens of international publications such as original articles, review articles, and book chapters. He is also the editor of the book Bone Grafting of InTechOpen.

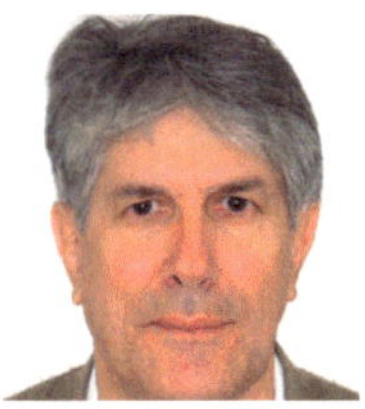

Professor João Batista de Miranda is the chairman of the Division of Knee Surgery and Inflammatory Diseases, at the Department of Orthopedic Surgery, Campinas State University (Unicamp), Brazil. He performs teaching activities with medical students, orthopedic fellows, and postgraduating researchers. He also develops research and clinical care. He is currently the superintendent of the Unicamp Teaching Hospital. Prof. Miranda obtained PhD with an experimental study on bone regeneration and on allografts. He has published several scientific articles in international journals and is coeditor of the book Bone Grafting of InTechOpen.

Contents

Preface

Bone is one of the few human tissues that has the ability to be completely regenerated after injury. Unlike other tissues, the majority of bony injuries heal without the formation of scar tissue, and bone is regenerated with its preexisting properties restored. The newly formed bone is eventually indistinguishable from the adjacent uninjured bone.

However, some situations compromise the regenerative capacity of the tissue, leading to the need for medical or dental intervention. There are conditions in which bone regeneration is required in large quantity, beyond the usual potential for self-healing, such as large bone defects created by trauma, infection, tumor resection, and skeletal abnormalities, or in cases in which the process is compromised, as in the avascular necrosis.

Although there are many techniques in use in clinical practice to deal with these problems, such as bone grafts, bone graft substitutes, and distraction osteogenesis, many of them still have limitations, making this field favorable to the emergence of new technologies.

The aim of this book is to present recent advances in this area, with chapters written by leading international researchers. The book is organized into three sections. The first part describes some of the techniques already available for clinical use nowadays. The second part presents the results of new research in the field and may be used in clinical practice in the near future. The third section deals specifically with research in tissue engineering, where major advances have occurred with the use of cells, scaffolds, and growth factors.

Alessandro Rozim Zorzi
Orthopedics and Traumatology Department,
Campinas State University (UNICAMP),
Brazil

João Batista de Miranda
Orthopedics and Traumatology Department,
Campinas State University (UNICAMP),
Brazil

Section 1

Clinical Approaches to Enhance Bone Regeneration

Chapter 1

Bone Regeneration: Current Status and Future Prospects

Hossein Ghanbari and Roghayyeh Vakili-Ghartavol

Additional information is available at the end of the chapter

http://dx.doi.org/10.5772/63912

Abstract

The ability of bone to heal with practically no scarring is the most extraordinary feature of it. However, perturbations of the fracture site could disrupt the repair process when defects reach a critical size, resulting in non-union. Current therapies include allografting, autografting, applying vascularized grafts, and other bone transport techniques. However, although commonplace in orthopaedic surgery, these treatments have some limitations.

Harvesting autografts is very expensive, typically from the iliac crest, associated with donor-site morbidity due to infection and haematoma and constrained by anatomical limitations. Allografts are limited by the possible risks of introducing infection or disease, while vascularized grafts are prohibitively expensive. So, due to technical difficulties and shortcoming of reconstructive surgery, the need for suitable fillers in large fracture reconstructive surgery is inevitable. Thus, recent tissue engineering approaches have been attempted to create new bone based on stem or precursor cells seeded onto biocompatible materials or scaffolds, with or without appropriate growth factors to improve clinical outcome. This chapter review the clinical necessity for tissue engineered bone, recent approaches attempting to create new bone, the main challenges of them and the novel strategies to overcome these barriers.

Keywords: bone fracture, regenerative medicine, stem cell, scaffold, growth factor, osteogenesis

1. Introduction

Reconstruction and regeneration of significant skeletal defects have amazed mankind for thousands of years. Grafting techniques were employed as early as 2000 BC when Khurits employed a piece of animal bone to reconstruct a small skull defect. In the modern age, Job van Meekeren, a Dutch surgeon, performed first documented bone graft in 1668. He utilized a xenograft to repair a skull defect in an injured soldier [1]. The understanding of orthopaedic science and bone grafts was further propelled in the seventeenth century by the work of Antoni van Leeuwenhoek who is famously known for his work on microscopy. Also, he primitively explained the microarchitecture of bone, what we now refer to as Haversian canals [2]. Hard-working examination of bone-grafting criteria and outcomes surfaced in the early 1900s by Vittorio Putti who determined the principles of grafting. Putti's work presented a foundation for grafting science in the orthopaedic field. Since then, researchers and surgeons have continued to smooth the science of bone grafting to allow for the most proper surgical intervention with the best outcomes [2, 3]. The current standard treatment is harvesting autologous grafts from other positions in the body (harvested primarily from the patient's iliac crest or other locations, such as the distal femur, proximal tibia, ribs and intramedullary canal) and transplantation into the massive fractures, or the transplantation of allografts, which have many obstacles, such as donor-site morbidity, limited tissue supply, infection, and poor integration [2, 4, 5]. Autografts are clinically approved therapies, which demonstrate the biological characteristics of osteogenesis, osteoconduction, and osteoinduction. Both grafts possess unique advantages and disadvantages; however, autografts gained desirability over allograft in the early 1900s with recognition of the advantage that vascularization provided to the integrity of the graft with the surrounding bone [6]. So, synthetic bone graft substitutes that were developed to overcome the inherent limitations of auto- and allograft represent an alternative strategy. These synthetic substitutes, or matrices, are made from a variety of materials, such as natural and synthetic polymers, ceramics, and composites that are designed to mimic the three-dimensional (3D) characteristics of autograft tissue while maintaining viable cell populations. Matrices also function as delivery vehicles for factors, chemotherapeutic agents, and antibiotics depending on the nature of the injury to be repaired. This junction of matrices, cells, and therapeutic molecules has collectively been termed tissue engineering (TE) [7]. Clinically, a bone regenerative therapeutic to treat patients must provide fundamental criteria, including safety, predictability, and reproducibility, in providing the clinical outcome. Also, as noted earlier, a tissue-regenerative therapy should exhibit four characteristics, including osteogenicity, osteoconductivity, osteoinductivity, and osteopromotivity [8, 9]. Osteogenesis refers to the process by which osteoprogenitor cells mature into osteoblasts, which subsequently mineralize and form bone tissue [9]. During osteoconduction process, bone formations occur on a surface. With respect to biomaterials, osteoconduction is defined by the ability of an implant to support the growth of bone at a defect site three dimensionally. Osteoinduction is the process of recruitment of immature osteoprogenitor cells to the site and the subsequent differentiation of them into osteoblasts under the influence of a diffusible bone morphogenetic factor. Finally, osteopromotion refers to the ability of a substance to enhance osteoinduction without being osteoinductive on its own [1, 9, 10].

2. Bone grafts

Fracture healing is performed based on a delicate balance between biology of fracture repair and biomechanical stability of fracture fixation, which are interrelated. Too many - attempts have been developing to minimize damage to the blood supply of the fracture blocks during surgery, but the sequential activation of cells and bioactive molecules necessary for fracture healing still remains disrupted. Moreover, a non-union often develops when this sequential activation is interfered. Some approaches suggested to overcome non-unions and some acute fractures include bone grafts and bone graft alternatives—specifically autologous bone grafts, allografts, synthetic bone grafts, and osteoinductive proteins. The ability of grafts to promote healing depends on their osteoconductive, osteoinductive, osteogenic, and osteopromotive qualities [11–13]. Each bone graft type and its alternative own some combination of these qualities. This section is going to compare benefits and potential limitations of available grafting strategies.

The iliac crest bone graft (ICBG), harvested from the anterior and posterior iliac crest, is the gold standard for cancellous autografts in cases in which fracture healing rather than void filling is needed. It is corticocancellous with osteoconductive, osteoinductive, and osteogenic effects. Also, the other benefit of ICBG is the availability of large amounts of bone without structural compromise to the extremity [14]. In a study, Takemoto et al. objected to consider whether there are variations in the expression of bone morphogenetic proteins (BMPs) and their receptors in different bone-graft-harvesting sites. They analysed autogenous marrow aspirates obtained from the iliac crest, the proximal humerus, and the proximal tibia for the mRNA levels of BMPs and their receptors. Their results suggested that ICBG is rich in colony-forming cells, and the number of progenitor cells directly promotes healing [15]. Despite the relative advantages of ICBG, it is not without disadvantages. The limitations, however, have been well documented in the literature and include donor-site morbidity, increased time in the operating room, and an increased length of hospital stay [16, 17]. So, for certain patients with compromised bone or inadequate volume for grafting, bone graft substitutes may be preferable.

Substitutes to bone grafting consist of bone bank allograft, osteoconductive materials, demineralized bone matrix (DBM), and osteoinductive proteins. The orthopaedic association has extensive experience with bone bank allograft, with the first clinical tissue bank opening in 1949 [18]. The main concerns of allografts include the risk of rejection, disease transmission, inconsistent incorporation, and late resorption. An alternative to bone bank allograft is DBM. DBM is made from an allograft with the inorganic materials removed. Researchers demonstrated that DBM implanted intramuscularly resulted in new bone formation [19]. Also, DBM has osteoconductive property but only weak osteoinductive feature. Furthermore, DBM offers an advantage over allografts or synthetic biomaterials that need incorporation by the host before they can support mechanical loads and would diminish the morbidity associated with harvesting autologous bone [20].

Synthetic osteoconductive materials have been widely used for bone graft in orthopaedic practice and include hydroxyapatite (HA), coralline hydroxyapatite, $CaSO_4$ and $CaPO_4$ cements, and collagraft [21]. Hydroxyapatite has a porous structure comparable to the cancellous bone and functions as an effective osteoconductive matrix and thus replicates the biological properties of bone extracellular matrix (ECM). The nominal composition of this mixture is $Ca_{10}(PO_4)_6(OH)_2$ with an atomic ratio for calcium-to-phosphate of 1.67 [22, 23]. Most studies have reported the mineralization and remodelling of this material can lead to the formation of mature bone [21]. Coralline hydroxyapatite is a similar substance, in which coral is converted to pure crystalline hydroxyapatite. It has good compressive strength but has low tensile strength and limited remodelling potential. Similar to hydroxyapatite, coralline hydroxyapatite functions strictly osteoconductive, but lacking osteogenic and osteoinductive properties. Calcium-based bone cements are osteoconductive and primarily used for filling metaphyseal defects. They possess sufficient compressive strength but lack resistance to shear and torsional forces and are very costly. They are also associated with resorption, leading to wound drainage [21]. The situations in which osteoinduction is the primary concern, BMPs are available. Detailed insights into BMPs will be provided later.

3. Molecular aspects of fracture healing

Fracture healing is a complex physiological process. Cascade of complex biological events involving intracellular and extracellular molecular signalling for bone induction and conduction remain unknown to a great extent. Indeed, it is a multistep repair process that follows a determined spatial and temporal sequence [24–26]. It was clearly demonstrated that known molecular mechanisms that regulate skeletal tissue formation during embryological development are replicated during the fracture-healing process [27]. Many growth and differentiation factors (GDFs), such as cytokines, hormones, and extracellular matrix, are local and systemic regulatory factors that interact with various cell types, including bone- and cartilage-forming primary cells, or even muscle mesenchymal cells, recruited at the fracture site or from the circulation. Advances in understanding cellular and molecular mechanisms will provide the tools for discovering the fracture-healing process. This section aims to contribute to promoting and inhibiting fracture healing and to prepare awareness of the complexity of involved signalling pathways.

3.1. Biology of fracture healing

The nature of the repair phase is dependent on mechanical conditions in the fracture-healing zone (primary or secondary bone healing) and the anatomical location of the fracture (metaphyseal-epiphyseal trabecular bone healing or diaphyseal callus healing). Indeed, fracture healing is a complex process, resulting in optimal skeletal repair and restoration of skeletal function. However, it is a well-orchestrated, regenerative process, which is initiated in response to injury. Repair process is promoted by the normal pathway of embryonic development repeated with the coordinated participation of several cell types [28]. Depending on several parameters involved in the fracture site, such as growth factors, nutrients, hormones, and oxygen tension, pH, the mechanical stability and the electrical environment, various components present at the injured tissue, such as the cortex, the periosteum, the external soft tissues and the bone marrow, contribute to the healing process [29–31]. Classical histology has divided fracture healing into direct (primary) and indirect (secondary) mode.

Direct strategy (known as primary cortical bone healing) occurs only when there is extremely low interfragmentary movement or if the bony fragments are under compression [32]. Most often compression plates and lag screws provide the required stability for direct healing [33]. Similar to the normal bone-remodelling process, fracture surfaces in contact and under compression are bridged by Haversian systems (or osteons) when such stability is achieved. Indeed, primary process involves a direct attempt by the cortex to regenerate new Haversian systems by the formation of discrete remodelling units known as 'cutting cones', in order to restore mechanical continuity [34]. Osteoclasts digest bone, causing tunnels from one side of the fracture to the other, which provides the in-growth of blood vessels. Subsequently, vascular endothelial cells and perivascular mesenchymal cells prepare the osteoprogenitor cells to differentiate into osteoblasts which create new osteons connecting both fragments [35, 36]. Healing by Haversian systems is slow, and notable time is necessary to gain sufficient strength by healing zone and, therefore, allow removal of load-bearing implants. Also, because it is not associated with a major influx of inflammatory cells, primary bone healing is less affected by systemic inflammation [37].

Another type of fracture healing is *indirect mode* that heals the majority of fractures. This mode of fracture healing occurs by either intramembranous ossification or endochondral ossification with the subsequent formation of a callus [38, 39]. This mode is usually enhanced by motion and inhibited by rigid fixation [38].

Intramembranous ossification forms bone directly without first forming cartilage. Migrated mesenchymal stromal cells that reside in the periosteum directly differentiate into osteoblasts that synthesize and deposit bone matrix. This process results in callus formation, characterized histologically as 'hard callus' [40]. In this type of healing, the bone marrow contribute to bone formation during the early phase of healing, when endothelial cells transform into polymorphic cells that subsequently express an osteoblastic phenotype [12]. Advanced studies have shown that flat bones such as bones from the skull, trabecular bones, and clavicle heal via intramembranous ossification [41].

By contrast, endochondral ossification involves the recruitment, proliferation, and differentiation of undifferentiated mesenchymal cells into a transient cartilaginous matrix, which calcifies into mature bone. This type of fracture healing is advocated to have the following identifiable stages: (1) an initial stage of haematoma formation and inflammation, (2) subsequent angiogenesis and formation of cartilage, (3) cartilage calcification, (4) cartilage removal, (5) bone formation, and (6) ultimately bone remodelling [42]. Also, it is contributed from the adjacent to the fracture periosteum and the external soft tissues, providing an early bridging callus, histologically described as 'soft callus' that stabilizes the fracture fragments [40]. Many studies have shown that diaphyseal fractures heal by endochondral mechanisms, forming a cartilaginous callus intermediate [41].

The classification of fracture healing into direct and indirect forms reflects the histological events that happen during the repair process. However, it is necessary to provide a further understanding of various signalling molecules and elucidate their contribution in the initiation and control of this physiological event at the molecular level.

3.2. Signalling molecules in bone regeneration and fracture repair

Various types of signalling factors influence the fracture healing, and continuous study of these factors can lead to promising new clinical treatments for bone repairing. To date, the delivery of signalling molecules for bone regeneration has been based primarily on factors that directly affect the bone formation pathways (osteoinduction) or that apply to increase the number of bone-forming progenitor cells. Overall, the signalling molecules can be classified into three groups, including the pro-inflammatory cytokines, the transforming growth factor-β (TGF-β) superfamily and other growth factors, and the angiogenic factors [43].

3.2.1. Pro-inflammatory cytokines

Pro-inflammatory cytokines, such as Interleukin-1 (IL-1), IL-6, IL-11, IL-18 and tumour necrosis factor-α (TNF-α), are critical for triggering the repair cascade [44]. They are secreted by macrophages, inflammatory cells, and cells of mesenchymal origin existing in the periosteum [43, 45, 46]. These molecules play key roles in the induction of downstream mediators to the fracture site by exerting a chemotactic effect on other inflammatory cells, augmenting ECM synthesis, stimulating angiogenesis, and recruiting endogenous fibrogenic cells to injury [47]. Furthermore, cytokines were found to regulate endochondral bone formation and remodelling [43, 47]. For example, TNF-α recruits mesenchymal stem cells (MSCs), promotes the induction of apoptosis in hypertrophic chondrocytes during endochondral ossification and incites osteoclastic function. Also, IL-1 mainly provided by osteoblasts and simplifies bone remodelling by stimulating proteases to degrade callus tissue [46]. The absence of TNF-α results in delayed resorption of mineralized cartilage, delayed endochondral bone formation by several weeks, and impaired fracture healing. Several studies have demonstrated that TNF-α signalling is unique to postnatal fracture repair [46].

3.2.2. Growth and differentiation factors

3.2.2.1. Transforming growth factor-β superfamily

It is a large group of regulatory polypeptides that includes bone morphogenetic proteins (BMPs), multiple isoforms of transforming growth factor-βs (TGF-βs), growth and differentiation factors (GDFs), activins (ACTs), inhibins (INHs), and glial-derived neurotrophic factors (GDNFs), as well as some proteins not included in the above families, such as Mullerian-inhibiting substance (MIS), also known as anti-Mullerian hormone (AMH), left-right determination factor (Lefty), and nodal growth differentiation factor (Nodal) (**Figure 1**) [48, 49]. Their isolation from bone extracts and further gene identification was accomplished in the 1980s, based on the previous results by Marshall R. Urist [19]. Transforming growth factor-β family encompasses at least 34 members in the human genome. These molecules originate from high-molecular-weight precursors, which are activated by proteolytic degradation. They can activate serine/threonine kinase membrane receptor on target cells. TGF-β ligand-bound receptor triggers an intracellular signal transmission via a canonical signalling pathway, which ultimately affects gene expression in the nucleus [47].

http://dx.doi.org/10.5772/63912

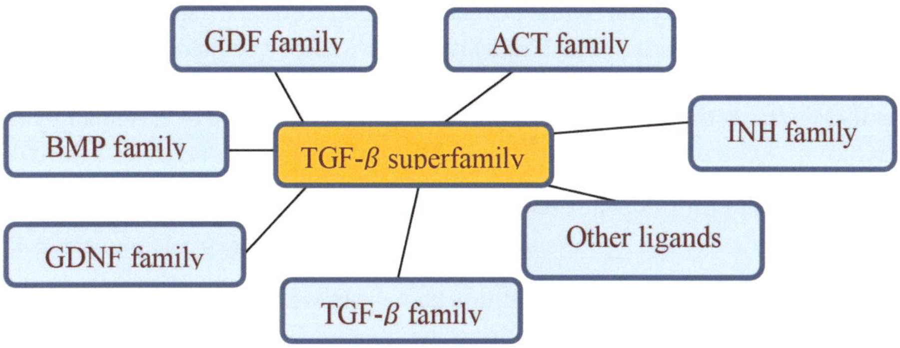

Figure 1. A schematic illustration of TGF-β superfamily. BMPs: bone morphogenetic proteins, TGF-β: transforming growth factor beta, GDF: growth and differentiation factor, GDNF: glial-derived neurotrophic factors, ACT: activin, INH: inhibin, other ligands include Mullerian-inhibiting substance (MIS) or anti-Mullerian hormone (AMH), left-right determination factor (Lefty), and nodal growth differentiation factor (Nodal).

Several members of the subfamilies of these morphogens including bone morphogenetic proteins (BMPs 1–8), growth and differentiation factors (GDF-1, 5, 8, 10) and transforming factor β (TGF-β1, TGF-β2, TGF-β3), have been shown to promote the various stages of intramembranous and endochondral bone ossification during fracture healing (the following parts provide details on the use of them in attempts at bone regeneration) [24]. Of course, it is difficult to determine the physiological role of many of the members of this superfamily because of their functional redundancy.

Bone morphogenetic proteins are secreted signalling molecules that belong to the TGF-β superfamily, acting as potent regulators during embryogenesis and bone and cartilage formation and repair. BMP ligands are divided into at least four separate subfamilies depending on their primary amino acid sequence similarity and functions [50]. The first group consists of BMP-2, BMP-4, and the second group includes BMP-5, BMP-6, and BMP-7. Group three includes GDF-5 (or BMP-14), GDF-6 (or BMP-13) and GDF-7 (or BMP-12), and finally, group four consists of BMP-3 (or osteogenin) and GDF-10 (or BMP-3b) [51, 52]. BMP-1 does not include in this list as a member of the TGF-β superfamily and it may carry out a role in modulating BMP functions by the proteolysis of BMP antagonists/binding proteins, such as chondrin and noggin [47, 53].

BMPs bind to type-II serine/threonine kinase receptors and thus provoke the assembly of type-I and type-II receptors in a hetero-oligomeric complex [54]. Subsequently, the Smad-signalling cascade is triggered into the cell. BMPs are pleiotropic morphogens and carry out an important role in regulating growth, differentiation, and apoptosis of various cell types, including osteoblasts, chondroblasts, epithelial cells, and neural cells [55]. Furthermore, it has been demonstrated that the active signalling molecule is usually formed by homodimerization through a disulphide bond [56]. However, in particular, experimental settings heterodimers have been shown to have enhanced osteoinductive activity regulating more efficiently differentiation and proliferation of mesenchymal cells to osteoblasts *in vitro* and *in vivo* than the corresponding homodimers (i.e., BMP-2/-5, BMP-4/-7, BMP-2/-6; BMP-2/-7) [57, 58]. In bone, BMPs are produced by different types of cells, including osteoprogenitors, mesenchymal cells, osteoblasts, and chondrocytes. BMPs are able to induce a sequential cascade of events for chondro-osteogenesis, including mesenchymal and osteoprogenitor cells proliferation and differentiation, chemotaxis, angiogenesis, and controlled synthesis of extracellular matrix [53, 55].

Regulatory effect of BMPs depends on the type of the targeted cell, its differentiation stage, the local concentration of the ligand and the interaction with other circulating factors [59].

BMPs are closely related structurally and functionally; however, each has a unique role and different temporal expression pattern during the fracture healing. The researchers demonstrated in several studies that BMPs could have a variety of osteogenic effects, mitogenic capacities, and temporal expressions in the rat and mouse [24, 60, 61].

Cheng et al. prepared a comprehensive analysis of the osteogenic activity of 14 types of BMPs and their results suggested an osteogenic hierarchical model of BMPs. BMP-2, BMP-6, and BMP-9 may act as the most potent to induce osteoblast differentiation of mesenchymal progenitor cells, while most BMPs (except BMP-3 and BMP-13) promote the terminal differentiation of committed osteoblastic precursors and osteoblasts [62]. Furthermore, BMPs are able to stimulate the synthesis and secretion of other bone and angiogenic growth factors such as insulin-like growth factor (IGF) and vascular endothelial growth factor (VEGF), respectively and also stimulate bone formation by directly activating endothelial cells to stimulate angiogenesis [63].

Recent studies have shown that the expression of the BMP antagonists, most importantly noggin, plays an important role in fracture healing regulation [64]. They could block BMP-2 interaction with its receptor [65].

Transforming growth factor-β family includes five isoforms such as TGF-β1, TGF-β2, and TGF-β3 [66, 67]. The main sources of TGF-β existing during the bone healing are practically all cells involved in healing process, incoming blood platelets, and the surrounding ECM releasing TGF-β following a mechanical injury causing tissue ischaemia and local change in pH, facilitating release of not only of TGF-β, but also other growth factors, such as VEGF, platelet-derived growth factor (PDGF), or BMP-2 [68, 69]. Intracellular signal transduction is exerted via type-I and type-II serine/threonine kinase receptors, activating the Smad cascade (Smad 2 and 3) [70]. TGF-β is a potent chemotactic stimulator of mesenchymal stem cells and it enhances proliferation of MSCs, preosteoblasts, chondrocytes, and osteoblasts. Indeed, its main role is thought to be during processes of proliferation, differentiation, and synthesis of cartilage and bone tissue, collectively mentioned as the bone-healing process [67, 71]. Also, it is able to induce the production of extracellular proteins, such as proteoglycans, fibronectin, collagen, osteonectin, osteopontin, thrombospondin, and alkaline phosphatase [72]. Moreover, TGF-β may trigger signalling for BMP synthesis by the osteoprogenitor cells, while it may inhibit activation, proliferation, and differentiation of osteoclasts and promote their apoptosis [60, 73].

http://dx.doi.org/10.5772/63912

Several studies have shown that TGF-β2 and possibly TGF-β3 had stronger effect in fracture-healing process than TGF-β1, as their expression peak during chondrogenesis. On the other hand, Joyce et al. injected TGF-β1 and TGF-β2 subperiosteally to newly born rats, at doses ranging from 20 to 200 ng, and their results showed that subperiosteal MSC starts to proliferate and differentiate at the injection site, promoting chondrogenesis and osteogenesis, and that TGF-β2 play more important roles than TGF-β1 [74]. Moreover, Beck et al., designed an experiment concerning local administration of TGF-β1 at doses ranging from 0.5 to 5 μg to rabbits with skull defect, caused stimulation, recruitment, and proliferation of osteoblasts at the defect site resulting in healing [75]. Despite different studies demonstrated that TGF-β induces cellular proliferation, its osteoinductive potential is limited by concern for its unforeseen side effects [71].

Platelet-derived growth factors (PDGFs) are homo- or heterodimeric polypeptides in which their A and B chains are linked by disulphide bonds. PDGF receptors exert their effect on cells by activating receptors that have tyrosine kinase activity [76]. PDGF's binding is affected by IL-1, TNF-a, and TGF-β1 affect [77]. It is synthesized by numerous cell types, including platelets, monocytes, macrophages, osteoblasts, and endothelial cells and is a major mitogen for cells of mesenchymal origin such as osteoblasts, fibroblasts, glial cells, and smooth muscle cells [78–80].

PDGF is released by platelets upon activation during the early callus phase of healing and acts as a potent chemotactic for inflammatory cells and a major proliferative and migratory stimulus for MSCs and osteoblasts. It has been demonstrated that treating with PDGF increased callus density and volume in tibial osteotomies in rabbits [47, 81]. However, its therapeutic potential still remains unclear.

Fibroblast growth factors (FGFs) consist of nine structurally related polypeptides. The acidic and basic FGFs are the most abundant FGFs in normal adult tissue [82]. FGF effect is exerted via binding to tyrosine kinase receptors [82].

FGFs are synthesized by monocytes, macrophages, osteoblasts, mesenchymal cells, and chondrocytes during bone healing. FGFs are able to induce growth and differentiation of a variety of cells, such as fibroblasts, osteoblasts, myocytes, and chondrocytes. They function during the early stages of fracture healing and play a critical role in angiogenesis and mesenchymal cell mitogenesis. α-FGF mainly affects chondrocyte proliferation and is probably crucial for chondrocyte maturation, while β-FGF is produced by osteoblasts and is recognized as a potent mitogen than a-FGF [71]. In a canine tibial osteotomy model, a single injection of FGF-2 resulted in an early increase in callus size [83].

Insulin-like growth factors (IGFs) consist of IGF-I (or somatomedin-C) and IGF-II (or skeletal growth factor) [84]. The sources of IGF-I and IGF-II are the bone matrix, osteoblasts and chondrocytes, and endothelial cells. The concentration of circulating IGF-I is mainly regulated by the growth hormone. Also, it has been demonstrated that the biological actions of IGFs is modulated in a cell-specific manner by IGF-binding proteins (IGFBPs) [71, 85].

IGF-I promotes bone matrix formation such as type-I collagen and non-collagenous matrix proteins by fully differentiated osteoblasts and acts more effective than IGF-II [71, 86]. IGF-II functions at a later stage of endochondral bone formation and incites type-I collagen production, cellular proliferation cartilage matrix synthesis [87]. The findings from various animal studies assessing the influence of IGF on skeletal repair have reported different results, so further studies are required [88].

3.2.3. Metalloproteinases and angiogenic factors

Conditions of fracture healing establish a demand on the surrounding tissues to increase blood flow so that can induce bone regeneration within the callus [89]. Also, endochondral ossification in normal fracture healing requires the following two processes: (1) molecular mechanisms that regulate the extracellular matrix remodelling and (2) the vascular penetration of new blood vessels into the resorbing matrix [90]. Thus, angiogenesis and matrix degradation are either concurrent or correlated processes during endochondral ossification. The final stages of endochondral ossification and bone remodelling are accomplished by the action of specific matrix metalloproteinases, which degrade the cartilage and bone, allowing the invasion of the blood vessels. Angiogenesis regulation requires the coordination of both separate pathways, including a vascular endothelial growth factor (VEGF)-dependent pathway and an angiopoietin-dependent pathway [91]. Numerous types of studies reported that VEGFs are required mediators of endothelial-cell-specific mitogens and neo-angiogenesis [92]. Whereas angiopoietin 1 and 2 are regulatory vascular morphogenetic molecules related to the formation of larger vessel and development of colateral branches from present vessels [43]. Street et al. showed that exogenous administration of VEGF can induce fracture repair [48]. Also, recent studies have reported that BMPs promote the expression of VEGF by osteoblasts and osteoblast-like cells. However, their contribution in bone repair is still not as well understood.

3.3. Role of mesenchymal stem cells in bone regeneration and fracture repair

Mesenchymal stem cells (MSCs) are non-haematopoietic stromal stem cells capable of extensive replication without differentiation. They have many sources including bone marrow, peripheral circulation, adipose, periosteum, muscle, vessel walls, tendon, umbilical cord blood, skin, and dental tissues. MSCs have the potential to commit and differentiate along several cell lineages giving rise to those cells that form mesenchymal tissues, including cartilage, bone, muscle, ligament, tendon, and marrow stroma and fat [93, 94]. MSCs can migrate to sites of injury and have been used widely in tissue engineering, stem cell transplantation and immunotherapy. There are different sets of molecules interacting with both local cells and circulating cells to coordinate the healing cascade, such as effectors of inflammation (IL-1, IL-6, TNF-a), mitogens (TGF-β, IGF, FGF, and PDGF), morphogens (BMPs), and angiogenic factors (VEGF and angiopoietins). The effects of these molecules on the proliferation and differentiation of MSCs have been widely investigated *in vitro* [47]. The results indicated that these signalling molecules can induce cell proliferation and differentiation, both MSC and other progenitor lineages. The temporal expression of this array of signalling molecules in models of fracture healing has been charted, but explicit data on how this microenvironment can regulate MSC activity is still needed.

4. Tissue engineering strategies for bone regeneration

As it was defined by Laurencin, tissue engineering (TE) is 'the application of biological, chemical, and engineering principles toward the repair, restoration, or regeneration of living tissue by using biomaterials, cells, and factors alone or in combination' [95].

Bone tissue engineering (BTE) is a dynamic and complex process that includes migration and recruitment of osteoprogenitor cells, followed by their proliferation, differentiation, matrix formation along with remodelling of the bone. In this section, we consider BTE as three interplaying components: (a) the extracellular matrix/scaffold, (b) the cells that reside in the matrix/scaffold, and (c) the environment that hosts the cells. However, major advances in BTE with scaffolds are achieved through biochemical factors, such as growth factors, genes, proteins, and drugs. Bone scaffolds are typically made of porous-degradable materials that prepare the mechanical support during repair and regeneration of diseased or damaged bone [7]. Also, physical factors, including substrate topography, stiffness, shear stress, and electrical forces, are other stimuli that have been proposed as one of the principal mediators of de novo tissue formation [96]. Box 1 highlights requirements for an ideal scaffold.

4.1. Biomolecule delivery

The strategy of concurrently modulating the chemical environments of the fracture site *in vivo* via controlled delivery/elution of biomolecule agents from an orthopaedic implant represents an elegant method of targeted therapeutics in bone regeneration [97, 98]. This strategy enables higher local concentration (localized delivery) of the bioactive agent to the fracture site, while the favourable bulk properties of the orthopaedic implant are unchanged. It also provides the chance to maximize the local growth-inducing potentials of bioactive agents at a desired rate without any local and systematic toxic effects to the host tissue that is attributed to other routes of delivery such as systemic or non-controllable local delivery. Soluble biochemical molecules that are integrated into scaffolds include proteins/growth factors, such as TGF-β, BMP, VEGF, IGF, and FGF, which have attracted much attention because of their potency in bone tissue repair. As described earlier, these growth factors are able to control osteogenesis, bone tissue regeneration, and ECM formation via recruiting and differentiating MSCs (osteoprogenitor) to specific lineages [99]. Therefore, various growth factors and other biomolecules are of special interest for bone tissue engineering and effective incorporation of them in scaffolds could reduce fracture healing time and thus facilitate in patient recovery [100, 101]. Also, bone is a highly vascularized tissue; therefore, the performance of a scaffold in bone engineering can be affected by its ability to induce new blood vessel formation. Because insufficient vascularization can lead to oxygen and nutrient deficiency, this may result in improper cell integration and cell death [102, 103]. On the other hand, in the *in vivo* conditions, supply of oxygen and nutrients are essential for the survival of growing cells and tissues within scaffolds. So, VEGF is used to induce a complex network of blood vessels throughout a scaffold [104].

Box 1. Requirements for an ideal scaffold

Biocompatibility is one of the primary requirements of bone scaffolds. It is a term that has been defined in many ways. Biocompatibility can be principally defined as the ability of scaffold to support normal cellular activity, such as molecular signalling pathways, without any local and systematic toxic effects to the host tissue [105]. An ideal bone scaffold must act as an osteoconductive substrate such that it permits the bone cells to adhere, proliferate, and form ECM on its surface and pores. Furthermore, the scaffold needs to induce bone formation within the defect through signalling systems and recruiting progenitor cells, a feature known as osteoinduction. Also, an ideal scaffold should be able to serve as a platform for formation of blood vessels in or around the implant during few weeks of implantation to promote nutrients and metabolic waste transportation [106].

Mechanical properties: An ideal bone scaffold should yield a close match to the host bone properties and also convenient load transfer is important. Mechanical properties of bone vary widely from cancellous to cortical bone. Cortical bone exhibits a Young's modulus between 15 and 20 GPa and that of cancellous bone is between 0.1 and 2 GPa. Compressive strength of cortical bone is between 100 and 200 MPa, and between 2 and 20 MPa for cancellous bone. Because of the large variation in mechanical property and geometry, it is difficult to design an 'ideal scaffold' for BTE [106].

Pore size and closed void volumes may concurrently play important roles in scaffold degradation patterns and associated bone healing [107]. It should be approximately 100 μm in diameter for successful cellular infiltration and nutrient and oxygen supply for cell survivability [102]. However, scaffolds with pore sizes between 200 and 350 μm are indicated to be optimum for bone tissue in-growth [108]. Moreover, recent papers have reported that multi-scale porous scaffolds which involve both micro- and macroporosities can act better than only macroporous scaffolds [109]. Unfortunately, porosity can reduce mechanical properties, such as compressive strength, and also increase the complexity for reproducible scaffold making. Researchers have developed porous scaffolds using polymers, ceramics, metals, and composites. Strength of different polymers matches close to the cancellous bone and dense bioceramic materials to that of cortical bone. However, scaffolds manufacturing ceramic-polymer composite are typically weaker than bone. Porous metallic scaffolds provide the mechanical necessities of bone, but fail to meet the required implant-tissue integration and also, there is potential concern regarding metal ion leaching [110].

Bioresorbability is another crucial requirement for scaffolds in BTE [105]. In addition to similar mechanical properties that of the host tissue, an ideal scaffold should be able to degrade with time *in vivo* by cellular and enzymatic activity, preferably at a controlled resorption rate in parallel with the production of new bone matrix. The degradation behaviour of the scaffolds is determined based on their applications; for example, 3–6 months for scaffolds in cranio-maxillofacial applications or 9 months or more for scaffolds in spinal fusion. Recently, design and development of multi-scale porous scaffolds having ideal composition, including related bioresorbability, targeted biomolecules, and mechanical properties are some challenging areas of research [106, 111].

4.2. Stem/progenitor cells applicable to bone tissue engineering

4.2.1. Mesenchymal stem cells

Mesenchymal stem cells have been isolated from a diverse host tissues throughout the adult organism including bone marrow [94] and an array of other postnatal tissues, such as adipose tissue [112], periodontal ligaments [113], synovium [114], blood [115] and the lung [116]. As the ultimate aim of regenerative medicine is to avoid *in vitro* expansion of cells and the associated complications, the adipose-derived stem cell indicates an ideal progenitor cell in bone tissue engineering.

Intriguingly, several studies have reported that 6×10^6 nucleated cells can be isolated from 1 mL bone marrow of which 0.001–0.01% are considered to be stem cells [94]. Contrastingly, adipose tissue aspiration yields 2×10^6 nucleated cells per 1 g, of which 10% are stem cells. Thus, one can easily distinguish the potential clinical implications of this abundant source of MSCs [117, 118]. In a study, researchers compared the in vivo osteogenic potential of adipose-derived, bone marrow-derived, and periosteal-derived MSCs in a guided bone regeneration model in pig calvarial defects to identify if there is a more desirable site from which to harvest MSCs for bone tissue engineering. They reported that regardless of the tissue source of MSCs, the speed and pattern of bone healing after cell transplantations into monocortical bone defects were comparable, indicating that the performance of autologous adipose-derived MSCs, periosteal-derived MSC, and bone marrow-derived MSC (BM-MSCs) following *ex vivo* cell expansion was not considerably different for the guided regeneration of bone defects [119].

4.2.2. Endothelial progenitor cells

Vascularization is a vital process for the survival of the implanted cells on the carrier material after implantation. Many studies demonstrated that close spatial and temporal association between blood vessels and bone cells is necessary to maintain skeletal integrity. Several studies have shown that new bone formation in porous scaffolds was considerably increased by the insertion of a vascular pedicle in the scaffold, while others have shown that fracture healing and new bone formation could be prohibited by the administration of angiogenesis inhibitors. Such that previous reports illustrated that the rate of delayed union or non-union of fracture can be as high as 46% in fracture patients with concomitant vascular injuries [120]. Because adequate vascularization making it possible to stem cells reach the site of tissue repair and allows the delivery of nutrients, oxygen, and morphogens and the removal of waste [121–124].

In 1997, Asahara and colleagues identified endothelial progenitor cells (EPCs) in the peripheral blood and reported their ability to initiate neovascularization [125]. EPC derived from purified hematopoietic progenitor cells, express endothelial-associated markers (i.e., cluster of differentiation molecule, CD34) and display endothelial phenotypical characteristics. They can enhance neovascularization by incorporation and differentiation, and by the secretion of angiogenic factors affecting resident endothelium [126].

The major role of EPCs in the ability of EPCs to proliferate and differentiate into endothelial cells and new vessel formation present them as an ideal therapeutic strategy for recovery of the ischemic environment of a critical-sized bone defect in bone tissue engineering. Furthermore, a research group reported that the frequency of EPCs increased in the bone marrow and peripheral blood in the early stages of fracture repair and further illustrated incorporation of EPCs into developing blood vessels at the site of bone injury. Further histological results demonstrated that neovascularization did not exclusively involve the EPC population; however, supporting the hypothesis that paracrine signalling from EPCs may also contribute to neovascularization at the ischemic site [127].

4.2.3. Induced pluripotent stem cells

Induced pluripotent stem (iPS) cells, a discovery that resulted in a Nobel Prize in 2012, are somatic cells from embryonic or adult fibroblasts that are reprogrammed with defined classical transcription factors (Oct4, Sox2, Klf4, and c-Myc) [121, 128]. By forcing expression of these transcription factors, iPS cells retain the capacities of embryonic stem cells, including self-renewal and pluripotentiality to differentiate into all three germ layers [129]. Using these biological properties, iPS cells with an incorporation of gene therapy will be able to not only treat degenerative syndromes and genetic disorders but also appear as a promising candidate for autologous cell transplantation in bone defects. [129, 130]. Also, iPS cells, without the challenges of immunological rejection and ethical controversy, are preferable to embryonic stem cells and seem to be a potential alternative stem cell source for bone tissue engineering.

5. Conclusion

Bone regeneration strategies can make convenient, efficacious alternative therapies for orthopaedic usages and is attractive on a several aspects including: (1) *in vitro* tissue engineering for transplantation would reduce the necessity for donor tissue as required skeletal cells could be expanded in the laboratory prior to implantation; (2) using scaffolds with similar mechanical characteristics to bone that could integrate with the surrounding native tissue has the potential to alleviate the rate of implant failure and the need for revision surgery; and (3) treatment of damaged tissue at an early stage with mesenchymal stem cells could decrease or even cure the disease, reducing the need for lifelong treatment and improving the quality of life of the patient. Clinical applications include for the support of bone stock, in maxillo-facial surgery as well fracture and non-union fractures [131]. However, it is clear that a single approach is not able to support many of the bone tissue requirements, and refined approaches targeted to a specific application site/problem will be needed.

Author details

Hossein Ghanbari* and Roghayyeh Vakili-Ghartavol

*Address all correspondence to: hghanbari@tums.ac.ir

Department of Medical Nanotechnology, School of Advanced Technologies in Medicine, Tehran University of Medical Science, Tehran, Iran

References

[1] Bose, S., M. Roy, and A. Bandyopadhyay, *Recent advances in bone tissue engineering scaffolds.* Trends in Biotechnology, 2012. 30(10): pp. 546–554.

[2] Griffin, K.S., et al., *Evolution of bone grafting: bone grafts and tissue engineering strategies for vascularized bone regeneration.* Clinical Reviews in Bone and Mineral Metabolism, 2015. 13(4): p. 232–244.

[3] Kairiyama, E., LEGAL SYSTEM FOR TISSUE BANKING IN LATIN AMERICA. Legal Basis of Global Tissue Banking: A Proactive Clinical Perspective. 2015. London, Research Transfer Ltd, p. 149–196.

[4] Laurencin, C.T., et al., *The ABJS Nicolas Andry Award: tissue engineering of bone and ligament: a 15-year perspective.* Clinical Orthopaedics and Related Research, 2006. 447: pp. 221–236.

[5] Belthur, M.V., et al., *Bone graft harvest using a new intramedullary system.* Clinical Orthopaedics and Related Research, 2008. 466(12): pp. 2973–2980.

[6] An, H.S., K. Lynch, and J. Toth, *Prospective comparison of autograft vs. allograft for adult posterolateral lumbar spine fusion: differences among freeze-dried, frozen, and mixed grafts.* Journal of Spinal Disorders & Techniques, 1995. 8(2): pp. 131–135.

[7] Khan, Y., et al., *Tissue engineering of bone: material and matrix considerations.* The Journal of Bone & Joint Surgery, 2008. 90(Supplement 1): pp. 36–42.

[8] Calori, G.M., et al., *Clinical effectiveness of Osigraft in long-bones non-unions.* Injury, 2015. 46: pp. S55–S64.

[9] Shrivats, A.R., M.C. McDermott, and J.O. Hollinger, *Bone tissue engineering: state of the union.* Drug Discovery Today, 2014. 19(6): pp. 781–786.

[10] Samavedi, S., A.R. Whittington, and A.S. Goldstein, *Calcium phosphate ceramics in bone tissue engineering: a review of properties and their influence on cell behavior.* Acta Biomaterialia, 2013. 9(9): pp. 8037–8045.

[11] Alberius, P., C. Dahlin, and A. Linde, *Role of osteopromotion in experimental bone grafting to the skull: a study in adult rats using a membrane technique.* Journal of Oral and Maxillofacial Surgery, 1992. 50(8): pp. 829–834.

[12] Scala, A., et al., *Sequential healing of the elevated sinus floor after applying autologous bone grafting: an experimental study in minipigs.* Clinical Oral Implants Research, 2015. 26(4): pp. 419–425.

[13] Sen, M. and T. Miclau, *Autologous iliac crest bone graft: should it still be the gold standard for treating nonunions?* Injury, 2007. 38(1): pp. S75–S80.

[14] Conway, J.D., *Autograft and nonunions: morbidity with intramedullary bone graft versus iliac crest bone graft.* Orthopedic Clinics of North America, 2010. 41(1): pp. 75–84.

[15] Hernigou, P., et al., *Percutaneous autologous bone-marrow grafting for nonunions.* The Journal of Bone & Joint Surgery, 2005. 87(7): pp. 1430–1437.

[16] Westrich, G.H., et al., *Anterior iliac crest bone graft harvesting using the corticocancellous reamer system.* Journal of Orthopaedic Trauma, 2001. 15(7): pp. 500–506.

[17] Gruskay, J.A., et al., *Short-term adverse events, length of stay, and readmission after iliac crest bone graft for spinal fusion.* Spine, 2014. 39(20): pp. 1718–1724.

[18] Giannoudis, P.V., et al., *Bone regeneration strategies: current trends but what the future holds.* Injury, 2013. 44(Suppl 1): pp. S1–S2.

[19] Urist, M.R., *Bone: formation by autoinduction.* Science, 1965. 150(3698): pp. 893–899.

[20] Einhorn, T.A., et al., *The healing of segmental bone defects induced by demineralized bone matrix. A radiographic and biomechanical study.* The Journal of Bone & Joint Surgery, 1984. 66(2): pp. 274–279.

[21] Egol, K.A., et al., *Bone grafting: sourcing, timing, strategies, and alternatives.* Journal of Orthopaedic Trauma, 2015. 29: pp. S10–S14.

[22] Erbe, E., et al., *Potential of an ultraporous β-tricalcium phosphate synthetic cancellous bone void filler and bone marrow aspirate composite graft.* European Spine Journal, 2001. 10(2): pp. S141–S146.

[23] Ghosh, S.K., et al., *In vivo response of porous hydroxyapatite and β-tricalcium phosphate prepared by aqueous solution combustion method and comparison with bioglass scaffolds.* Journal of Biomedical Materials Research Part B: Applied Biomaterials, 2008. 86(1): pp. 217–227.

[24] Cho, T.J., L.C. Gerstenfeld, and T.A. Einhorn, *Differential temporal expression of members of the transforming growth factor β superfamily during murine fracture healing.* Journal of Bone and Mineral Research, 2002. 17(3): pp. 513–520.

[25] Einhorn, T.A., *The cell and molecular biology of fracture healing.* Clinical Orthopaedics and Related Research, 1998. 355: pp. S7–S21.

[26] McClung, M.R., et al., *Romosozumab in postmenopausal women with low bone mineral density.* New England Journal of Medicine, 2014. 370(5): pp. 412–420.

[27] Lee, K.-B., et al., *Temporal regulation of mRNAs for select bone morphogenetic proteins (BMP), BMP receptors and their associated SMAD proteins during bovine early embryonic development: effects of exogenous BMP2 on embryo developmental progression.* Reproductive Biology and Endocrinology, 2014. 12(1): p. 67.

[28] Ferguson, C., et al., *Does adult fracture repair recapitulate embryonic skeletal formation?* Mechanisms of development, 1999. 87(1): pp. 57–66.

[29] Tingstad, E.M., et al., *Effect of immediate weightbearing on plated fractures of the humeral shaft.* Journal of Trauma and Acute Care Surgery, 2000. 49(2): pp. 278–280.

[30] Misra, A., R. Kapur, and N. Maffulli, *Complex proximal humeral fractures in adults—a systematic review of management.* Injury, 2001. 32(5): pp. 363–372.

[31] Carter, D., M. Van der Meulen, and G. Beaupre, *Mechanical factors in bone growth and development.* Bone, 1996. 18(1): pp. S5–S10.

[32] Claes, L., S. Recknagel, and A. Ignatius, *Fracture healing under healthy and inflammatory conditions.* Nature Reviews Rheumatology, 2012. 8(3): pp. 133–143.

[33] Claes, L., S. Recknagel, and A. Ignatius, Fracture healing under healthy and inflammatory conditions. Nature Reviews Rheumatology, 2012. 8(3): p. 133–143.

[34] Campbell, E.J., G.M. Campbell, and D.A. Hanley, *The effect of parathyroid hormone and teriparatide on fracture healing.* Expert Opinion on Biological Therapy, 2015. 15(1): pp. 119–129.

[35] Perren, S.M., *Evolution of the internal fixation of long bone fractures. The scientific basis of biological internal fixation: choosing a new balance between stability and biology.* The Bone & Joint Journal, 2002. 84(8): pp. 1093–1110.

[36] Lee, F.Y.I., et al., *Programmed removal of chondrocytes during endochondral fracture healing.* Journal of Orthopaedic Research, 1998. 16(1): pp. 144–150.

[37] Israel, D.I., et al., *Heterodimeric bone morphogenetic proteins show enhanced activity in vitro and in vivo.* Growth Factors, 1996. 13(3–4): pp. 291–300.

[38] Mckibbin, B. *The biology of fracture healing in long bones.* The Journal of Bone and Joint Surgery, 1978. 60-B(2): pp. 150–162 (Citeseer).

[39] Claes, L., et al., *Moderate soft tissue trauma delays new bone formation only in the early phase of fracture healing.* Journal of Orthopaedic Research, 2006. 24(6): pp. 1178–1185.

[40] Tsiridis, E., N. Upadhyay, and P. Giannoudis, *Molecular aspects of fracture healing: which are the important molecules?* Injury, 2007. 38(1): pp. S11–S25.

[41] Sánchez-Duffhues, G., et al., *Bone morphogenetic protein signaling in bone homeostasis.* Bone, 2015. 80: pp. 43–59.

[42] Ogasawara, A., et al., *Molecular basis for affected cartilage formation and bone union in fracture healing of the streptozotocin-induced diabetic rat.* Bone, 2008. 43(5): pp. 832–839.

[43] Gerstenfeld, L.C., et al., *Fracture healing as a post-natal developmental process: Molecular, spatial, and temporal aspects of its regulation.* Journal of Cellular Biochemistry, 2003. 88(5): pp. 873–884.

[44] Zhao, Y.-p., et al., *The promotion of bone healing by progranulin, a downstream molecule of BMP-2, through interacting with TNF/TNFR signaling.* Biomaterials, 2013. 34(27): pp. 6412–6421.

[45] Kondegowda, N.G., et al., *Osteoprotegerin and denosumab stimulate human beta cell proliferation through inhibition of the receptor activator of NF-kB ligand pathway.* Cell Metabolism, 2015. 22(1): pp. 77–85.

[46] Mountziaris, P.M. and A.G. Mikos, *Modulation of the inflammatory response for enhanced bone tissue regeneration.* Tissue Engineering Part B: Reviews, 2008. 14(2): pp. 179–186.

[47] Dimitriou, R., E. Tsiridis, and P.V. Giannoudis, *Current concepts of molecular aspects of bone healing.* Injury, 2005. 36(12): pp. 1392–1404.

[48] Street, J., et al., *Vascular endothelial growth factor stimulates bone repair by promoting angiogenesis and bone turnover.* Proceedings of the National Academy of Sciences, 2002. 99(15): pp. 9656–9661.

[49] Javelaud, D. and A. Mauviel, *Mammalian transforming growth factor-βs: smad signaling and physio-pathological roles.* The International Journal of Biochemistry & Cell Biology, 2004. 36(7): pp. 1161–1165.

[50] Lissenberg-Thunnissen, S.N., et al., *Use and efficacy of bone morphogenetic proteins in fracture healing.* International Orthopaedics, 2011. 35(9): pp. 1271–1280.

[51] Daluiski, A., et al., *Bone morphogenetic protein-3 is a negative regulator of bone density.* Nature Genetics, 2001. 27(1): pp. 84–88.

[52] Shen, B., et al., *BMP-13 emerges as a potential inhibitor of bone formation.* International Journal of Biological Sciences, 2009. 5(2): p. 192.

[53] Reddi, A., *Bone morphogenetic proteins: from basic science to clinical applications.* The Journal of Bone & Joint Surgery, 2001. 83(1 suppl 1): pp. S1–S6.

[54] Upton, P.D. and N.W. Morrell, *TGF-β and BMPR-II pharmacology—implications for pulmonary vascular diseases.* Current Opinion in Pharmacology, 2009. 9(3): pp. 274–280.

[55] Sakou, T., *Bone morphogenetic proteins: from basic studies to clinical approaches.* Bone, 1998. 22(6): pp. 591–603.

[56] Carreira, A., et al., *Bone morphogenetic proteins facts, challenges, and future perspectives.* Journal of Dental Research, 2014: p. 0022034513518561.

[57] Little, S.C. and M.C. Mullins, *Bone morphogenetic protein heterodimers assemble heteromeric type I receptor complexes to pattern the dorsoventral axis.* Nature Cell Biology, 2009. 11(5): pp. 637–643.

[58] Sieber, C., et al., *Recent advances in BMP receptor signaling.* Cytokine & Growth Factor Reviews, 2009. 20(5): pp. 343–355.

[59] Groeneveld, E. and E. Burger, *Bone morphogenetic proteins in human bone regeneration.* European Journal of Endocrinology, 2000. 142(1): pp. 9–21.

[60] Bostrom, M.P., *Expression of bone morphogenetic proteins in fracture healing.* Clinical Orthopaedics and Related Research, 1998. 355: pp. S116–S123.

[61] Bostrom, M.P., et al., *Immunolocalization and expression of bone morphogenetic proteins 2 and 4 in fracture healing.* Journal of Orthopaedic Research, 1995. 13(3): pp. 357–367.

[62] Cheng, H., et al., *Osteogenic activity of the fourteen types of human bone morphogenetic proteins (BMPs).* The Journal of Bone & Joint Surgery, 2003. 85(8): pp. 1544–1552.

[63] Deckers, M.M., et al., *Bone morphogenetic proteins stimulate angiogenesis through osteoblast-derived vascular endothelial growth factor A.* Endocrinology, 2002. 143(4): pp. 1545–1553.

[64] Groppe, J., et al., *Structural basis of BMP signaling inhibition by Noggin, a novel twelve-membered cystine knot protein.* The Journal of Bone & Joint Surgery, 2003. 85(suppl 3): pp. 52–58.

[65] Gazzerro, E., V. Gangji, and E. Canalis, *Bone morphogenetic proteins induce the expression of noggin, which limits their activity in cultured rat osteoblasts.* Journal of Clinical Investigation, 1998. 102(12): p. 2106.

[66] Fujii, D., et al., *Transforming growth factor β gene maps to human chromosome 19 long arm and to mouse chromosome 7.* Somatic Cell and Molecular Genetics, 1986. 12(3): pp. 281–288.

[67] Poniatowski, Ł.A., et al., *Transforming growth factor beta family: insight into the role of growth factors in regulation of fracture healing biology and potential clinical applications.* Mediators of Inflammation, 2015. 2015: p. 137823.

[68] Wahlström, O., et al., *Variation of pH in lysed platelet concentrates influence proliferation and alkaline phosphatase activity in human osteoblast-like cells.* Platelets, 2007. 18(2): pp. 113–118.

[69] Wahlström, O., et al., *Acidic preparations of platelet concentrates release bone morphogenetic protein-2.* Acta Orthopaedica, 2008. 79(3): pp. 433–437.

[70] Heldin, C.-H., K. Miyazono, and P. Ten Dijke, *TGF-β signalling from cell membrane to nucleus through SMAD proteins.* Nature, 1997. 390(6659): pp. 465–471.

[71] Lieberman, J.R., A. Daluiski, and T.A. Einhorn, *The role of growth factors in the repair of bone.* The Journal of Bone & Joint Surgery, 2002. 84(6): pp. 1032–1044.

[72] Massague, J., *The transforming growth factor-beta family.* Annual Review of Cell Biology, 1990. 6(1): pp. 597–641.

[73] Mundy, G.R., *Regulation of bone formation by bone morphogenetic proteins and other growth factors.* Clinical Orthopaedics and Related Research, 1996. 324: pp. 24–27.

[74] Joyce, M.E., et al., *Transforming growth factor-beta and the initiation of chondrogenesis and osteogenesis in the rat femur.* The Journal of Cell Biology, 1990. 110(6): pp. 2195–2207.

[75] Beck, L.S., et al., *TGF-β1 induces bone closure of skull defects: temporal dynamics of bone formation in defects exposed to rhTGF-β1.* Journal of Bone and Mineral Research, 1993. 8(6): pp. 753–761.

[76] Andrae, J., R. Gallini, and C. Betsholtz, *Role of platelet-derived growth factors in physiology and medicine.* Genes & Development, 2008. 22(10): pp. 1276–1312.

[77] Solheim, E., *Growth factors in bone.* International Orthopaedics, 1998. 22(6): pp. 410–416.

[78] Heldin, C.-H. and B. Westermark, *Mechanism of action and in vivo role of platelet-derived growth factor.* Physiological Reviews, 1999. 79(4): pp. 1283–1316.

[79] Andrew, J., et al., *Platelet-derived growth factor expression in normally healing human fractures.* Bone, 1995. 16(4): pp. 455–460.

[80] Graham, S., et al., *Investigating the role of PDGF as a potential drug therapy in bone formation and fracture healing.* Expert Opinion on Investigational Drugs, 2009. 18(11): pp. 1633–1654.

[81] Nash, T., et al., *Effect of platelet-derived growth factor on tibial osteotomies in rabbits.* Bone, 1994. 15(2): pp. 203–208.

[82] Wang, J.-S., *Basic fibroblast growth factor for stimulation of bone formation in osteoinductive and conductive implants.* Acta Orthop Scand Suppl, 1996. 269: pp. 1–33.

[83] Nakamura, T., et al., *Recombinant human basic fibroblast growth factor accelerates fracture healing by enhancing callus remodeling in experimental dog tibial fracture.* Journal of Bone and Mineral Research, 1998. 13(6): pp. 942–949.

[84] Kawai, M. and C.J. Rosen, *The insulin-like growth factor system in bone: basic and clinical implications.* Endocrinology and Metabolism Clinics of North America, 2012. 41(2): pp. 323–333.

[85] Shimasaki, S. and N. Ling, *Identification and molecular characterization of insulin-like growth factor binding proteins (IGFBP-1,-2,-3,-4,-5 and -6).* Progress in Growth Factor Research, 1991. 3(4): pp. 243–266.

[86] Canalis, E., *Effect of insulinlike growth factor I on DNA and protein synthesis in cultured rat calvaria.* Journal of Clinical Investigation, 1980. 66(4): p. 709.

[87] Prisell, P.T., et al., *Expression of insulin-like growth factors during bone induction in rat.* Calcified Tissue International, 1993. 53(3): pp. 201–205.

[88] Barnes, G.L., et al., *Growth factor regulation of fracture repair.* Journal of Bone and Mineral Research, 1999. 14(11): pp. 1805–1815.

[89] Einhorn, T.A. and C.A. Lee, *Bone regeneration: new findings and potential clinical applications.* Journal of the American Academy of Orthopaedic Surgeons, 2001. 9(3): pp. 157–165.

[90] Vu, T.H., et al., *MMP-9/gelatinase B is a key regulator of growth plate angiogenesis and apoptosis of hypertrophic chondrocytes.* Cell, 1998. 93(3): pp. 411–422.

[91] Suri, C., et al., *Requisite role of angiopoietin-1, a ligand for the TIE2 receptor, during embryonic angiogenesis.* Cell, 1996. 87(7): pp. 1171–1180.

[92] Ferrara, N. and T. Davis-Smyth, *The biology of vascular endothelial growth factor*. Endocrine Reviews, 1997. 18(1): pp. 4–25.

[93] Bruder, S.P., D.J. Fink, and A.I. Caplan, *Mesenchymal stem cells in bone development, bone repair, and skeletal regenaration therapy*. Journal of Cellular Biochemistry, 1994. 56(3): pp. 283–294.

[94] Pittenger, M.F., et al., *Multilineage potential of adult human mesenchymal stem cells*. Science, 1999. 284(5411): pp. 143–147.

[95] Laurencin, C.T., et al., *Tissue engineering: orthopedic applications*. Annual Review of Biomedical Engineering, 1999. 1(1): pp. 19–46.

[96] Fernandez-Yague, M.A., et al., *Biomimetic approaches in bone tissue engineering: integrating biological and physicomechanical strategies*. Advanced Drug Delivery Reviews, 2015. 84: pp. 1–29.

[97] Chang, Y.-Y., et al., *Analyses of antibacterial activity and cell compatibility of titanium coated with a Zr–C–N film*. PLoS One, 2013. 8(2): p. e56771.

[98] Nakahara, I., et al., *Interfacial shear strength of bioactive-coated carbon fiber reinforced polyetheretherketone after in vivo implantation*. Journal of Orthopaedic Research, 2012. 30(10): pp. 1618–1625.

[99] Cao, H. and N. Kuboyama, *A biodegradable porous composite scaffold of PGA/β-TCP for bone tissue engineering*. Bone, 2010. 46(2): pp. 386–395.

[100] Cao, X. and D. Chen, *The BMP signaling and in vivo bone formation*. Gene, 2005. 357(1): pp. 1–8.

[101] Pollak, M., *The insulin and insulin-like growth factor receptor family in neoplasia: an update*. Nature Reviews Cancer, 2012. 12(3): pp. 159–169.

[102] Rouwkema, J., N.C. Rivron, and C.A. van Blitterswijk, *Vascularization in tissue engineering*. Trends in Biotechnology, 2008. 26(8): pp. 434–441.

[103] Bramfeld, H., et al., *Scaffold vascularization: a challenge for three-dimensional tissue engineering*. Current Medicinal Chemistry, 2010. 17(33): pp. 3944–3967.

[104] Jain, R.K., et al., *Engineering vascularized tissue*. Nature Biotechnology, 2005. 23(7): pp. 821–823.

[105] Williams, D.F., *On the mechanisms of biocompatibility*. Biomaterials, 2008. 29(20): pp. 2941–2953.

[106] Olszta, M.J., et al., *Bone structure and formation: a new perspective*. Materials Science and Engineering: R: Reports, 2007. 58(3): pp. 77–116.

[107] Petrie Aronin, C.E., et al., *Comparative effects of scaffold pore size, pore volume, and total void volume on cranial bone healing patterns using microsphere-based scaffolds*. Journal of Biomedical Materials Research Part A, 2009. 89(3): pp. 632–641.

[108] Murphy, C.M., M.G. Haugh, and F.J. O'Brien, *The effect of mean pore size on cell attachment, proliferation and migration in collagen–glycosaminoglycan scaffolds for bone tissue engineering.* Biomaterials, 2010. 31(3): pp. 461–466.

[109] Woodard, J.R., et al., *The mechanical properties and osteoconductivity of hydroxyapatite bone scaffolds with multi-scale porosity.* Biomaterials, 2007. 28(1): pp. 45–54.

[110] Rezwan, K., et al., *Biodegradable and bioactive porous polymer/inorganic composite scaffolds for bone tissue engineering.* Biomaterials, 2006. 27(18): pp. 3413–3431.

[111] Lichte, P., et al., *Scaffolds for bone healing: concepts, materials and evidence.* Injury, 2011. 42(6): pp. 569–573.

[112] Zuk, P.A., et al., *Human adipose tissue is a source of multipotent stem cells.* Molecular Biology of the Cell, 2002. 13(12): pp. 4279–4295.

[113] Seo, B.-M., et al., *Investigation of multipotent postnatal stem cells from human periodontal ligament.* The Lancet, 2004. 364(9429): pp. 149–155.

[114] De Bari, C., et al., *Multipotent mesenchymal stem cells from adult human synovial membrane.* Arthritis & Rheumatism, 2001. 44(8): pp. 1928–1942.

[115] Zvaifler, N.J., et al., *Mesenchymal precursor cells in the blood of normal individuals.* Arthritis Research, 2000. 2(6): pp. 477–488.

[116] Sabatini, F., et al., *Human bronchial fibroblasts exhibit a mesenchymal stem cell phenotype and multilineage differentiating potentialities.* Laboratory Investigation, 2005. 85(8): pp. 962–971.

[117] Aust, L., et al., *Yield of human adipose-derived adult stem cells from liposuction aspirates.* Cytotherapy, 2004. 6(1): pp. 7–14.

[118] Zhu, Y., et al., *Adipose-derived stem cell: a better stem cell than BMSC.* Cell Biochemistry and Function, 2008. 26(6): pp. 664–675.

[119] Stockmann, P., et al., *Guided bone regeneration in pig calvarial bone defects using autologous mesenchymal stem/progenitor cells – a comparison of different tissue sources.* Journal of Cranio-Maxillofacial Surgery, 2012. 40(4): pp. 310–320.

[120] Dickson, K., S. Katzman, and G. Paiement, *The importance of the blood supply in the healing of tibial fractures.* Contemporary Orthopaedics, 1995. 30(6): pp. 489–493.

[121] Akita, S., et al., *Capillary vessel network integration by inserting a vascular pedicle enhances bone formation in tissue-engineered bone using interconnected porous hydroxyapatite ceramics.* Tissue Engineering, 2004. 10(5–6): pp. 789–795.

[122] Kim, W.S. and H.K. Kim, *Tissue engineered vascularized bone formation using in vivo implanted osteoblast-polyglycolic acid scaffold.* Journal of Korean Medical Science, 2005. 20(3): pp. 479–482.

[123] Hausman, M., M. Schaffler, and R. Majeska, *Prevention of fracture healing in rats by an inhibitor of angiogenesis.* Bone, 2001. 29(6): pp. 560–564.

[124] Mori, S., et al., *Antiangiogenic agent (TNP-470) inhibition of ectopic bone formation induced by bone morphogenetic protein-2.* Bone, 1998. 22(2): pp. 99–105.

[125] Asahara, T., et al., *Isolation of putative progenitor endothelial cells for angiogenesis.* Science, 1997. 275(5302): pp. 964–966.

[126] Rouwkema, J., et al., *The use of endothelial progenitor cells for prevascularized bone tissue engineering.* Tissue Engineering Part A, 2009. 15(8): pp. 2015–2027.

[127] Matsumoto, T., et al., *Fracture induced mobilization and incorporation of bone marrow-derived endothelial progenitor cells for bone healing.* Journal of Cellular Physiology, 2008. 215(1): pp. 234–242.

[128] Takahashi, K. and S. Yamanaka, *Induction of pluripotent stem cells from mouse embryonic and adult fibroblast cultures by defined factors.* Cell, 2006. 126(4): pp. 663–676.

[129] Takahashi, K. and S. Yamanaka, *Induced pluripotent stem cells in medicine and biology.* Development, 2013. 140(12): pp. 2457–2461.

[130] Yoshida, Y. and S. Yamanaka, *iPS cells: a source of cardiac regeneration.* Journal of Molecular and Cellular Cardiology, 2011. 50(2): pp. 327–332.

[131] Rose, F.R. and R.O. Oreffo, *Bone tissue engineering: hope vs hype.* Biochemical and Biophysical Research Communications, 2002. 292(1): pp. 1–7.

Chapter 2

Acoustic Therapy as Mechanical Stimulation of Osteogenesis

Carlos Vinícius Buarque de Gusmão,
José Marcos Alves and William Dias Belangero

Additional information is available at the end of the chapter

http://dx.doi.org/10.5772/63745

Abstract

Acoustic therapy is a branch of mechanotherapy. This modality of treatment can be used for osteogenesis-related orthopaedic disorders. Because bone cells are responsive to acoustic forces, specially designed devices were developed to generate acoustic forces in the form of low-intensity pulsed ultrasound, extracorporeal shock waves or radial pressure waves. With the developed devices, it became possible to provide patients an alternative, or adjunctive, treatment for pathologies involving bone homeostasis, that is, the balance of bone formation and bone resorption. The so-called acoustic therapy (low-intensity pulsed ultrasound stimulation, LIPUS; extracorporeal shock wave therapy, ESWT; and radial pressure wave therapy, RPWT) acts through physical phenomena produced when acoustic waves are transmitted into living tissue and converted to biological reactions, thereby activating signalling pathways that drive a cellular response in favour of osteogenesis. In this chapter, an extensive review of the literature was performed to provide the reader the "state of the art" about the physical phenomena, molecular events and clinical uses of acoustic forces for osteogenesis-related orthopaedics disorders.

Keywords: osteogenesis, low-intensity pulsed ultrasound stimulation (LIPUS), extracorporeal shock wave therapy (ESWT), radial pressure wave therapy (RPWT), acoustic forces, mechanotransduction, mechanical loading

1. Introduction

Mechanical stimulation of bone cells modulates a myriad of molecular signalling pathways involved in osteogenesis. There are distinct forms of mechanical forces, such as centrifuge force, gravitational force, electromagnetic force, hydrostatic force and acoustic force. Acoustic forces comprise a modality of mechanical load that can be represented basically by three different types of acoustic waves: ultrasound wave, shock wave and radial pressure wave. Those waves may be applied to patients suffering from orthopaedics disorders, especially those related to osteogenesis; for instance, delayed union, nonunion, osteoporosis and acute fractures.

The application of mechanical devices for medical purposes is termed mechanotherapy. Accordingly, the use of acoustic devices, which is a category of mechanical devices, for medical purposes will be termed here acoustic therapy and will be further divided into three subcategories: low-intensity pulsed ultrasound stimulation (LIPUS), extracorporeal shock wave therapy (ESWT) and radial pressure wave therapy (RPWT). This chapter discusses the physical phenomena, biological events and clinical indications of acoustic therapy on bone tissue (**Table 1**).

Abbreviations	Meanings	Abbreviations	Meanings
ActR	activin receptor	MCP	monocyte chemoattractant protein
ALP	alkaline phosphatase	MIP	macrophage-inflammatory protein
AT1	angiotensin II type 1 receptor	Msx	Msh homeobox
ATP	adenosine triphosphate	mTOR	mechanistic target of rapamycin
Bax	Bcl-2-associated X protein	NADPH	nicotinamide adenine dinucleotide phosphate
BMP	bone morphogenetic protein	NO	nitric oxide
BMPR	bone morphogenetic protein receptor	NOS	nitric oxide synthase
Ca^{2+}	calcium ion	OPG	osteoprotegerin
cbfa	core binding factor subunit alpha-1, also known as Runx2	PGE_2	prostaglandin E_2
CDK	cyclin-dependent kinase	PPARγ2	peroxisome proliferator-activated receptor γ2
c-fos	FBJ murine osteosarcoma viral oncogene homolog	PTHr	parathyroid hormone receptor
c-jun	Jun proto-oncogene	Rac	Ras-related C3 botulinum toxin substrate
c-myc	avian myelocytomatosis viral oncogene homolog	RANK	receptor activator of nuclear factor kappa B
cox	cyclooxygenase	RANKL	receptor activator of nuclear factor kappa B ligand
CXCR	C-X-C chemokine receptor	RANTES	regulated upon activation, normal T-cell-expressed and secreted
Dlx	distal-less homeobox	Ras	portmanteau of "rat" and "sarcoma"
egr	early growth response	rhBMP-2	recombinant human BMP-2

http://dx.doi.org/10.5772/63745

Abbreviations	Meanings	Abbreviations	Meanings
ERK	extracellular signal-regulated kinase	RPWT	radial pressure wave therapy
ESWT	extracorporeal shock wave therapy	Runx	runt-related transcription factor
FAK	focal adhesion kinase	SDF	stromal cell-derived factor
FGF	fibroblast growth factor	Smad	portmanteau of "small body size" and "decapentaplegic"
HIF	hypoxia-inducible factor	SOST	sclerostin gene
IGF	insulin-like growth factor	TCF/LEF	T-cell factor/Lymphoid enhancer binding factor
IL-8	interleukin-8	TGF	transforming growth factor
ILK	integrin-linked kinase	TSC	transforming growth factor-beta-stimulated clone
IRS	insulin receptor substrate	Tyr	tyrosine residue
LIPUS	low-intensity pulsed ultrasound stimulation	VEGF	vascular endothelial growth factor
LRP	low-density lipoprotein receptor-related protein	Wnt	wingless-related integration site
MAPK	mitogen-activated protein kinase		

Table 1. Abbreviations used throughout text.

2. From concepts to acoustic devices

Bone modelling refers to changes in bone structure and density in response to increased loads. Bone remodelling is defined as, the almost obligatory, bone resorption that follows bone formation irrespective of mechanical loads. The first to describe that bone deposition occurs preferably on sites of compressive loads, whereas bone resorption occurs preferably on sites of tensile loads was Julius Wolff, whose observations were the foundation of Wolff's law (1892) [1].

Later, Frost realized that different ranges of intensities (magnitudes) of bone deformation elicited different biological responses. Based on that, he published the mechanostat model (1964), in which low-frequency cyclic (less than 5–10 Hz), or static, loads lower than 50–100 μstrain (desuse range) lead to bone resorption, loads from 50–100 to 1000–1500 μstrain (physiological range) do not change bone mass, loads from 1000–1500 to 3000 μstrain (overuse range) induce osteogenesis and loads greater than 3000 μstrain (pathological overuse range) may lead to fracture or stress fracture. Strain stands for relative deformation of a cell or tissue. It should be noted that the ranges of intensities proposed by Frost refer to bone tissue, not to bone cells, which normally need higher strains to elicit an osteogenic response [1–3]. For detailed information, see reference [3].

Based on Wolff's law and mechanostat model concepts, mechanical devices were developed to purposely stimulate osteogenesis. LIPUS and ESWT are applied by acoustic devices approved in many countries for clinical use in the management of bone healing disorders. On the other hand, currently, RPWT lacks evidence for its use to induce osteogenesis, but it is used to address soft tissue orthopaedic disorders.

2.1. LIPUS device

Low-intensity pulsed ultrasound was developed by Duarte, and its use for accelerating fracture healing was published in 1983. Most commonly used device generates 1.5 MHz ultrasound in a pulse wave mode (duty cycle of 20%, 200 μs burst width with repetitive frequency of 1 KHz) and average intensity 30 mW/cm^2. Low-intensity ultrasound waves are produced from a piezoelectric crystal within an unfocused, circular transducer. Its effective radiating area is 3.88 cm^2, peak rarefactional pressure at specimen (nonderated) is 0.076 MPa and focal length is ~130 mm [4–6].

2.2. ESWT devices

ESWT originally was developed for lithotripsy in order to break up and disrupt stones within genitourinary tract. Its use for osteogenesis initiated after the observation that shock waves provoked osteogenic response on the pelvis of animals during lithotripsy experiments [7].

There are three main techniques for generation of shock waves. Irrespective of the technique, production of shock waves requires the conversion of electrical energy into acoustic energy. All three devices (electrohydraulic, electromagnetic and piezoelectric) are used in orthopaedics, and there is no evidence that a certain device provides better results than the other [7–10].

2.2.1. Electrohydraulic device

This is the first generation of orthopaedic shock wave devices. A high-voltage electrical discharge is applied across electrode tips—a spark gap—within a water-filled semi-ellipsoid reflector. The resultant spark heats and vaporizes the surrounding water, which, in turn, generates a gas bubble filled with water vapour that expands and produces a shock wave. The wave is reflected by the metallic surface of the semi-ellipsoid and is focused into the therapeutic zone [7, 9, 11].

Electrohydraulic shock wave devices usually are characterized by relatively large axial diameters of the focal volume and high total energy within that volume. The spark gap wears out after about 50,000 shots (impulses) and needs to be replaced [7, 11].

Technical specifications vary according to manufacturer (not all manufacturers provide complete data): energy flux density varies from 0.01 to 1.80 mJ/mm^2, focal zones vary from 0 to 95 mm (fx[-6dB]) and from 4.8 to 25 mm (fz[-6dB]), frequency varies from 0.5 to 360 Hz, and penetration depth is up to 84 mm [12–15].

2.2.2. *Electromagnetic device*

Within this device, there is an electromagnetic coil and a metal membrane besides the coil both embedded in a water medium. A high current pulse is released through the coil, generating a strong magnetic field, which repels the membrane rapidly away from the coil, therefore pushing the surrounding water to produce a shock wave. The shock wave is focused with an acoustic lens to the therapeutic zone. The lens can be used for several hundred thousand impulses with no need to replace the elements [7, 9, 11].

A variation of the electromagnetic device uses a repelling membrane formed as a cylinder and the sound waves are reflected by a surrounding parabolic reflector [11].

Technical specifications vary according to the manufacturer (not all manufacturers provide complete data): energy density flux varies from 0.01 to 0.55 mJ/mm^2, frequency varies from 1 to 8 Hz shock waves, penetration depth is up to 80 mm and focal zone varies from 0 to 65 mm [16, 17].

2.2.3. *Piezoelectric device*

Within this device, a few hundred to some thousand piezoelectric crystals—usually more than a thousand—are arranged in a spherical surface filled with water. A high pulse discharge is applied to the crystals, which immediately contract and expand (piezoelectric effect) generating a shock wave in the surrounding fluid. The emitted energy of each crystal is fairly weak, but reaches higher energy at the focus where all shock waves gather together. The focal zone is relatively small and cigar shaped. Because of the spherical shape of the device's surface, this device has an extremely precise focus and a high energy density within a well-confined focal volume. In addition, the large aperture of the source allows for almost pain-free treatment because of the low-pressure at the skin entry zone [7, 9, 11].

Technical specifications vary according to the manufacturer (not all manufacturers provide complete data): energy flux density ranges from 0.03 to 0.4 mJ/mm^2, frequency ranges from 1 to 8 Hz, pressure ranges from 11.5 to 82.2 MPa, focal size ranges from 1.2 to 4.8 mm (fx[-6dB] = fy[-6dB]) and from 1.2 to 14.1 mm (fz[-6dB]) and penetration depth ranges from 5 to 40 mm [18–20].

2.2.4. *RPWT*

Radial pressure waves are produced pneumatically (ballistically). A projectile is accelerated with compressed air, or an electromagnetic field, within a guiding tube (cylindrical piston) and strikes a metal applicator placed on the patient's skin. The projectile produces stress waves in the applicator that transforms their kinetic energy into a radially expanding pressure—or pulse—wave towards tissue [21, 22].

Technical specifications vary according to model and manufacturer (not all manufacturers provide complete data): energy density flux is up to 0.55 mJ/mm^2, frequency ranges from 1 to 22 Hz, pressure ranges from 1.0 to 5.0 bar and penetration depth is up to 60 mm [23–26].

3. Physical phenomena elicited by acoustic waves in biological tissues

3.1. Forms of acoustic waves

Low-intensity pulsed ultrasound, shock waves and radial pressure waves are different forms of acoustic waves. Their distinct physical parameters are expected to produce different physical phenomena when transmitted into biological tissues.

3.1.1. Low-intensity pulsed ultrasound

Sound is the vibration (rapid motion) of molecules within a compressible medium such as air or water. It can only propagate in compressible media. When sound waves (acoustic waves) reach molecules, molecules may get closer—compression—or farther—rarefaction. By alternating compression and rarefaction, sound travels in waves transporting energy from one location (transmitter) to another (receiver). Because sound waves produce mechanical motion of molecules, they are mechanical waves. When the frequency of a sound wave is above the typical human audible range (greater than 20 kHz), this sound wave is called ultrasound. Ultrasound is an acoustic radiation that can be transmitted as high-frequency pressure waves (1–12 MHz) [4, 6, 7, 27, 28].

Spatial average temporal average (ISATA) lower than 150 mW/cm^2 is generally regarded as the intensity spectrum of LIPUS. ISATA refers to the spatial average intensity over both the on time and the off time of the pulse. Nevertheless, there is no clear-cut upper intensity boundary to define an ultrasound wave as low-intensity ultrasound. LIPUS studies have been conducted with intensity level between 5 and 1000 mW/cm^2, with frequency between 45 kHz and 3 MHz, in continuous or burst mode and with daily exposure times between 1 and 20 min. In spite of that, most used parameters for LIPUS are as originally described by its creator: intensity of 30 mW/cm^2, frequency of 1.5 MHz, pulse (burst mode) of 1 KHz with duty cycle of 20% and daily exposure times of 20 min [4, 29, 30].

3.1.2. Shock waves

They are also acoustic pressure waves, or sonic pulses. In general, a shock wave can be described as a single pulse with a wide frequency range up to 20 MHz (typically in the range from 16 Hz to 20 MHz), high positive pressure amplitude up to 120 MPa (often 50–80 MPa), low tensile wave up to 10 MPa with short duration (about 1 μs), small pulse width at -6dB, short life cycle of approximately 10 μs and a short rise time of the positive pressure amplitude (lower than 10 ns). The reader may find studies with measured rise times of shock wave devices in the range of 30 ns as a result of the limited time resolution of piezoelectric hydrophones. However, optical hydrophones, which are more sensitive measure devices, displayed measure rise times below 10 ns for electrohydraulic devices [7, 9, 22].

The energy density (maximum amount of acoustical energy transmitted through an area per pulse) of ESWT is up to 1.5 mJ/mm^2 and the pulse energy (sum of all energy densities across the beam profile multiplied by the area of the beam profile) is up to 100 mJ. Arbitrarily, energy levels up to 0.08–0.12 mJ/mm^2 in the focal zone are defined as low-energy ESWT, energy levels between 0.08 and 0.28 mJ/mm^2 are defined as medium-energy ESWT and energy levels greater than 0.28 mJ/mm^2 are defined as high-energy ESWT (some authors consider 0.12 mJ/mm^2 the cut-off from low- to high-energy ESWT) [7–9, 22, 31, 32].

3.1.3. *Ultrasound vs shock waves*

Shock waves differ from regular sound waves in that the wave front, where compression takes place, is a region of sudden change in stress and density. Shock waves travel faster than sound, and their speed increases as the amplitude (pressure) is raised. On the other hand, the intensity of a shock wave decreases faster than does of a sound wave. As a consequence, wavelets at high pressure lead to deformation of the wave so that the wave crest assumes a sawtooth appearance, which is different from the sinusoidal appearance of a regular sound wave. Furthermore, shock waves differ from ultrasound waves since the former is uniphasic with high peak pressure (in the order of a hundred MPa), and the latter is biphasic with very low peak pressure (in the order of a hundredth of MPa) [7, 22].

3.1.4. *Radial pressure waves*

Considering the physical definition of shock waves, radial pressure waves are wrongly termed unfocused shock waves in the literature. The rise time of the positive pressure waves produced by currently available devices are much greater than 10 ns, varying from 600 to 800 ns. Also, the maximum peak positive pressure of a radial pressure wave device varies from 0.1 to 7 Mpa, and the pulse duration varies from 1 to 5 ms. Since the time taken for the radial wave to rise is too long, the curve of the concave surface of the ray is too wide for it to be possible to focus the energy; therefore, radial waves cannot be focused, unlike ESWT. Moreover, the air pressure-accelerated projectile has a speed from 2 to 20 m/s, which is 2 orders of magnitude slower than sound speed in water or tissue. Shock waves are produced when the projectile speed is comparable or higher than sound speed (i.e. supersonic). In addition, the distinction between RPWT as "low-energy therapy" and ESWT as "high-energy therapy" is not correct. Most protocols of RPWT use energy density lower than 0.20 mJ/mm^2, but the device can reach up to 0.55 mJ/mm^2. Accordingly, ESWT has a wide range of energy density protocols varying from 0.02 mJ/mm^2 to more than 0.60 mJ/mm^2 [8, 21, 22, 26, 33].

3.2. Attenuation of acoustic energy

When an acoustic wave is transmitted into a biological tissue, a portion of the acoustic energy is reflected, another portion is attenuated (lost) and the other portion is refracted and continues propagating. Much from the attenuated portion is absorbed by irreversible conversion of acoustical energy into heat mainly via viscous friction, and less is scattered by inhomogeneities within tissue that redirect some sonic energy to regions outside the original wave-propagation path. If the density of the inhomogeneity is high, multiple scattering may occur. Therefore, acoustic energy may scatter several times until it is completely absorbed by tissue and converted to heat [27, 34, 35].

Bone has one of the highest attenuation coefficients among biologic tissues. Besides, as frequency increases, penetration decreases and attenuation increases. Therefore, acoustic waves tend to produce heat preferentially in bones and joints. Accordingly, tissue damage and pain may be produced if the intensity of acoustic energy is high enough. For instance, continuous unfocused ultrasound waves in the range of 4000–5000 mW/cm^2 at 1 MHz for 5 min increase temperature by 1.8–4.3°C at different areas of bone within 1–3 cm of distance. On the other hand, ultrasound at intensities of 20–50 mW/cm^2, which is LIPUS, produces negligible variation of tissue temperature (0.01 ± 0.005°C). Moreover, reports using very high ultrasound intensities (5000–25,000 mW/cm^2) showed delayed bone healing and necrosis, whereas ultrasound at intensities of 200–3000 mW/cm^2 has been shown to increase callus formation and accelerate fracture healing [4, 27, 35–38].

Extracorporeal shock waves and radial pressure waves also increase temperature of tissues either by absorption or by cavitation (see Section 3.3). However, no reports were found about temperature raise within biological tissues subjected to ESWT and RPWT. In spite of that, thermal effects may be responsible for decreased cell viability immediately after ESWT with some energy densities and number of impulses [39–44].

3.3. Cavitation bubbles

When near gas or vapour bubbles, a portion of the refracted acoustic wave may generate cavitation bubbles at locations termed "nucleation sites". Cavitation refers to a range of complex phenomena that involve the creation, oscillation, growth and collapse of bubbles within a liquid or liquid-like medium. Cavitation bubbles have never been confirmed in living tissues; therefore, the following information is based on mathematical simulations and in vitro studies [3, 27, 37].

The occurrence and behaviour of cavitation depend on the acoustic pressure; the existence of microheterogeneities in liquids such as free gas, solid particles or a combination of both; whether the acoustic field is focused or unfocused, or pulsed or continuous; and the nature and state of the material and its boundaries. Cavitation does not occur with ultrasound intensities below 500 mW/cm^2. Consequently, LIPUS does not produce the phenomenon of cavitation. On the other hand, the biological effects of ESWT and RPWT are triggered mainly by the phenomenon of cavitation [4, 27, 30, 38, 45].

Bubbles are gas-filled spheres in a liquid under constant hydrostatic pressure when there are no acoustic waves. In response to a sound field in which the acoustic pressure varies sinusoidally in time with a given frequency, the bubble radius oscillates (expands and contracts) with radial displacement and velocity, which vary sinusoidally in time with the same frequency of the wave. When there is lower level pressure amplitude in synchrony with bubble motion, the immediately surrounding liquid moves in and out creating a small steady flow of fluid called microstreaming. This is called stable cavitation and may occur with low-energy ESWT and some RPWT. Stable cavitation occurs near a solid boundary (e.g. bone) and creates shear stress near the bubble surface that can also mechanically stimulate cells [7, 45].

Shock waves and radial pressure waves generate cavitation bubbles during the tensile phase of the acoustic wave due to its tensile forces that exceed the dynamic tensile strength of water. During the growth phase of the bubble, a huge amount of energy is delivered to the bubble. Following a number of shock, or radial pressure, wave pulses (sometimes after the first impulse), the bubble collapses (i.e. experiences an extremely rapid contraction), which is called inertial cavitation. As the bubble collapses, four phenomena can be observed [7, 27, 35, 45, 46]:

1. Release of energy in the form of high temperature, which can produce free radicals that may damage cells. However, the production of free radicals has not been confirmed in living tissue.
2. Secondary shock wave emission into the fluid that produces a direct mechanical effect on tissue.
3. The bubble may aggregate with surrounding bubbles, may fragment or may repeat the growth/collapse cycle several times.
4. When bubble collapse is not perfectly symmetric, a liquid jet can form. The liquid jet traverses the bubble and impacts on the surface of tissue perpendicularly at considerable speed.

Additionally, during the positive pressure phase of a second shock, or radial pressure, wave pulse, may also push the liquid of the surrounding medium towards one of the walls of a preformed bubble. That wall goes under deformation and reaches the opposite wall of the same bubble to originate a water jet in the same direction of the propagation of the shock wave. The formation of a water jet usually occurs in the vicinity of boundary areas between materials of differing density, such as bone and cartilage, in the direction of the boundary area. The generated water jet is faster with increasing softness of the interface and more damaging than jets from inertial cavitation. In addition, the presence of a hard biomaterial (e.g. bone and cartilage) causes the bubble to collapse towards it. Besides, as the bubble expands, the interface between the medium and the biomaterial is pushed away from the bubble; however, when the bubble collapses, the interface moves slightly towards the bubble. It should be noted that inertial cavitation bubbles near softer material, such as fat, skin and muscle, tend to collapse by splitting into two or three smaller bubbles without the formation of water jets [7, 21, 38, 46, 47].

3.4. Acoustic radiation pressure

This is the proposed mechanism by which LIPUS stimulates living tissues. The authors also believe this is the main mechanism by which ESWT and RPWT stimulate living tissues. Acoustic radiation pressure tends to increase in proportion to intensity, is generally relatively small in magnitude and produces forces and motions at much lower frequencies than those of the incident acoustic wave. While the tensile phase of the shock and radial pressure waves generates cavitations, the positive pressure phase of those waves produces acoustic radiation pressure [9, 35, 37, 45].

Radiation pressure is a universal phenomenon in any wave motion involving sound. It is exerted on surface or media interfaces and acts in the direction of propagation of the wave thereby producing direct and indirect mechanical stress. Direct mechanical stress is produced by strain. Following mechanical deformation, bone exhibits electrical activity and cellular activation. It is unclear, however, whether the main responsible for bone electrical activity is piezoelectricity, streaming potentials, or ion channels and ATP receptor activities (see 3.4.1) [4, 28, 34, 45].

Indirect mechanical stress is produced by acoustic streaming and modal conversion. When acoustic waves are refracted from water to soft tissues, waves propagate longitudinally (in the same direction of the beam source) due to impedance similarity. Differently, when acoustic waves are refracted to materials with impedance mismatch, such as bones, modal conversion occurs, that is, shear waves (waves at right angles to the direction of the beam source) are produced along with longitudinal waves. Shear waves may produce direct mechanical deformation to tissue, called shear stress [7, 27, 36, 45].

Acoustic radiation pressure decreases with the distance of the wave from its source; hence, radiation pressure gradients are formed within the fluid. As a result, fluid flow originates, which is called acoustic streaming. The flow is directed away from the transducer with gradual build up of the axial streaming speed with distance from the transducer and a peak of velocity in the focal region. The fluid flow continues beyond the focal region and returns to the transducer as recirculation vortices. Fluid flow can also build up again in the acoustic beam after a membrane. Acoustic streaming and microstreaming are often used as synonyms in the literature. Although both produce fluid flow which can modulate osteogenesis, they are distinct phenomena. As described above, acoustic streaming results from radiation pressure gradients, whereas microsteaming is generated by stable cavitation bubbles. Furthermore, not only mechanical deformation but also acoustic streaming increases cell membrane permeability and generates streaming potentials. It has not been shown, however, whether acoustic streaming directly affects cell membrane permeability, or triggers cellular reactions that increase membrane permeability [30, 37, 45, 48]. For a detailed explanation of streaming potentials, see reference [3].

3.4.1. Electric potentials

Bone exhibits electrical activity when subjected to mechanical forces. The opposite is also true: bone undergoes deformation when exposed to electric potentials. For instance, ESWT induces transient cell membrane hyperpolarization. There are three possible contributors to electric potentials on bone. First, mechanically induced activity of ion channels and ATP receptors promotes ion transport between the intra and extracellular environments resulting in membrane action potentials; second, piezoelectricity, which is the generation of electricity when asymmetric crystalline materials—as those that form the extracellular matrix of bone—are subjected to strain; and finally, streaming potentials that result from mechanically induced flow of fluid containing high conductivity ions [3, 4, 44, 49].

4. Mechanosensation and mechanotransduction

4.1. Strain amplification

The various cell types that populate bone—osteoblasts, osteocytes, osteoclasts, periosteal cells (fibroblasts and progenitor cells) and bone marrow cells (include mesenchymal stem cells)—are responsive to mechanical stimulation. Bone is a hard material that can handle up to 2% of strain (i.e. 20,000 μstrain) without failure (fracture). However, based on in vitro studies, bone cells need strains up to 10% in order to direct their response to osteogenesis. In addition, a large amount of energy is lost during wave propagation within bone by means of attenuation and reflection; as such, bone cells may be exposed to low pressure waves. A possible explanation would be that strains are amplified at tissue level, so that cells are exposed to higher strain intensities. At the moment, that hypothesis could not be proved. Nevertheless, the following mathematic-based model supports that explanation [1–3, 41, 43, 44, 50–57].

The model for strain amplification was based on the microanatomy of osteocytes, which are the main mechanosensors of bone. Cytoplasmic processes of osteocytes are separated from their canalicular wall by a pericellular space filled with albumin-rich fluid. Moreover, cytoplasmic processes are anchored to their canalicular wall by transverse fibrils. When mechanically induced fluid flow collides with fibrils, hoop strains are generated on the membrane-cytoskeleton system of cytoplasmic processes. Hoop strains produce forces which are 20–100 times higher than at bone's surface. The magnitude of hoop strains depends on the relationship between fluid and transverse fibrils within pericellular space, and between cell membrane and cytoskeleton constituents (i.e. actin filaments and fimbrins) [3, 57–61].

4.2. Mechanoreceptors

Several structures at cell membrane act as "mechanoreceptors." Mechanically-induced structural deformation of mechanoreceptors triggers their activation. Sequentially, a cascade of biological reactions initiates and results in osteogenesis. Known mechanoreceptors of bone cells include integrins, ATP receptors, ion channels, growth factors (includes hormones) receptors, low-density lipoprotein receptors, frizzled proteins, G proteins and connexins. Among those mechanoreceptors, only integrins were proved to have a role in mechanosensation of ESWT. Regarding mechanosensation of LIPUS, integrins, ATP receptors, growth factors receptors, low-density lipoprotein receptors and frizzled proteins have established participation. In the following sections, the molecular events triggered by LIPUS and ESWT are described. To date, RPWT effects on bone cells have not been investigated properly. It should be noted that acoustic loading refers only to LIPUS, ESWT or RPWT, and mechanical loading refers to any type of mechanical forces that may, or not, be acoustic loads. **Tables 2** and **3** enlist molecular events related to LIPUS and ESWT [1, 10, 50, 55, 62–66].

4.2.1. Integrins

Mechanoreceptors convert mechanical deformations into biological reactions, a process called mechanotransduction. Among mechanoreceptors, it is believed that integrins are vital for mechanotransduction. Evidence suggests the activation of all others mechanoreceptors and a multitude of signalling pathways are integrin-dependent. Therefore, osteogenic response of bone cells (adhesion, migration, differentiation and proliferation) depends on integrins. The expression of α2, α5, β1, β3 integrins subunits are increased by mechanical loading. Furthermore, clusters of α5β1 and αvβ3 integrins formed at the deformation site—also known as focal adhesions—attract a number of cytoplasmic proteins and trigger a cascade of reactions [3, 10, 37, 43, 50, 53, 55, 60, 67–71].

Signalling pathways	LIPUS	ESWT
α5β1 and αvβ3 integrins/FAK/Scr/Grb2/Sos/Ras/Raf-1/MEK/ERK/IKKα,β/IκBα/NFκB/cox-2/PGE_2	X	
α5β1 and αvβ3 integrins/FAK/Scr/Grb2/Sos/Ras/Raf-1/MEK/ERK/IKKα,β/IκBα/NFκB/iNOS/NO	X	
α5β1 integrin/FAK/Scr/Grb2/Sos/Ras/Raf/MEK/ERK		X
α5β1 and αvβ3 integrins/FAK/PI3K/Akt/NFκB/cox-2/PGE_2	X	
α5β1 integrin/β-catenin	X	X
AT1/ERK-1,2	X	
Ras/Rac1/NADPH/superoxide/ERK/cbfa1		X
Ras/Rac1/NADPH/superoxide/HIF-1α/VEGF		X
α5β1 and αvβ3 integrins/FAK/PI3K/Akt/Bcl-2	X	

Table 2. Signalling pathways triggered by acoustic stimulation.

Biological effects	LIPUS	ESWT
Increased expression of α5 and β1 integrins	X	X
Increased expression of α2 and β3 integrins	X	
β1 and β3 integrins clustering	X	
α5β1-mediated FAK activation	X	X
αvβ3-mediated FAK activation	X	
Increased IRS-1 activity	X	
Increased $P2X_7$receptor activation and activation, and ATP release	X	
$P2Y_1$ receptor activation		
mTOR activation	X	
Bax expression	X	X
ILK phosphorylation	X	

http://dx.doi.org/10.5772/63745

Biological effects	LIPUS	ESWT
IκBα degradation	X	
Increased parathyroid hormone receptor-1 expression	X	
Increased iNOS, NO, cox-2 and PGE_2 production	X	X
Increased HIF-1α and VEGF expression	X	X
RANKL production	X	
Increased IGF-1 production	X	
Increased TGF-β1 production		X
Increased cyclin E2/CDK2 activation		X
Increased bone sialoprotein expression	X	X
Increased osterix expression	X	
Increased osteopontin expression	X	X
Increased osteocalcin expression	X	X
Increased ALP activity	X	X
Increased type I collagen expression	X	X
Increased bone nodule formation	X	X
Increased CBFA1 expression (core binding factor alfa-1)	X	X
Increased SDF-1 (serum and bone) and CXCR4 expression	X	
Increased c-fos, c-jun, c-myc, TSC-22 (transforming growth factor-beta stimulated clone), SOST, FGF-23, Msx2, Dlx	X	
Increased BMP-2	X	X
Increased BMP-4, BMP-7, BMPR-IA, BMPR-IB, ActR-I, BMPR-II, ActR-IIA, ActR-IIB, Smad1	X	
Increased FGF-2		X
Increased egr-1 (early growth response)	X	
Decreased PPARγ activity	X	
Increased superoxide production		X
Osteoblast differentiation	X	
Osteoblast proliferation	X	X
Osteoblast adhesion		X
Osteoblast migration		X
Bone marrow cells proliferation	X	X
Bone marrow cells osteogenic differentiation		X
Mesenchymal stem cell migration and differentiation	X	

Table 3. Biological effects of LIPUS and ESWT.

4.2.2. *ATP receptors*

ATP receptors promote the exchange of calcium from intracellular deposits to extracellular environment, or from extracellular environment to intracellular environment. ATP receptors complex with integrins and G proteins, and some ($P2X_7$ and $P2Y_1$) are activated by mechanical loading. By means that need to be explored, mechanically induced activation of $P2X_7$ and $P2Y_1$ induce osteogenic differentiation—represented by increased expression of cbfa-1, osterix, type I collagen, bone sialoprotein, osteopontin and osteocalcin—and osteoblasts proliferation [3, 64, 72].

4.2.3. *Wnt pathways*

Activation of Wnt canonical pathways involves the formation of complexes between Wnt1, or Wnt3a, Frizzled proteins and LRP-5/6, which may be integrin dependent. Those complexes prevent cytoplasmic β-catenin degradation, which, in turn, translocates to nucleus, where it activates members of the TCF/LEF family to promote osteogenesis. Acoustic stimulation increases expression of Wnt1, Wnt3a, β-catenin and Frizzled proteins 2/4. It also activates β-catenin in an integrin-dependent manner. Wnt5a, which plays a role in Wnt non-canonical pathway, is responsive to mechanical stimulation, but its responsiveness to acoustic stimulation is yet to be evaluated [3, 10, 73].

4.2.4. *Growth factors and hormones crosstalk*

Different growth factors and hormones induce osteogenesis that includes bone cells proliferation, migration and adhesion to stimulation sites, angiogenesis and osteogenic differentiation. Mechanical stimulation possesses the same effect and affects growth factors and hormones signalling. Acoustic stimulation increases the expression of BMP-2/4/7 and related receptors (BMPR-IA, BMPR-IB, ActR-I, BMPR-II, ActR-IIA, ActR-IIB), FGF-2, IGF-1, PTHr-1, TGF-β1 and VEGF. Nevertheless, the exact signaling pathways of those factors are still not fully understood [37, 44, 54, 66, 74–80].

BMP-2, BMP-4 and BMP-7 play important roles in osteogenesis following fracture. They stimulate mesenchymal cell proliferation and osteogenic differentiation, induce osteoprogenitor cell migration, modulate osteoclast activity and promote angiogenesis. Their mechanism of action involves Smad-1, which is activated by BMP receptors; then Smad-1 translocates to nucleus where it upregulates transcription of osteogenic factors as cbfa1. Acoustic stimulation activates Smad-1, but it has not been proved whether BMP receptors activity is responsible to Smad-1 acoustically induced activation [66, 75].

Similar to BMPs, TGF-β1 induces cellular proliferation, osteogenic differentiation, mineralization and angiogenesis. Acoustic force-induced TGF-β1 production depends on superoxide production which is possibly promoted by Ras/Rac-1/NADPH oxidase pathway. Superoxide is a free radical that, in contrary to common knowledge, is harmless to bone cells when produced by a certain range of acoustic pressure (that is yet to be determined). Moreover, superoxide promotes ERK activation, which induces osteogenic differentiation through cbfa-1 transcription [79, 81].

Angiogenesis is vital for fracture healing. BMPs, TGF-β1 and VEGF induce angiogenesis. Among those factors, VEGF seems to be the most important for angiogenesis. HIF-1α is a transcription factor that regulates VEGF expression and is activated by acoustic stimulation. In addition, superoxide and Ras mediate HIF-1α activation and VEGF expression. However, VEGF expression is not dependent on BMP-2, TGF-β1, IGF-1, cox-2, PGE_2 and Ca^{2+} influx. Interestingly, LIPUS-induced VEGF expression depends on NO production, whereas ESWT-induced VEGF expression does not [81–83].

4.2.5. *Differentiation markers and transcriptional factors*

A variety of differentiation markers are modulated by acoustic stimulation, such as cbfa-1, osterix, bone sialoprotein, osteopontin, osteocalcin, type I collagen and ALP. Contrarily, the unique report investigating RPWT effects in osteoblasts showed decreased expression of cbfa-1, osterix, type I collagen, bone sialoprotein and osteocalcin. RPWT is commonly used for orthopaedic pathologies of soft tissues with satisfactory results, but no reports were found for bone-related orthopaedic disorders. Therefore, further investigations are required to determine the biological effects of RPWT on bone [33, 43, 44, 75, 76].

Regarding cellular proliferation, there are some transcriptional factors that are affected by acoustic forces, such as c-fos, c-jun, c-myc, egr-1, TSC-22, SOST, FGF-23, Dlx, Msx2 and cyclin E2/CDK2 [37, 39, 43, 55, 68, 69, 84–86].

4.2.6. *Signalling for migration*

Cells must migrate to the healing site so that new bone can be generated. SDF-1 is an important chemotactic factor mostly produced by immature osteoblasts in the endosteal region near stem cells population. SDF-1 normally is released from the fracture site to attract mesenchymal stem cells which will differentiate into osteoblasts. SDF-1 binds to CXCR4, a seven transmembrane G-protein coupled receptor, and triggers a cascade of reactions leading to cellular migration and survival. Reports have shown that acoustic loading increases expression of SDF-1 and CXCR4, thereby resulting in mesenchymal stem cells migration to the fracture site. In spite of that, more investigation is needed to clarify the exact cascade of reactions triggered by SFD-1/CXCR4 [56, 87–89].

4.2.7. *Signalling for bone remodelling*

Bone remodelling is an important step of bone healing. This important stage follows bone formation and is governed by osteoclasts—bone cells of the granulocyte/monocyte lineage—that resorb extracellular matrix. In order to attract osteoclast progenitor cells to the healing site, osteoblasts express MCP-1, MIP-1, RANTES and IL-8. Osteoblasts also express, or secrete, RANKL, which induces osteoclasts differentiation through their native RANK; and secrete OPG, a decoy receptor of RANKL, which antagonizes RANKL-mediated osteoclastogenesis. Acoustic loading in the form of LIPUS affects osteoclastogenesis by increasing the expression of MCP-1, MIP-1b, RANKL and OPG in osteoblasts through AT1. Increased RANKL expression is also dependent on integrins activity. Moreover, acoustic forces increase the expression of MIP-2, which may also be involved in osteoclastogenesis. On the other hand, it has been shown that low-energy ESWT decreases OPG and RANKL expression in osteoblasts; RPWT does not change OPG expression, but decreases RANKL; and LIPUS does not change the expression of OPG (contradictory results) and RANTES in osteoblasts. Those data show that acoustic deformation affects osteoclastogenesis; however, the exact influence on osteoclastogenesis needs to be better elucidated [33, 43, 50, 55].

4.2.8. Proteins with few data

There is another list of proteins whose activation has been shown to be influenced by acoustic waves, but there is poor information about their role in mechanotransduction and osteogenesis:

1. AT1 is classically involved in arterial pressure control. This receptor was identified in bone cells, but its role is yet to be determined. AT1 is required for mechanically induced ERK-1/2 activation [50].

2. Bax is a key component for apoptosis induced through interactions with pore proteins on the mitochondrial membrane. Bax mechanism of activation is complex and not fully understood, but may be modulated by acoustic deformation in favour of cell survival. Bax activation is also integrin dependent [43, 70].

3. IRS-1 activity increased in intact and healthy bones of rats subjected to acoustic stimulation. IRS-1 is involved in insulin-mediated and IGF-1-mediated bone formation, but its mechanism of activation following acoustic loading is yet to be determined [90].

4. p38 is a MAPK that regulates cell proliferation and differentiation. Because conflicting results were found for p38 activation following LIPUS and ESWT, more investigation is required. Some studies report increased activity, while others report unchanged activity [68, 81, 91, 92].

5. PPARγ2 is expressed in mesenchymal stem cells. Upon acoustic stimulation, PPARγ2 drives those cells to differentiate into osteogenic lineage [68].

5. Optimization of biological responses

As previously described, acoustic loads can be exerted by different types of waves, such as LIPUS, ESWT and RPWT. Changing some physical properties (e.g. magnitude and frequency) and mode of application (e.g. axial distance, incidence angle and number of cycles) of acoustic waves can elicit different cellular responses. No studies explored the subject with RPWT.

5.1. Magnitude and number of cycles

According to mechanostat model, for strains within the overuse range, bone formation increases as a proportion of the load magnitude. Loads within the pathological overuse range stimulate osteogenesis, but also damage tissue until bone breaks (about 15,000–20,000 μstrain). Furthermore, cellular response also increases as a proportion of the number of cycles [3].

LIPUS at intensities between 2 and 150 mW/cm^2 were compared. Higher intensities produced greater bone formation, faster healing rate, and better torsional stiffness and failure torque. The best results were found for 30 mW/cm^2. Average temperature at the soft tissue was 1.74°C higher for 150 mW/cm^2 in comparison with 30 mW/cm^2. Temperature elevation may affect some enzymes like collagenase I and cause tissue damage, resulting in worse biological response. LIPUS commonly is applied as a daily 20-min treatment; therefore, the number of cycles are not changed [29, 93, 94].

On the contrary, there is no exact protocol for ESWT that determines the best response to stimulation. ESWT at magnitudes ranging from 0.05 to 0.62 mJ/mm^2 positively affects osteogenesis. The number of impulses of shock waves corresponds to the number of cycles of ESWT. In studies, number of impulses varies from 250 to more than 4000. Moreover, biological response is different when treatment is performed in vitro, or in vivo with small animals (e.g. rodents), or in vivo with large animals (e.g. goats) and humans. For most in vitro studies, 500 impulses promote the best cellular response; above this threshold, cellular damage surpasses bone formation. On the other hand, the best intensity (mJ/mm^2) could not be found, suggesting that, for cells directly exposed to ESWT, the number of cycles affects cellular response more than the intensity of energy density itself. On the other hand, most in vivo studies in animals show that better responses are elicited by higher energy densities up to 0.47 mJ/mm^2 in comparative studies, while number of cycles (impulses) was not proved to have the same influence [54, 95–98].

5.2. Frequency

Normally, load frequencies within the range of 1–30 Hz at physiological and overuse ranges progressively induce osteogenesis. Higher frequencies (17–90 Hz), in the form of vibration, induce osteogenesis but at a much lower strain range (about 5 μstrain; i.e. strain in the order of 10^{-5}). LIPUS is a low magnitude and high frequency wave, which, based on mathematical and experimental models, produces strains in the order of 10^{-5} at 1.5 MHz. Because of high frequency, those strains promote the same effects as strains in the order of 10^{-1} (i.e. 10% = 100,000 μstrain) at 1 Hz on cells, and the estimated intracellular strain on organelles is about 0.5% (i.e. 5000 μstrain). Accordingly, it was shown that LIPUS increased transcriptional factors (c-fos, c-jun and c-myc) as frequency increased, resulting in maximum response at 5 MHz (within a range from 2 to 8 Mhz). Those calculations were obtained for strains at cellular level. For strains at bone level, it is believed that the model for strain amplification (see Section 4.1) may apply firstly, followed by the estimative presented here. No investigations were found about the role of frequency on ESWT and RPWT [3, 99–101].

5.3. Axial distance

Energy distribution varies according to the distance from the transducer and the surface (axial distance). For LIPUS, two zones were defined according to axial distance: near field (close to transducer) and far field (about 130 mm away from transducer). There is also a mid-near field, when the surface is about 60 mm away from transducer. Within near field, energy distribution of LIPUS beam is not uniform. As such, there are many peaks of acoustic pressure (maxima and minima) across the beam diameter. As the distance from transducer increases, the number of peaks of acoustic pressure across the beam diameter decreases (less maxima and minima). When surface is at far field, a regular beam is formed [5, 102].

As LIPUS transducer is placed transcutaneously during treatment, superficial and deeper cells are exposed to different acoustic fields. Although LIPUS promotes osteogenesis within near, mid-near and far fields, axial distance affects the biological effects of LIPUS. Mid-near field LIPUS elicited greater callus formation in a fractured-femur rat model; on the other hand, in that same model, femurs subjected to far field LIPUS exhibited higher peak torque and torsional stiffness. Those results indicate that, mid-near field LIPUS is optimal for cellular proliferation, while far field LIPUS stands for osteogenic differentiation (bone mineralization). Reinforcing that, mid-near LIPUS incited more NO production whereas far field LIPUS promoted increased ALP activity and mineralization in preosteoblasts. Moreover, both mid-near and far field LIPUS produced increased β-catenin nuclear translocation [5, 102].

During ESWT, maximal intensity of energy density is obtained at the focus. Consequently, superficial and deeper cells are exposed to different acoustic fields. However, no studies were found on this subject for ESWT and RPWT.

5.4. Incidence angle

As previously described, acoustic waves transmitted into bone can be decomposed in longitudinal waves and shear waves. The magnitude of each wave depends on the incidence angle of the acoustic wave. Accordingly, two critical angles were determined. The first critical angle is defined as the angle of incidence after which incident acoustic waves travel along the medium surface and only shear waves are refracted to that medium. In that case, longitudinal waves do not travel into the medium. The second critical angle is defined as the angle at which acoustic waves are totally reflected and shear waves travel along the medium surface, but not into the medium. For LIPUS, the first critical angle is 22°, and the second critical angle is 48°. Between the first and second critical angles, at 35°, the amount of transmitted shear waves is maximized, and an optimal cellular response is obtained. Those critical angles were not determined for ESWT and RPWT [36].

5.5. Different sources of acoustic waves

As previously described, the method for producing low-intensity pulsed ultrasound waves is unique, but there are three generation methods for extracorporeal shock waves. No clinical studies compare the effectiveness between the three methods, but one experimental research compared osteoblasts responses to electrohydraulic and electromagnetic ESWT. It was found greater cell viability and osteocalcin expression for electrohydraulic-stimulated cells, and greater expression of type I procollagen-C enzyme, and TGF-β1 production for electromagnetic-stimulated cells. These findings can be attributed to the difference in the pressure distribution at the focal zone between the electrohydraulic and electromagnetic generators [40].

5.6. Combined therapy

Mechanical stimulation can be combined with different types of acoustic waves or with growth factors.

5.6.1. ESWT and LIPUS

Electromagnetic ESWT and LIPUS combined therapy applied to periosteal cells showed no difference regarding cell proliferation, cell viability and ALP activity in comparison with ESWT alone, but, in comparison with LIPUS alone, showed worse results for early response (after 6 days) and better results for late response (after 18 days) [42].

5.6.2. LIPUS and growth factors

BMPs are known osteogenic factors. Their combined therapy (BMP-7 or rhBMP-2) with LIPUS enhances bone formation, osteogenic differentiation and biomechanical properties of bone [103, 104].

Bisphosphonates are anti-osteoclastic agents that increase or maintain bone mineral density in osteoporotic patients. Combined therapy with LIPUS is not better than alendronate or LIPUS alone to increase bone healing. On the other hand, combined therapy with LIPUS enhances bone mineral density more than separate treatment [105].

1,25-Dihydroxyvitamin D3 increases the expression of VEGF in osteoblasts and modulates cellular proliferation and differentiation. Combined treatment with LIPUS, however, does not ameliorate cellular response in comparison with LIPUS or 1,25-dihydroxyvitamin D3 alone [106].

Statins (e.g. simvastatin, mevastatin and lovastatin) stimulate osteogenesis through Ras/Smad/ERK/BMP-2 pathway. Combined therapy with LIPUS does not increase bone formation rate more than statins or LIPUS alone [77].

No studies were found on the subject for ESWT and RPWT.

6. Acoustic therapy

Clinical applications for acoustic therapy include nonunions and delayed unions. Debatable applications include acceleration of fracture healing, acceleration of segmental defects healing, enhancement of bone density and quality, management of stress fracture, enhancement of bone-tendon junction healing and management of avascular necrosis of the femoral head.

LIPUS has a unique protocol of treatment, which consists of daily 20-min sessions at 30 mW/cm^2. On the contrary, ESWT has no established protocol regarding energy levels, frequency, number of sessions and number of cycles (impulses). This heterogeneity makes it difficult for the clinician to adopt the best approach for ESWT. No studies were found on the subject for RPWT.

6.1. Delayed union and nonunion

Normally, patients with nonunion and delayed union are managed surgically for revision of a primary surgery or for biological stimulation. Those managed surgically for biological stimulation may be the best candidates for a non-invasive approach with acoustic therapy, since there is no problem with hardware and fracture reduction. Those experiencing technical problems related to the first procedure (gross bone instability, broken hardware, malalignment) should be subjected to revision surgery combined with acoustic therapy to provide also biological stimulation.

LIPUS exhibits healing rate from 67 to 92% and may challenge surgical treatment for delayed union and nonunion. Patients aged 70–79 years feature decreased healing rates (83.3 vs 86.2%), and older than 80 years feature even lower healing rates (77.8 vs 86.2%). LIPUS may also be an alternative approach to treat conservatively congenital pseudarthrosis of the tibia. Mean body mass index, open fracture, multiple prior surgical procedures, time to initiate treatment with LIPUS, type of surgical procedure, comorbidities and number of smoking years represented no risk factor for failure with LIPUS in a cohort of 767 patients. Smaller cohorts present some conflicting data: decreased healing rate was found in late treated (more than 12 months) nonunions and smokers. Moreover, atrophic nonunions may be a risk factor for decreased healing rates. Interestingly, LIPUS combined with iliac crest autograft exhibits synergistic effect to overcome spinal pseudarthrosis created by nicotine administration, although LIPUS alone cannot [94, 107–114].

ESWT also shows healing rates that may challenge surgical treatment for nonunion and delayed union, with successful rates ranging from 63.6 to 95% using electrohydraulic or electromagnetic devices. No reports explored the effectiveness of piezoelectric devices, and RPWT. Energy density varied from 0.25 to 0.70 mJ/mm^2, 1000–10000 impulses, single or multiple sessions. Technical parameters depended on bone size and authorship. Specifically for scaphoid pseudarthrosis, energy density varied from 0.05 to 0.12 mJ/mm^2 depending on patient's pain tolerance. Some studies also investigated serum level of BMP-2, NO, TGF-β1 and VEGF, which were higher in treated individuals. Again, atrophic nonunions, smoking and treatment performed at late stages (after 12 months) provided decreased healing rates [115–124].

6.2. Accelerated healing of bone defects and fractures

The potential benefits of LIPUS and ESWT to accelerate healing of bone defects and fractures have been shown in various animal studies, but there is not sufficient clinical evidence to support their routine use.

LIPUS promoted earlier callus formation, promoted larger callus width, increased biomechanical strength, reduced adverse outcomes (nonunion and delayed union), accelerated maturation of newly formed bone and healing time in distraction osteogenesis and reduced time for fracture healing. LIPUS reduced 18–36 days of healing time in conservatively treated fractures, and decreased about 30% of the healing time for surgically managed closed comminuted diaphyseal tibial and femoral fractures (irrespective of implant choice). Open fractures and patients older than 60 years had pronounced benefit from LIPUS treatment. LIPUS' effectiveness increases as soon as treatment is initiated. In addition, fractures of the metatarsal, radius, scaphoid, ankle, fibula and ulna exhibited better healing rates. Smoking, diabetes, vascular insufficiency, osteoporosis, cancer, rheumatoid arthritis and obesity are risk factors for failure. A large cohort of 4190 patients showed 96% healing rate, which is greater than literature averages (93%). In that study, patients between 20 and 29 years old had greater healing rate than patients over 30 years old. Furthermore, LIPUS has no reported adverse effects [37, 56, 86, 125–132].

Only electrohydraulic devices investigated the beneficial effects of ESWT for bone defects and fracture healing. Energy density varied from 0.16 to 0.62 mJ/mm^2, 500–6000 impulses, single or multiple sessions. Increased callus formation; biomechanical properties; ALP activity; and expression of BMPs, IGF-1, eNOS, TGF-β1 and VEGF were reported. Patients subjected to ESWT exhibited better pain scores and decreased nonunion rates, but no difference of fracture-related complications rate. Reported complications include skin petechiae, scarring to the muscle at the treatment site (only for small animals) and subcutaneous swelling. No neuronal damage has been reported even for vertebral exposure (study with small animals) [54, 80, 91, 95, 98, 133–136].

6.2.1. *Diabetes*

Diabetes is a systemic disease that affects bone healing. Therefore, diabetic individuals are at risk of developing delayed unions, nonunions and pseudarthrosis. Those individuals may also exhibit impaired biomechanical strength of newly formed bone. LIPUS does not increase cellular proliferation during fracture healing in diabetic animals but increases bone healing and biomechanical properties. Additionally, LIPUS increases the expression of TGF-β1 and VEGF but not the expression of IGF-1 and PDGF-β. There are no reports on ESWT and RPWT in diabetic animals or individuals [137, 138].

6.2.2. *Osteoporosis*

Fracture healing slows and endochondral ossification is impaired with senescence. At the molecular aspect, fracture-induced cox-2 expression in aged rats is lower than youngsters. Thankfully, bone cells keep their mechanosensitivity; as such, acoustic stimulation accelerates fracture healing. It has been shown that LIPUS accelerates fracture healing in estrogen-deficient osteoporotic bone and regains biomechanical strength so that it becomes comparable to non-osteoporotic bones also subjected to LIPUS. Furthermore, LIPUS increases the activity of ALP, and the expression of aggrecan, BMP-2/4/6, cbfa-1, cox-2, FGF-2, OPG, osteocalcin, osterix, RANKL, TGF-α1, VEGF and types I, II and X collagen. The effects of ESWT and RPWT were not investigated for fractures in osteoporotic bones [139–141].

6.2.3. Bone-implant osseointegration

Osseointegration of implants is an important step for recovery of biomechanical strength of bone. Facilitation of this biological process may decrease recovery time and the risk of hardware failure. LIPUS accelerates osseointegration of titanium screws in tibias and femurs, porous hydroxyapatite ceramic and miniscrew implants. Histologically, LIPUS-induced osseointegration provides denser trabecular microstructure at implant-bone interface and thicker newly formed bone. Those findings suggest acoustic therapy may be used as adjunctive therapy to increase hardware lifetime (e.g. for arthroplasties) and decrease recovery time. No reports were found on the subject for ESWT and RPWT [142–144].

6.2.4. Bone graft substitutes

Bone graft substitutes provide an osteoconductive scaffold for filling large osseous defects, and they are an alternative for autologous bone graft, which adds morbidity to the patient. Acoustic therapy provides osteoinductive stimulation for bone. Therefore, combination of acoustic therapy and bone graft substitutes may be a finer alternative to treat fractures associated with large defects. A report showed LIPUS increased bone formation in ulna defect filled with β-tricalcium phosphate (bone graft substitute). In addition, LIPUS did not alter resorption rate of the bone graft substitute. The influence of ESWT and RPWT on large osseous defects filled with bone graft substitutes needs to be explored [86].

6.2.5. Bone-tendon junction

Healing at bone-tendon junction is crucial for tendon repairs (e.g. quadriceps tendon repair, rotator cuff repair, calcaneal tendon repair) and ligament reconstruction (e.g. anterior cruciate ligament of the knee reconstruction and medial patellofemoral ligament reconstruction) to ensure early recovery and improved biomechanical strength. Acoustic therapy may be used as adjunctive therapy in those situations since LIPUS and ESWT were found to enhance healing of bone-tendon junction. Histologically, those acoustic therapies promoted better remodelling of the newly formed trabecular bone, increased bone mineral density and improved tendon-to-bone collagen fibre reconnection [145–147].

6.2.6. Stress fractures

Stress fractures are pathological overuse injuries common in athletes and military recruits. Those injuries result from repetitive loading beyond the regenerative capacity of bone, and represent failure of the adaptive mechanisms of bone to mechanical loads. Results regarding this subject are variable.

LIPUS at 30 mW/cm^2 used to treat incomplete stress injury of the posteromedial tibia, fibula, or second to fourth metatarsals was ineffective to accelerate recovery during a 4-week treatment. On the other hand, LIPUS at 100 mW/cm^2 accelerated stress fracture healing of ulnae even in the presence of non-steroidal anti-inflammatory drugs, which normally delay fracture healing. In addition, athletes with delayed or nonunions of stress fractures of tibia or fifth metatarsus experienced bone healing within 6–14 weeks of exposure to electromagnetic ESWT [148–150].

6.3. Intact bone

Despite fractures, bone is subject to other diseases that alter its biomechanical strength, such as osteoporosis; or produce disabling pain, such as avascular necrosis of the femoral head. Acoustic therapy may be used for prevention and treatment of some bone disorders.

6.3.1. *Healthy bone*

It is not known how healthy and intact bone reacts to acoustic loading. Most studies focus on pathological conditions, such as fractures and osteoporosis. The understanding of the normal response of bone to acoustic loads within the physiological range and overuse range is required to ameliorate the comprehension of tissue behaviour in pathological situations, and to prevent some disorders; for instance, stress fractures and osteoporosis.

Intact and healthy bones subjected to LIPUS experience increased density of trabecular spongiosa, and increased activity of FAK, ERK-1/2 and IRS-1. Electrohydraulic ESWT (from 0.15 to 0.47 mJ/mm^2, 500–6000 impulses, single session), in turn, promotes angiogenesis, increased cellular population and bone formation, increased activity of ERK-1/2 and Akt, and increased TGF-β1 production, but no difference on biomechanical tests was found following ESWT exposure [54, 79, 90, 95, 151–153].

6.3.2. *Osteoporosis*

Studies demonstrated that LIPUS does not increase bone mineral density of osteoporotic bones and does not prevent osteoporosis as measured by dual energy X-ray absorptiometry. However, in those studies the exposure to LIPUS occurred within a short time (from 4 to 12 weeks), and the population of some investigations was heterogeneous. Additionally, histological and molecular analysis of osteoporotic bones subjected to LIPUS showed increased bone formation, normal density of trabecular spongiosa, decreased disruption of trabecular spongiosa and greater expression of cbfa-1 (although lower than controls) [37, 153–157]. Therefore, the authors believe LIPUS possesses beneficial effects for treating osteoporosis.

Electromagnetic ESWT exhibited more pronounced effects on osteoporotic intact bones than LIPUS since ESWT showed increased bone mineral density and decreased bone loss [158].

6.3.3. *Immature bone*

Concern exists about possible negative effects of ESWT on ephiphyseal plaque in skeletally immature individuals; therefore, ESWT is not formally indicated for children. Contrarily, LIPUS is not contraindicated for skeletally immature individuals. Two studies addressed the effects of ESWT on epiphyseal plaques of animals. It was found that electrohydraulic or electromagnetic ESWT, from 0.38 to 0.60 mJ/mm^2, 1500–3000 impulses, single or multiple sessions, did not harm epiphyseal plaque cells and did not impair growth. Furthermore, histological analysis revealed increased number of chondrocytes in the proliferative zone and increased thickness of the epiphyseal plaque, suggesting a possible role for growth stimulation. No studies were found for LIPUS that could suggest a possible role for growth stimulation in skeletally immature individuals [96, 97].

6.3.4. Avascular necrosis of the femoral head

Patients who develop avascular necrosis of the femoral head experience groin pain and disability, and further may necessitate joint replacement. A novel possible approach for initial stages of that condition, when bone collapse and osteoarthritis have not established yet, is acoustic therapy. Experimental studies with avascular necrosis of the femoral head models showed that LIPUS and electrohydraulic ESWT increase neovascularization, osteogenesis, osteogenic differentiation of bone marrow cells, decreased size of fat cells—which substitute dead bone—and biomechanical strength of bone. Increased expression of proliferative factors, such as BMP-2, FGF, IGF-1, NO and VEGF, was also found. Furthermore, a clinical and an experimental research revealed that electrohydraulic ESWT may be more effective than core decompression and non-vascularized fibular grafting in patients with early-stage disease; reverts osteonecrosis by one stage; decelerates, or stops, disease' progression; and decreases pain and functional disability [10, 38, 149, 159, 160].

7. Future directions

Undoubtedly, acoustic devices are useful tools to stimulate osteogenesis. Nevertheless, there is a wide list of topics that require further investigations: physical phenomena elicited by acoustic forces need to be proved in vivo, signalling molecules need to be assigned to specific signalling pathways, the control of cellular response to acoustic loads needs to be clarified, RPWT and piezoelectric ESWT influence on bone biology lack investigations, clinical protocols for ESWT and RPWT should be established and, finally, randomized controlled trials addressing acoustic therapy should be performed. As a conclusion, a lot of research is expected within the next years to clarify the unanswered questions about the relationship of bone tissue and acoustic forces.

Author details

Carlos Vinícius Buarque de Gusmão[1*], José Marcos Alves[2] and William Dias Belangero[1]

*Address all correspondence to: vigusmao@yahoo.com

1 Department of Orthopedics and Traumatology, State University of Campinas (UNICAMP), Campinas, São Paulo, Brazil

2 Department of Electrical Engineering, College of Engineering og São Carlos, University of São Paulo (USP), São Carlos, São Paulo, Brazil

References

[1] Duncan RL, Turner CH. Mechanotransduction and the functional response of bone to mechanical strain. Calcif Tissue Int. 1995;57(5):344–58. DOI: 10.1007/bf00302070

[2] Frost HM. Bone's mechanostat: a 2003 update. Anat Rec A Discov Mol Cell Evol Biol. 2003;275(2):1081–101. DOI: 10.1002/ar.a.10119

[3] Buarque de Gusmão CV, Mariolani JRL, Belangero WD. Mechanotransduction and osteogenesis. In: Yunfeng Lin, editor. Osteogenesis. InTech Open. 2012. 153–82. DOI: 10.5772/34504

[4] Duarte LR. The stimulation of bone growth by ultrasound. Arch Orthop Trauma Surg. 1983;101(3):153–9.

[5] Fung CH, Cheung WH, Pounder NM, Harrison A, Leung KS. Osteocytes exposed to far field of therapeutic ultrasound promotes osteogenic cellular activities in pre-osteoblasts through soluble factors. Ultrasonics. 2014;54(5):1358–65. DOI: 10.1016/j.ultras.2014.02.003

[6] Martinez de Albornoz P, Khanna A, Longo UG, Forriol F, Maffulli N. The evidence of low-intensity pulsed ultrasound for in vitro, animal and human fracture healing. Br Med Bull. 2011;100:39–57. DOI: 10.1093/bmb/ldr006

[7] Ogden JA, Tóth-Kischkat A, Schultheiss R. Principles of shock wave therapy. Clin Orthop Relat Res. 2001;(387):8–17. DOI: 10.1097/00003086-200106000-00003

[8] Schmitz C, Császár NB, Milz S, Schieker M, Maffulli N, Rompe JD, Furia JP. Efficacy and safety of extracorporeal shock wave therapy for orthopedic conditions: a systematic review on studies listed in the PEDro database. Br Med Bull. 2015;116(1):115–38. DOI: 10.1093/bmb/ldv047

[9] Shrivastava SK, Kailash. Shock wave treatment in medicine. J Biosci. 2005;30(2):269–75. DOI: 10.1007/BF02703708

[10] Xu JK, Cheng HJ, Li XD, Huang ZL, Xu H, Yang HL, Hu J. Optimal intensity shock wave promotes the adhesion and migration of rat osteoblasts via integrin β1-mediated expression of phosphorilated focal adhesion kinase. J Biol Chem. 2012;287(31):26200–12. DOI: 10.1074/jbc.M112.349811

[11] Wilbert DM. A comparative review of extracorporeal shock wave generation. BJU Int. 2002;90(5):507–11. DOI: 10.1046/j.1464-4096.2002.02961.x

[12] Tissue Regeneration Technologies. Orthogold 280^{ASWT} [Internet]. 2009. Available from: http://www.trtllc.com/uploads/5/9/7/2/59724091/orthogold_280_brochure.pdf [Accessed: 2016/03/05]

[13] Tissue Regeneration Technologies. Applicator information of dermagold100 and orthogold100 [Internet]. 2009. Available from: http://www.trtllc.com/uploads/5/9/7/2/59724091/_focal_zones_dg100_og100_mts[1].pdf [Accessed: 2016/03/05]

[14] Medispec. Orthospec [Internet]. 2012. Available from: http://www.medispec.com/wp-content/uploads/2012/05/Orthospec.pdf [Accessed: 2016/03/05]

[15] Sanuwave. OrthoPACE [Internet]. Available from: http://www.eswt.hk/img/ortho-PACE%20Presentation%20(Introduction).pdf [Accessed: 2016/03/05]

[16] Storz Medical. DUOLITH VET [Internet]. 2016. Available from: https://www.storz-medical.com/images/brochures/VETERINARY_en/ [Accessed: 2016/03/05]

[17] Dornier MedTech. Epos Ultra [Internet]. Available from: http://www.dornier.com/unitedstates/linkservid/8B1C9B5A-D1EE-4AAB-A43B6FEFD6101674/showMeta/0/ [Accessed: 2016/03/05] Electro Medical Systems.

[18] Technical Data [Internet]. 2016. Available from: http://www.ems-company.com/en/medical/products/swiss-dolorclast/swiss-duoclast/technical-data [Accessed: 2016/03/05]

[19] Richard Wolf. PiezoWave [Internet]. 2014. Available from: http://www.godrmenge.com/wp-content/uploads/2014/02/Piezo-wave-technical-data.pdf [Accessed: 2016/03/05]

[20] Elvation Medical GmbH. Piezo Shockwave Technology [Internet]. 2013. Available from: http://www.hospimed.cz/wp-content/uploads/2013/05/Piezo_Wave_Broschuere_en.pdf [Accessed: 2016/03/05]

[21] Császár NB, Angstman NB, Milz S, Sprecher CM, Kobel P, Farhat M, Furia JP, Schmitz C. Radial shock wave devices generate cavitation. PLoS ONE. 2015;10(10):e0140541. DOI: 10.1371/journal. pone.0140541

[22] Schmitz C, Császár NB, Rompe JD, Chaves H, Furia JP. Treatment of chronic plantar fasciopathy with extracorporeal shock waves (review). J Orthop Surg Res. 2013;8:31. DOI: 10.1186/1749-799X-8-31

[23] Storz Medical. Masterpuls [Internet]. Available from: https://www.storzmedical.com/images/brochures/MASTERPULS_MP50_MP100_MP200_en [Accessed: 2016/03/05]

[24] Storz Medical. Extracorporeal shock wave therapy in veterinary medicine [Internet]. Available from: https://www.storzmedical.com/images/brochures/VETERINARY_en [Accessed: 2016/03/05]

[25] BTL. Shockwave Therapy [Internet]. Available from: http://kreja.eu/img/cms/BTL_udarni_globinski_valovi_katalog.pdf [Accessed: 2016/03/05]

[26] Electro Medical Systems. Technical Data [Internet]. 2016. Available from: http://www.ems-company.com/en/medical/products/swiss%20dolorclast/swiss%20dolor-clast%20classic/technical%20data [Accessed: 2016/03/05]

[27] O'Brien WD Jr. Ultrasound-biophysics mechanisms. Prog Biophys Mol Biol. 2007;93(1–3):212–55.

[28] Sarvazyan AP, Rudenko OV, Nyborg WL. Biomedical applications of radiation force of ultrasound: historical roots and physical basis. Ultrasound Med Biol. 2010;36(9): 1379–94. DOI: 10.1016/j.ultrasmedbio.2010.05.015

[29] Fung CH, Cheung WH, Pounder NM, de Ana FJ, Harrison A, Leung KS. Effects of different therapeutic ultrasound intensities on fracture healing in rats. Ultrasound Med Biol. 2012;38(5):745–52. DOI:10.1016/j.ultrasmedbio.2012.01.022

[30] Padilla F, Puts R, Vico L, Raum K. Stimulation of bone repair with ultrasound: a review of the possible mechanic effects. Ultrasonics. 2014;54(5):1125–45. DOI: 10.1016/j.ultras.2014.01.004

[31] Lei H, Liu J, Li H, Wang L, Xu Y, Tian W, Lin G, Xin Z. Low-intensity shock wave therapy and its application to erectile dysfunction. World J Mens Health. 2013;31(3): 208–14. DOI: 10.5534/wjmh.2013.31.3.208

[32] Neufeld SK, Cerrato R. Plantar fasciitis: evaluation and treatment. J Am Acad Orthop Surg. 2008;16(6):338–46.

[33] Notarnicola A, Tamma R, Moretti L, Fiore A, Vicenti G, Zallone A, Moretti B. Effects of radial shock waves therapy on osteoblasts activities. Musculoskelet Surg. 2012;96(3): 183–9. DOI: 10.1007/s12306-012-0213-4

[34] Chung SL, Pounder NM, de Ana FJ, Qin L, Leung KS, Cheung WH. Fracture healing enhancement with low intensity pulsed ultrasound at a critical application angle. Ultrasound Med Biol. 2011;37(7):1120–33. DOI: 10.1016/j.ultrasmedbio.2011.04.017

[35] Nyborg WL. Biological effects of ultrasound: development of safety guidelines. Part II: general review. Ultrasound Med Biol. 2001;27(3):301–33. DOI: 10.1016/S0301-5629(00)00333-1

[36] Wu J, Nyborg WL. Ultrasound, cavitation bubbles and their interaction with cells. Adv Drug Deliv Rev. 2008;60(10):1103–16. DOI: 10.1016/j.addr.2008.03.009

[37] Claes L, Willie B. The enhancement of bone regeneration by ultrasound. Prog Biophys Mol Biol. 2007;93(1–3):384–98. DOI: 10.1016/j.pbiomolbio.2006.07.021

[38] Ma HZ, Zeng BF, Li XL. Upregulation of VEGF in subchondral bone of necrotic femoral heads in rabbits with use of extracorporeal shock waves. Calcif Tissue Int. 2007;81(2): 124–31. DOI: 10.1007/s00223-007-9046-9

[39] Hofmann A, Ritz U, Hessmann MH, Alini M, Rommens PM, Rompe JD. Extracorporeal shock wave-mediated changes in proliferation, differentiation, and gene expression of human osteoblasts. J Trauma. 2008;65(6):1402–10. DOI: 10.1097/TA.0b013e318173e7c2

[40] Martini L, Giavaresi G, Fini M, Borsari V, Torricelli P, Giardino R. Early effects of extracorporeal shock wave treatment on osteoblast-like cells: a comparative study

between electromagnetic and electrohydraulic devices. J Trauma. 2006;61(5):1198–206. DOI: 10.1097/01.ta.0000203575.96896.34

[41] Tam KF, Cheung WH, Lee KM, Qin L, Leung KS. Delayed stimulatory effect of low-intensity shockwaves on human periosteal cells. Clin Orthop Relat Res. 2005;438:260–5. DOI: 10.1097/01.blo.0000169080.23281.f5

[42] Tam KF, Cheung WH, Lee KM, Qin L, Leung KS. Osteogenic effects of low-intensity pulsed ultrasound, extracorporeal shockwaves and their combination – an in vitro comparative study on human periosteal cells. Ultrasound Med Biol. 2008;34(12):1957–65. DOI: 10.1016/j.ultrasmedbio.2008.06.005

[43] Tamma R, Dell'endice S, Notarnicola A, Moretti L, Patella S, Patella V, Zallone A, Moretti A. Extracorporeal shock waves stimulate osteoblast activities. Ultrasound Med Biol. 2009;35(12):2093–100. DOI: 10.1016/j.ultrasmedbio.2009.05.022

[44] Wang FS, Wang CJ, Huang HJ, Chung H, Chen RF, Yang KD. Physical shock wave mediates membrane hyperpolarization and Ras activation for osteogenesis in human bone marrow stromal cells. Biochem Biophys Res Commun. 2001;287(3):648–55. DOI: 10.1006/bbrc.2001.5654

[45] Humphrey VF. Ultrasound and matter-Physical interactions. Prog Biophys Mol Biol. 2007;93(1–3):195–211.DOI: 10.1016/j.pbiomolbio.2006.07.024

[46] Zhonga P, Lin H, Xi X, Zhu S, Bhogte ES. Shock wave-inertial microbubble interaction: methodology, physical characterization, and bioeffect study. J Acoust Soc Am. 1999;105(3):1997–2009. DOI: 10.1121/1.426733

[47] Ohl SW, Klaseboer E, Khoo BC. The dynamics of a non-equilibrium bubble near biomaterials. Phys Med Biol. 2009;54(20):6313–36. DOI: 10.1088/0031-9155/54/20/019

[48] Choi MJ, Doh DH, Hwang TG, Cho CH, Paeng DG, Rim GH, Coleman AJ. Acoustic streaming in lithotripsy fields: preliminary observation using a particle image velocimetry method. Ultrasonics. 2006;44(2):133–45. DOI: 10.1016/j.ultras.2005.09.004

[49] Anderson JC, Eriksson C. Electrical properties of wet collagen. Nature. 1968;218(5137): 166–8.

[50] Bandow K, Nishikawa Y, Ohnishi T, Kakimoto K, Soejima K, Iwabuchi S, Kuroe K, Matsuguchi T. Low-intensity pulsed ultrasound (LIPUS) induces RANKL, MCP-1, and MIP-1b expression in osteoblasts through the angiotensin II type 1 receptor. J Cell Physiol. 2007;211(2):392–8. DOI: 10.1002/jcp.20944

[51] Buckwalter JA, Glimcher MJ, Cooper RR, Recker R. Bone biology. I: structure, blood supply, cells, matrix, and mineralization. Instr Course Lect. 1996;45:371–86.

[52] Hausdorf J, Sievers B, Schmitt-Sody M, Jansson V, Maier M, Mayer-Wagner S. Stimulation of bone growth factor synthesis in human osteoblasts and fibroblasts after

extracorporeal shock wave application. Arch Orthop Trauma Surg. 2011;131(3):303–9. DOI: 10.1007/s00402-010-1166-4

[53] Hou CH, Lin J, Huang SC, Hou SM, Tang CH. Ultrasound stimulates NF-kB activation and iNOS expression via the Ras/Raf/MEK/ERK signaling pathway in cultured preosteoblasts. J Cell Physiol. 2009;220(1):196–203. DOI: 10.1002/jcp.21751

[54] Kearney CJ, Lee JY, Padera RF, Hsu HP, Spector M. Extracorporeal shock wave-induced proliferation of periosteal cells. J Orthop Res. 2011;29(10):1536–43. DOI: 10.1002/jor.21346

[55] Watabe H, Furuhama T, Tani-Ishii N, Mikuni-Takagaki Y. Mechanotransduction activates α5β1 integrin and PI3K/Akt signaling pathways in mandibular osteoblasts. Exp Cell Res. 2011;317(18):2642–9. DOI: 10.1016/j.yexcr.2011.07.015

[56] Wei FY, Leung KS, Li G, Qin J, Chow SK, Huang S, Sun MH, Qin L, Cheung WH. Low-intensity pulsed ultrasound enhanced mesenchymal stem cell recruitment through stromal derived factor-1 signaling in fracture healing. PloS One. 2014;9(9):e106722. DOI: 10.1371/journal.pone.0106722

[57] You L, Cowin SC, Schaffler MB, Weinbaum S. A model for strain amplification in the actin cytoskeleton of osteocytes due to fluid drag on pericellular matrix. J Biomech. 2001;34(11):1375–86. DOI: 10.1016/S0021-9290(01)00107-5

[58] Bonewald LF. Mechanosensation and transduction in osteocytes. Bonekey Osteovision. 2006;3(10):7–15. DOI: 10.1138/20060233

[59] Galli C, Passeri G, Macaluso GM. Osteocytes and WNT: the mechanical control of bone formation. J Dent Res. 2010;89(4):331–43. DOI: 10.1177/0022034510363963

[60] Li L, Yang Z, Zhang H, Chen W, Chen M, Zhu Z. Low-intensity pulsed ultrasound regulates proliferation and differentiation of osteoblasts through osteocytes. Biochem Biophys Res Commun. 2012;418(2):296–300. DOI: 10.1016/j.bbrc.2012.01.014

[61] Taylor AF, Saunders MM, Shingle DL, Cimbala JM, Zhou Z, Donahue HJ. Mechanically stimulated osteocytes regulate osteoblastic activity via gap junctions. Am J Physiol Cell Physiol. 2007;292(1):C545–52.

[62] Cherian PP, Siller-Jakson AJ, Gu S, Wang X, Bonewald LF, Sprague E, Jiang JX. Mechanical strain opens connexin 43 hemichannels in osteocytes: a novel mechanism for the release of prostaglandin. Mol Biol Cell. 2005;16(7):3100–6. DOI: 10.1091/mbc.E04-10-0912

[63] Godin LM, Suzuki S, Jacobs CR, Donahue HJ, Donahue SW. Mechanically induced intracellular calcium waves in osteoblasts demonstrate calcium fingerprints in bone cell mechanotransduction. Biomech Model Mechanobiol. 2007;6(6):391–8. DOI: 10.1007/s10237-006-0059-5

[64] Manaka S, Tanabe N, Kariya T, Naito M, Takayama T, Nagao M, Liu D, Ito K, Maeno M, Suzuki N, Miyazaki M. Low-intensity pulsed ultrasound-induced ATP increases

bone formation via the P2X7 receptor in osteoblast-like MC3T3-E1 cells. FEBS Lett. 2015;589(3):310–8. DOI: 10.1016/j.febslet.2014.12.013

[65] Reich KM, McAllister TN, Gudi S, Frangos JA. Activation of G proteins mediates flow-induced prostaglandin E2 production in osteoblasts. Endocrinology. 1997;138(3):1014–8. DOI: 10.1210/endo.138.3.4999

[66] Suzuki A, Takayama T, Suzuki N, Kojima T, Ota N, Asano S, Ito K. Daily low-intensity pulsed ultrasound stimulates production of bone morphogenetic protein in ROS 17/2.8 cells. J Oral Sci. 2009;51(1):29–36.

[67] Kokubu T, Matsui N, Fujioka H, Tsunoda M, Mizuno K. Low intensity pulsed ultrasound exposure increases prostaglandin E2 production via the induction of cyclooxygenase-2 mRNA in mouse osteoblasts. Biochem Biophys Res Commun. 1999;256(2): 284–7. DOI: 10.1006/bbrc.1999.0318

[68] Kusuyama J, Bandow K, Shamoto M, Kakimoto K, Ohnishi T, Matsuguchi T. Low intensity pulsed ultrasound (LIPUS) influences the multilineage differentiation of mesenchymal stem and progenitor cell lines through ROCK-Cot/Tpl2-MEK-ERK Signaling Pathway. J Biol Chem. 2014;289(15):10330–44. DOI: 10.1074/jbc.M113.546382

[69] Naruse K, Miyauchi A, Itoman M, Mikuni-Takagaki Y. Distinct anabolic response of osteoblast to low-intensity pulsed ultrasound. J Bone Miner Res. 2003;18(2):360–9. DOI: 10.1359/jbmr.2003.18.2.360

[70] Pawlowski J, Kraft AS. Bax-induced apoptotic cell death. Proc Natl Acad Sci U S A. 2000;97(2):529–31. DOI: 10.1073/pnas.97.2.529

[71] Tang CH, Yang RS, Huang TH, Lu DY, Chuang WJ, Huang TF, Fu WM. Ultrasound stimulates cyclooxygenase-2 expression and increases bone formation through integrin, focal adhesion kinase, phosphatidylinositol 3-kinase, and Akt pathway in osteoblasts. Mol Pharmacol. 2006;69(6):2047–57. DOI: 10.1124/mol.105.022160

[72] Alvarenga EC, Rodriges R, Caricatti-Neto A, Silva-Filho FC, Paredes-Gamero EJ, Ferreira AT. Low-intensity pulsed ultrasound-dependent osteoblast proliferation occurs by via activation of the P2Y receptor: role of the P2Y1 receptor. Bone. 2010;46(2): 355–62. DOI: 10.1016/j.bone.2009.09.017

[73] Olkku A, Leskinen JJ, Lammi MJ, Hynynen K, Mahonen A. Ultrasound-induced activation of Wnt signaling in human MG-63 osteoblastic cells. Bone. 2010;47(2):320–30. DOI: 10.1016/j.bone.2010.04.604

[74] Chen YJ, Kuo YR, Yang KD, Wang CJ, Huang HC, Wang FS. Shock wave application enhances pertussis toxin protein-sensitive bone formation of segmental femoral defect in rats. J Bone Miner Res. 2003;18(12):2169–79. DOI: 10.1359/jbmr.2003.18.12.2169

[75] Huang W, Hasegawa T, Imai Y, Takeda D, Akashi M, Komori T. Low-intensity pulsed ultrasound enhances bone morphogenetic protein expression of human mandibular

fracture haematoma-derived cells. Int J Oral Maxillofac Surg. 2015;44(7):929–35. DOI: 10.1016/j.ijom.2015.03.001

[76] Imai Y, Hasegawa T, Takeda D, Akashi M, Lee SY, Niikura T, Shibuya Y, Kurosaka M, Komori T. The osteogenic activity of human mandibular fracture haematoma-derived cells is stimulated by low-intensity pulsed ultrasound in vitro. Int J Oral Maxillofac Surg. 2014;43(3):367–72. DOI: 10.1016/j.ijom.2013.07.746

[77] Ishihara Y, Ueki K, Sotobori M, Marukawa K, Moroi A. Bone regeneration by statin and low-intensity pulsed ultrasound (LIPUS) in rabbit nasal bone. J Craniomaxillofac Surg. 2014;42(3):185–93. DOI: 10.1016/j.jcms.2013.05.002

[78] Notarnicola A, Tamma R, Moretti L, Panella A, Dell'endice S, Zallone A, Moretti B. Effect of shock wave treatment on platelet-rich plasma added to osteoblast cultures. Ultrasound Med Biol. 2011;37(1):160–82. DOI: 10.1016/j.ultrasmedbio.2010.10.016

[79] Wang FS, Wang CJ, Sheen-Chen SM, Kuo YR, Chen RF, Yang KD. Superoxide mediates shock wave induction of ERK-dependent osteogenic transcription factor (CBFA1) and mesenchymal cell differentiation toward osteoprogenitors. J Biol Chem. 2002;277(13): 10931–7. DOI: 10.1074/jbc.M104587200

[80] Wang FS, Yang KD, Kuo YR, Wang CJ, Huang HJ, Chen YJ. Temporal and spatial expression of bone morphogenetic proteins in extracorporeal shock wave-promoted healing of fracture defect. Bone. 2003;32(4):387–96. DOI: 10.1016/S8756-3282(03)00029-2

[81] Wang FS, Wang CJ, Chen YJ, Chang PR, Huang YT, Sun YC, Huang HC, Yang YJ, Yang KD. Ras induction of superoxide activates ERK-dependent angiogenic transcription factor HIF-1alpha and VEGF-A expression in shock wave-stimulated osteoblasts. J Biol Chem. 2004;279(11):10331–7. DOI: 10.1074/jbc.M308013200

[82] Wang FS, Kuo YR, Wang CJ, Yang KD, Chang PR, Huang YT, Huang HC, Sun YC, Yang YJ, Chen YJ. Nitric oxide mediates ultrasound-induced hypoxia-inducible factor-1alpha activation and vascular endothelial growth factor-A expression in human osteoblasts. Bone. 2004;35(1):114–23. DOI: 10.1016/j.bone.2004.02.012

[83] Yin TC, Wang CJ, Yang KD, Wang FS, Sun YC. Shockwaves enhance the osteogenetic gene expression in marrow stromal cells from hips with osteonecrosis. Chang Gung Med J. 2011;34(4):367–74.

[84] Sena K, Leven RM, Mazhar K, Sumner DR, Virdi AS. Early gene response to low-intensity pulsed ultrasound in rat osteoblastic cells. Ultrasound Med Biol. 2005;31(5): 703–8. DOI: 10.1016/j.ultrasmedbio.2005.01.013

[85] Takayama T, Suzuki N, Ikeda K, Shimada T, Suzuki A, Maeno M, Otsuka K, Ito K. Low-intensity pulsed ultrasound stimulates osteogenic differentiation in ROS 17/2.8 cells. Life Sci. 2007;80(10):965–71. DOI: 10.1016/j.lfs.2006.11.037

[86] Walsh WR, Langdown AJ, Auld JW, Stephens P, Yu Y, Vizesi F, Bruce WJM, Pounder N. Effect of low intensity pulsed ultrasound on healing of an ulna defect filled with a

bone graft substitute. J Biomed Mater Res B Appl Biomater. 2008;86(1):74–81. DOI: 10.1002/jbm.b.30989

[87] Kumagai K, Takeuchi R, Ishikawa H, Yamaguchi Y, Fujisawa T, Kuniya T, Takagawa S, Muschler GF, Saito T. Low-intensity pulsed ultrasound accelerates fracture healing by stimulation of recruitment of both local and circulating osteogenic progenitors. 2012;30(9):1516–21. DOI: 10.1002/jor.22103

[88] Lim K, Kim J, Seonwoo H, Park SH, Choung PH, Chung JH. In vitro effects of low-intensity pulsed ultrasound stimulation on the osteogenic differentiation of human alveolar bone-derived mesenchymal stem cells for tooth tissue engineering. Biomed Res Int. 2013;2013:269724. DOI: 10.1155/2013/269724

[89] Lapidot T, Kollet O. The essential roles of the chemokine SDF-1 and its receptor CXCR4 in human stem cell homing and repopulation of transplanted immune-deficient NOD/SCID and NOD/SCID/B2m(null) mice. Leukemia. 2002;16(10):1992–2003. DOI: 10.1038/sj.leu.2402684

[90] de Gusmão CV, Pauli JR, Saad MJ, Alves JM, Belangero WD. Low-intensity ultrasound increases FAK, ERK-1/2, and IRS-1 expression of intact rat bones in a noncumulative manner. Clin Orthop Relat Res. 2010;468(4):1149–56. DOI: 10.1007/s11999-009-1146-6

[91] Chen YJ, Kuo YR, Yang KD, Wang CJ, Sheen Chen SM, Huang HC, Yang YJ, Yi-Chih S, Wang FS. Activation of extracellular signal-regulated kinase (ERK) and p38 kinase in shock wave-promoted bone formation of segmental defect in rats. Bone. 2004;34(3): 466–77. DOI: 10.1016/j.bone.2003.11.013

[92] Nakao J, Fujii Y, Kusuyama J, Bandow K, Kakimoto K, Ohnishi T, Matsuguchi. Low-intensity pulsed ultrasound (LIPUS) inhibits LPS-induced inflammatory responses of osteoblasts through TLR4–MyD88 dissociation. Bone. 2014;58:17–25. DOI: 10.1016/j.bone.2013.09.018

[93] Angle SR, Sena K, Sumner DR, Virdi AS. Osteogenic differentiation of rat bone marrow stromal cells by various intensities of low-intensity pulsed ultrasound. Ultrasonics. 2011;51(3):281–8. DOI: 10.1016/j.ultras.2010.09.004

[94] Zura R, Della Rocca GJ, Mehta S, Harrison A, Brodie C, Jones J, Steen RG. Treatment of chronic (<1 year) fracture nonunion: heal rate in a cohort of 767 patients treated with low-intensity pulsed ultrasound (LIPUS). Injury. 2015:46(10):2036–41. DOI: 10.1016/j.injury.2015.05.042

[95] Narasaki K, Shimizu H, Beppu M, Aoki H, Takagi M, Takashi M. Effect of extracorporeal shock waves on callus formation during bone lengthening. J Orthop Sci. 2003;8(4):474–81. DOI: 10.1007/s00776-003-0664-4

[96] Oztemur Z, Ozturk H, Ozyurek S, Kaloglu C, Golge UH, Bulut O. The long-term effects of extracorporeal shock waves on the epiphysis of the adolescent rat. J Orthop Sci. 2013;18(1):159–64. DOI: 10.1007/s00776-012-0321-x

[97] Ozturk H, Bulut O, Oztemur Z, Kaloglu C, Kol IO. Effect of high-energy extracorporeal shock waves on the immature epiphysis in a rabbit model. Arch Orthop Trauma Surg. 2008;128(6):627–31. DOI: 10.1007/s00402-007-0388-6

[98] Wang CJ, Yang KD, Wang FS, Hsu CC, Chen HH. Shock wave treatment shows dose-dependent enhancement of bone mass and bone strength after fracture of the femur. Bone. 2004;34(1):225–30. DOI: 10.1016/j.bone.2003.08.005

[99] Louw TM, Budhiraja G, Viljoen HJ, Subramanian A. Mechanotransduction of ultrasound is frequency dependent below the cavitation threshold. Ultrasound Med Biol. 2013;39(7):1303–19. DOI: 10.1016/j.ultrasmedbio.2013.01.015

[100] Mizrahi N, Zhou EH, Lenormand G, Krishnan R, Weihs D, Butler JP, Weitz DA, Fredberg JJ, Kimmel E. Low intensity ultrasound perturbs cytoskeleton dynamics. Soft Matter. 2012;8(8):2438–43. DOI: 10.1039/C2SM07246G

[101] Or M, Kimmel E. Modeling linear vibration of cell nucleus in low intensity ultrasound field. Ultrasound Med Biol. 2009;35(6):1015–25. DOI: 10.1016/j.ultrasmedbio.2008.11.011

[102] Fung CH, Cheung WH, Pounder NM, de Ana FJ, Harrison A, Leung KS. Investigation of rat bone fracture healing using pulsed 1.5 MHz, 30 mW/cm(2) burst ultrasound – axial distance dependency. Ultrasonics. 2014;54(3):850–9. DOI: 10.1016/j.ultras.2013.10.013

[103] Angle SR, Sena K, Sumner DR, Virkus WW, Virdi AS. Combined use of low intensity pulsed ultrasound and rhBMP-2 to enhance bone formation in a rat model of critical-size defect. J Orthop Trauma. 2014;28(10):605–11. DOI: 10.1097/BOT.0000000000000067

[104] Lee SY, Koh A, Niikura T, Oe K, Koga T, Dogaki Y, Kurosaka M. Low-intensity pulsed ultrasound enhances BMP-7-induced osteogenic differentiation of human fracture hematoma-derived progenitor cells in vitro. J Orthop Trauma. 2013;27(1):29–33. DOI: 10.1097/BOT.0b013e3182519492

[105] Aonuma H, Miyakoshi N, Kasukawa Y, Kamo K, Sasaki H, Tsuchie H, Segawa T, Shimada Y. Effects of combined therapy of alendronate and low-intensity pulsed ultrasound on metaphyseal bone repair after osteotomy in the proximal tibia of aged rats. J Bone Miner Metab. 2014;32(3):232–9. DOI: 10.1007/s00774-013-0492-3

[106] Ito M, Azuma Y, Ohta T, Komoriya K. Effects of ultrasound and 1,25-dihydroxyvitamin D3 on growth factor secretion in co-cultures of osteoblasts and endothelial cells. Ultrasound Med Biol. 2000;26(1):161–6. DOI: 10.1016/S0301-5629(99)00110-6

[107] Farkash U, Bain O, Gam A, Nyska M, Sagiv P. Low-intensity pulsed ultrasound for treating delayed union scaphoid fractures: case series. J Orthop Surg Res. 2015;10:72. DOI: 10.1186/s13018-015-0221-9

[108] Gebauer D, Mayr E, Orthner E, Ryaby JP. Low-intensity pulsed ultrasound: effects on nonunions. Ultrasound Med Biol. 2005;31(10):1391–402. DOI: 10.1016/j.ultrasmedbio.2005.06.002

[109] Jingushi S, Mizuno K, Matsushita T, Itoman M. Low-intensity pulsed ultrasound treatment for postoperative delayed union or nonunion of long bone fractures. J Orthop Sci. 2007;12(1):35–41. DOI: 10.1007/s00776-006-1080-3

[110] Liao JC, Chen WJ, Niu CC, Chen LH. Effects of low-intensity pulsed ultrasound on spinal pseudarthrosis created by nicotin administration: a model of lumbar posterolateral pseudarthrosis in rabbits. J Ultrasound Med. 2015;34(6):1043–50. DOI: 10.7863/ultra.34.6.1043

[111] Nolte PA, van der Krans A, Patka P, Janssen IM, Ryaby JP, Albers GH. Low-intensity pulsed ultrasound in the treatment of nonunions. J Trauma. 2001;51(4):693–703.

[112] Okada K, Miyakoshi N, Takahashi S, Ishigaki S, Nishida J, Itoi E. Congenital pseudoarthrosis of the tibia treated with low-intensity pulsed ultrasound stimulation (LIPUS). Ultrasound Med Biol. 2003;29(7):1061–4. DOI: 10.1016/S0301-5629(03)00906-2

[113] Rutten S, Nolte PA, Guit GL, Bouman DE, Albers GH. Use of low-intensity pulsed ultrasound for posttraumatic nonunions of the tibia: a review of patients treated in the Netherlands. J Trauma. 2007;62:902–8. DOI: 10.1097/01.ta.0000238663.33796.fb

[114] Watanabe Y, Matsushita T, Bhandari M, Zdero R, Schemitsch EH. Ultrasound for fracture healing: current evidence. J Orthop Trauma 2010;24(Suppl 1):S56–61. DOI: 10.1097/BOT.0b013e3181d2efaf

[115] Bara T, Synder M. Nine-year experience with the use of shock waves for treatment of bone union disturbances. Ortop Traumatol Rehabil. 2007;9(3):254–8.

[116] Cacchio A, Giordano L, Colafarina O, Rompe JD, Tavernese E, Ioppolo F, Flamini S, Spacca G, Santilli V. Extracorporeal shock-wave therapy compared with surgery for hypertrophic long-bone nonunions. J Bone Joint Surg Am. 2009;91(11):2589–97. DOI: 10.2106/JBJS.H.00841

[117] Furia JP, Juliano PJ, Wade AM, Schaden W, Mittermayr R. Shock wave therapy compared with intramedullary screw fixation for nonunion of proximal fifth metatarsal metaphyseal-diaphyseal fractures. J Bone Joint Surg Am. 2010;92(4):846–54. DOI: 10.2106/JBJS.I.00653

[118] Kuo SJ, Su IC, Wang CJ, Ko JY. Extracorporeal shockwave therapy (ESWT) in the treatment of atrophic non-unions of femoral shaft fractures. Int J Surg. 2015;24(Pt B): 131–4. DOI: 10.1016/j.ijsu.2015.06.075

[119] Notarnicola A, Moretti L, Tafuri S, Gigliotti S, Russo S, Musci L, Moretti B. Extracorporeal shockwaves versus surgery in the treatment of pseudoarthrosis of the carpal scaphoid. Ultrasound Med Biol. 2010;36(8):1306–13. DOI: 10.1016/j.ultrasmedbio.2010.05.004

[120] Rompe JD, Rosendahl T, Schöllner C, Theis C. High-energy extracorporeal shock wave treatment of nonunions. Clin Orthop Relat Res. 2001;387:102–11.

[121] Schaden W, Fischer A, Sailler A. Extracorporeal shock wave therapy of nonunion or delayed osseous union. Clin Orthop Relat Res. 2001;387:90–4.

[122] Wang CJ, Chen HS, Chen CE, Yang KD. Treatment of nonunions of long bone fractures with shock waves. Clin Orthop Relat Res. 2001;387:95–101.

[123] Wang CJ, Yang KD, Ko JY, Huang CC, Huang HY, Wang FS. The effects of shockwave on bone healing and systemic concentrations of nitric oxide (NO), TGF-b1, VEGF and BMP-2 in long bone non-unions. Nitric Oxide. 2009;20(4):298–303. DOI: 10.1016/j.niox.2009.02.006

[124] Xu ZH, Jiang Q, Chen DY, Xiong J, Shi DQ, Yuan T, Zhu XL. Extracorporeal shock wave treatment in nonunions of long bone fractures. Int Orthop. 2009;33(3):789–93. DOI: 10.1007/s00264-008-0553-8

[125] Bashardoust Tajali S, Houghton P, MacDermid JC, Grewa R. Effects of low-intensity pulsed ultrasound therapy on fracture healing: a systematic review and meta-analysis. Am J Phys Med Rehabil. 2012;91(4):349–67. DOI: 10.1097/PHM.0b013e31822419ba

[126] Dudda M, Hauser J, Muhr G, Esenwein SA. Low-intensity pulsed ultrasound as a useful adjuvant during distraction osteogenesis: a prospective, randomized controlled trial. J Trauma. 2011;71(5):1376–80. DOI: 10.1097/TA.0b013e31821912b2

[127] Griffin XL, Parsons N, Costa ML, Metcalfe D. Ultrasound and shockwave therapy for acute fractures in adults. Cochrane Database Syst Rev. 2014;6:CD008579. DOI: 10.1002/14651858.CD008579.pub3

[128] Hannemann PF, Mommers EH, Schots JP, Brink PR, Poeze M. The effects of low-intensity pulsed ultrasound and pulsed electromagnetic fields bone growth stimulation in acute fractures: a systematic review and meta-analysis of randomized controlled trials. Arch Orthop Trauma Surg. 2014;134(8):1093–106. DOI: 10.1007/s00402-014-2014-8

[129] Kinami Y, Noda T, Ozaki T. Efficacy of low-intensity pulsed ultrasound treatment for surgically managed fresh diaphyseal fractures of the lower extremity: multi-center retrospective cohort study. J Orthop Sci. 2013;18(3):410–8. DOI: 10.1007/s00776-013-0358-5

[130] Lubbert PH, van der Rijt RH, Hoorntje LE, van der Werken C. Low-intensity pulsed ultrasound (LIPUS) in fresh clavicle fractures: a multi-centre double blind randomised controlled trial. Injury. 2008;39(12):1444–52. DOI: 10.1016/j.injury.2008.04.004

[131] Snyder BM, Conley J, Koval KJ. Does low-intensity pulsed ultrasound reduce time to fracture healing? A meta-analysis. Am J Orthop. 2012;41(2):E12–9.

[132] Zura R, Mehta S, Della Rocca GJ, Jones J, Steen RG. A cohort study of 4,190 patients treated with low-intensity pulsed ultrasound (LIPUS): findings in the elderly versus all patients. BMC Musculoskelet Disord. 2015;16:45. DOI: 10.1186/s12891-015-0498-1

[133] Hsu RW, Tai CL, Chen CY, Hsu WH, Hsueh S. Enhancing mechanical strength during early fracture healing via shockwave treatment: an animal study. Clin Biomech (Bristol Avon). 2003:18(6):S33–9. DOI: 10.1016/S0268-0033(03)00082-2

[134] Lee TC, Huang HY, Yang YL, Hung KS, Cheng CH, Lin WC, Wang CJ. Application of extracorporeal shock wave treatment to enhance spinal fusion: a rabbit experiment. Surg Neurol. 2008;70(2):129–34. DOI: 10.1016/j.surneu.2007.05.050

[135] Wang CJ, Liu HC, Fu TH. The effects of extracorporeal shockwave on acute high-energy long bone fractures of the lower extremity. Arch Orthop Trauma Surg. 2007;127(2):137–42. DOI: 10.1007/s00402-006-0236-0

[136] Wang CJ, Wang FS, Yang KD. Biological effects of extracorporeal shockwave in bone healing: a study in rabbits. Arch Orthop Trauma Surg. 2008;128(8):879–84. DOI: 10.1007/s00402-008-0663-1

[137] Coords M, Breitbart E, Paglia D, Kappy N, Gandhi A, Cottrell J, Cedeno N, Pounder N, O'Connor JP, Lin SS. The effects of low-intensity pulsed ultrasound upon diabetic fracture healing. J Orthop Res. 2011;29(2):181–8. DOI: 10.1002/jor.21223

[138] Gebauer GP, Lin SS, Beam HA, Vieira P, Parsons JR. Low-intensity pulsed ultrasound increases the fracture callus strength in diabetic BB Wistar rats but does not affect cellular proliferation. J Orthop Res. 2002;20(3):587–92. DOI: 10.1016/S0736-0266(01)00136-X

[139] Cheung WH, Chin WC, Qin L, Leung KS. Low intensity pulsed ultrasound enhances fracture healing in both ovariectomy-induced osteoporotic and age-matched normal bones. J Orthop Res. 2012;30(1):129–36. DOI: 10.1002/jor.21487

[140] Cheung WH, Chow SK, Sun MH, Qin L, Leung KS. Low-intensity pulsed ultrasound accelerated callus formation, angiogenesis and callus remodelling in osteoporotic fracture healing. Ultrasound Med Biol. 2011;37(2):231–8. DOI: 10.1016/j.ultrasmedbio.2010.11.016

[141] Naruse K, Sekiya H, Harada Y, Iwabuchi S, Kozai Y, Kawamata R, Kashima I, Uchida K, Urabe K, Kannichi S, Itoman M, Mikuni-Takagaki Y. Prolonged endochondral bone healing in senescence is shortened by low-intensity pulsed ultrasound in a manner dependent on cox-2. Ultrasound Med Biol. 2010;36(7):1098–108. DOI: 10.1016/j.ultrasmedbio.2010.04.011

[142] Ganzorig K, Kuroda S, Maeda Y, Mansjur K, Sato M, Nagata K, Tanaka E. Low-intensity pulsed ultrasound enhances bone formation around miniscrew implants. Arch Oral Biol. 2015;60(6):902–10. DOI: 10.1016/j.archoralbio.2015.02.014

[143] Iwai T, Harada Y, Imura K, Iwabuchi S, Murai J, Hiramatsu K, Myoui A, Yoshikawa H, Tsumaki N. Low-intensity pulsed ultrasound increases bone ingrowth into porous

hydroxyapatite ceramic. J Bone Miner Metab. 2007;25(6):392–9. DOI: 10.1007/s00774-007-0777-5

[144] Liu Q, Liu X, Liu B, Hu K, Zhou X, Ding Y. The effect of low-intensity pulsed ultrasound on the osseointegration of titanium dental implants. Br J Oral Maxillofac Surg. 2012;50(3):244–50. DOI:10.1016/j.bjoms.2011.03.001

[145] Lu H, Zheng C, Wang Z, Chen C, Chen H, Hu J. Effects of low-intensity pulsed ultrasound on new trabecular bone during bone-tendon junction healing in a rabbit model: a synchrotron radiation micro-CT study. PLoS ONE. 2015;10(4):e0124724. DOI: 10.1371/journal.pone.0124724

[146] Qin L, Wang L, Wong MW, Wen C, Wang G, Zhang G, Chan KM, Cheung WH, Leung KS. Osteogenesis induced by extracorporeal shockwave in treatment of delayed osteotendinous junction healing. J Orthop Res. 2010;28(1):70–6. DOI: 10.1002/jor.20948

[147] Walsh WR, Stephens P, Vizesi F, Bruce W, Huckle J, Yu Y. Effects of low-intensity pulsed ultrasound on tendon-bone healing in an intra-articular sheep knee model. Arthroscopy. 2007;23(2):197–204. DOI: 10.1016/j.arthro.2006.09.003

[148] Gan TY, Kuah DE, Graham KS, Markson G. Low-intensity pulsed ultrasound in lower limb bone stress injuries: a randomized controlled trial. Clin J Sport Med. 2014;24(6): 457–60. DOI: 10.1097/JSM.0000000000000084

[149] Li J, Waugh LJ, Hui SL, Burr DB, Warden SJ. Low-intensity pulsed ultrasound and nonsteroidal anti-inflammatory drugs have opposing effects during stress fracture repair. J Orthop Res. 2007;25(12):1559–67. DOI: 10.1002/jor.20461

[150] Moretti B, Notarnicola A, Garofalo R, Moretti L, Patella S, Marlinghaus E, Patella V. Shock waves in the treatment of stress fractures. Ultrasound Med Biol. 2009;35(6):1042–9. DOI: 10.1016/j.ultrasmedbio.2008.12.002

[151] Faria LD. Electrohydraulic extracorporeal shock wave therapy increases ERK-1/2 and Akt activities in rat intact tíbia and fíbula for 21 days following primary stimulation [dissertation]. Campinas, São Paulo, Brazil: State University of Campinas; 2015. 61 p.

[152] Wang FS, Yang KD, Chen RF, Wang CJ, Sheen-Chen SM. Extracorporeal shock wave promotes growth and differentiation of bone-marrow stromal cells towards osteoprogenitors associated with induction of TGF-β1. J Bone Joint Surg Br. 2002;84(3):457–61. DOI: 10.1302/0301-620X.84B3.11609

[153] Wu S, Kawahara Y, Manabe T, Ogawa K, Matsumoto M, Sasaki A, Yuge L. Low-intensity pulsed ultrasound accelerates osteoblast differentiation and promotes bone formation in an osteoporosis rat model. Pathobiology. 2009;76(3):99–107. DOI: 10.1159/000209387

[154] Carvalho DC, Cliquet Júnior A. The action of low-intensity pulsed ultrasound in bones of osteopenic rats. Artif Organs. 2004;28(1):114–8.

[155] Leung KS, Lee WS, Cheung WH, Qin L. Lack of efficacy of low-intensity pulsed ultrasound on prevention of postmenopausal bone loss evaluated at the distal radius in older Chinese women. Clin Orthop Relat Res. 2004;427:234–40. DOI: 10.1097/01.blo.0000137557.59228.4d

[156] Warden SJ, Bennell KL, Forwood MR, Mcmeeken JM, Wark JD. Skeletal effects of low-intensity pulsed ultrasound on the ovariectomized rodent. Ultrasound Med Biol. 2001;27(7):989–98.

[157] Warden SJ, Bennell KL, Matthews B, Brown DJ, Mcmeeken JM, Wark JD. Efficacy of low-intensity pulsed ultrasound in the prevention of osteoporosis following spinal cord injury. Bone. 2001;29(5):431–6.

[158] Tam KF, Cheung WH, Lee KM, Qin L, Leung KS. Showckwave exerts osteogenic effect on osteoporotic bone in an ovariectomized goat model. Ultrasound Med Biol. 2009;35(7):1109–18. DOI: 10.1016/j.ultrasmedbio.2009.01.001

[159] Wang CJ, Yang YJ, Huang CC. The effects of shockwave on systemic concentrations of nitric oxide level, angiogenesis and osteogenesis factors in hip necrosis. Rheumatol Int. 2011;31(7):871–7. DOI: 10.1007/s00296-010-1384-7

[160] Zhu H, Cai X, Lin T, Shi Z, Yan S. Low-intensity pulsed ultrasound enhances bone repair in a rabbit model of steroid-associated osteonecrosis. Clin Orthop Relat Res. 2015;473(5):1830–9. DOI: 10.1007/s11999-015-4154-8

Chapter 3

Distraction Osteogenesis in the Treatment of Maxillary Hypoplasia

Sultan Olmez-Gurlen

Additional information is available at the end of the chapter

http://dx.doi.org/10.5772/62545

Abstract

The aim of this chapter is to review literature reporting on the use of internal distraction osteogenesis and rigid external distraction osteogenesis and to determine the biomechanical effects of internal distractors in the treatment of maxillary hypoplasia, especially in patients with cleft lip and palate (CLP), and compare the results with non-cleft patient. The standard osteotomy used for distraction osteogenesis of the hypoplastic maxilla is LeFort I. An advancement of more than 10 mm in patients with no cleft and 6 mm in patients with CLP is beyond the limit of LeFort I osteotomy, and in such cases distraction osteogenesis for advancement of the maxilla can be used. Distraction osteogenesis (DO) is a biological process involving the formation of new bone between viable bone segments that are gradually separated by incremental traction. The external and internal usage of distraction osteogenesis in the treatment of maxillary hypoplasia in patients with cleft lip and palate is a reliable, reproducible and stable alternative method to conventional one-step LeFort I advancement techniques. Biomechanical evaluation of internal maxillary distraction osteogenesis produces mathematical results to help the surgeon and the orthodontist to understand better the therapeutic effects on the maxillofacial bones and sutures of the craniofacial system.

Keywords: maxillary advancement, distraction osteogenesis, cleft lip and palate, finite element analysis, maxillary hypoplasia

1. Introduction

Distraction osteogenesis (DO) is an effective method used for bone regeneration. Advancement of the maxilla by use of rigid external distraction (RED) device has been performed successfully and many other internal devices have been introduced for better results regarding the patient's comfort [1].

Patients with cleft lip and palate and maxillary hypoplasia usually present with a collapsed maxillary dental arch and impaired forward and downward growth of the maxilla [2–4]. Two factors have been proposed for the growth deficiency [2]: One such factor is the intrinsic factor, mainly introduced by developmental deficiency leading to the formation of a cleft and the growth potential of midfacial skeleton. The other factor is the iatrogenic factor, including surgical repair. Therefore, management of cleft-related maxillary hypoplasia is more complex due to the larger degree of malocclusion and advancement, the risk of post-surgical relapse and the potential velopharyngeal incompetence following maxillary advancement [1, 5].

The general aim of this chapter is to present a brief review of sagittal distraction osteogenesis in sagittal maxillofacial advancement and the biomechanical effects of maxillary sagittal distraction osteogenesis both in patients with unilateral cleft lip and palate and in patients with no cleft.

2. Traditional treatment options for maxillary hypoplasia

Patients with maxillary hypoplasia secondary to orofacial cleft present multiple challenging problems. Traditional orthodontic/orthopaedic approaches to treat these patients, while sometimes successful in obtaining stable occlusal relationships, often fall short of expectations with respect to facial balance and aesthetics.

Usual treatment sequence can be explained as follows: (1) at the ages of 5–7 years orthodontic expansion apparatus can be used such as Quad Helix, Spring jet appliance or Hyrax type palatal expanders (**Figure 1**); (2) protraction with facial mask is used at 8 years or later (**Figure 2**); (3) bone grafting harvested from iliac crest is performed at 7–9 years of age (**Figure 3**). To overcome three-dimensional constriction of the maxilla due to the previous surgical scars, different types of therapeutic concepts are used [6].

The patient with complete unilateral cleft lip and palate shown below (**Figures 1–4**) was a rare case that could be treated in terms of only orthodontics and orthopaedics. However, most of

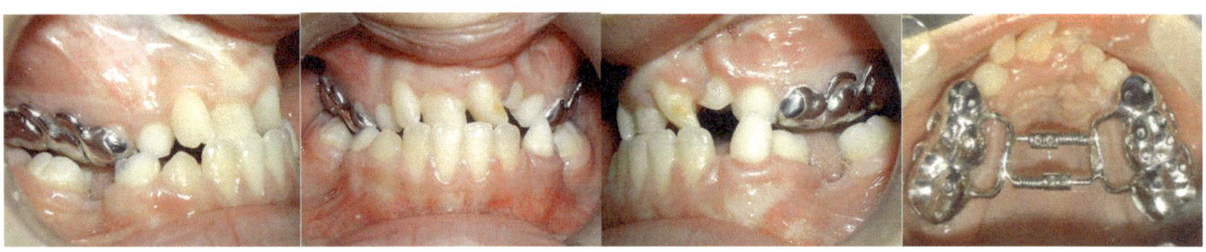

Figure 1. An alternative type of maxillary expansion apparatus (Modified spring jet appliance) used in UCLP patients to achieve appropriate transversal dimension in the maxillary arch.

http://dx.doi.org/10.5772/62545

the patients need surgical intervention to overcome both intrinsic and iatrogenic factors that caused serious maxillary hypoplasia.

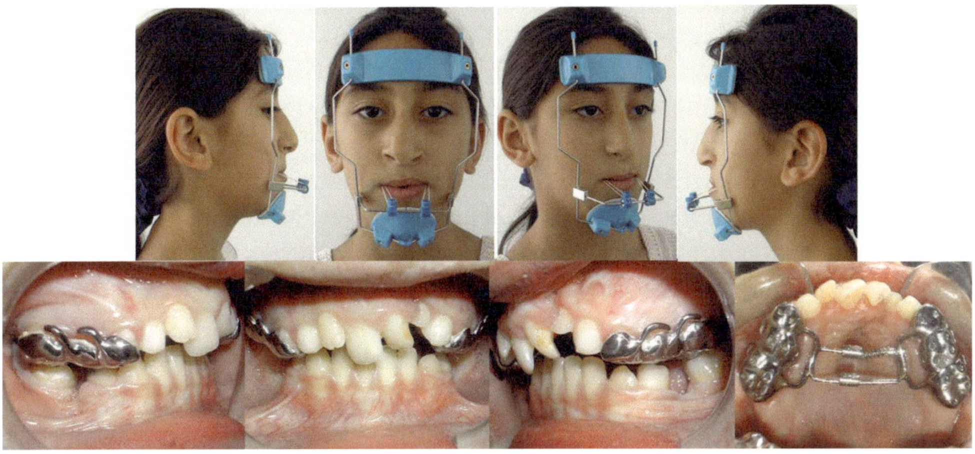

Figure 2. Maxillary sagittal protraction with Delaire type facial mask.

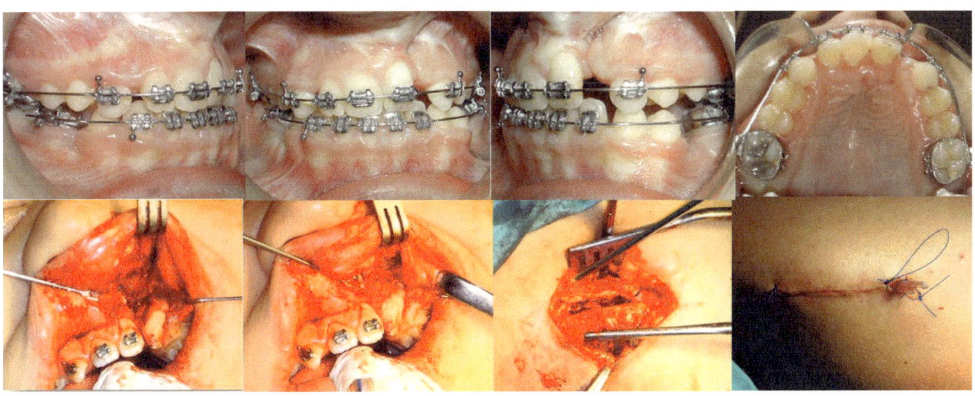

Figure 3. Secondary alveolar bone grafting harvested from iliac crest of the patient.

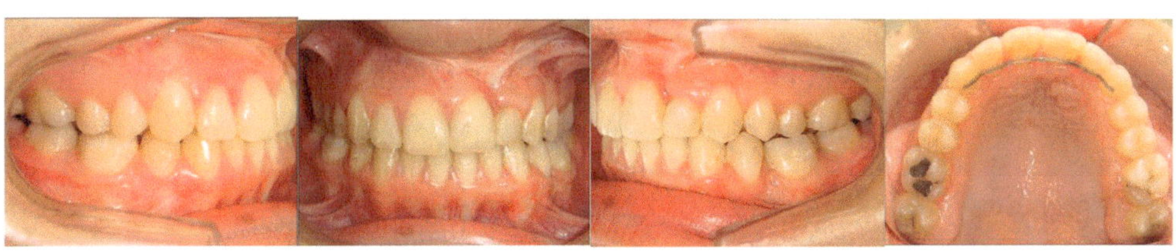

Figure 4. Clinical appearance of the patient one year after both orthopaedic and orthodontic treatment (**Figures 1–4** reprinted [6]).

3. Conventional LeFort I osteotomy

In the treatment of severe hypoplastic cleft palate with conventional LeFort I osteotomy, the major advancement and the extreme discrepancies made stabilization difficult, and the added effect of palatal scarring can result in significant surgical relapse [7].

4. Distraction osteogenesis

"Distraction osteogenesis" (DO) is a biological process involving the formation of new bone between viable bone segments that are gradually separated by incremental traction. Soft tissue envelope (mucosa, muscle, tendon, skin, cartilage, blood vessels and peripheral nerves) beside bone has been also observed to form under tension stress [8, 9]. Experimental studies also have demonstrated formation of the mature lamellar bone by distraction osteogenesis [7, 10, 11].

4.1. History of distraction osteogenesis

Manipulation of the bone segments was first described by Codivilla in 1905 [12]. Gavriel Awramowitch Ilizarov performed several studies to advance the technique in orthopaedic therapy in 1950s [13–16]. Ilizarov performed this technique in two steps and observed the bone regeneration between the two time periods.

Application of mandibular lengthening in maxillofacial complex with the usage of external fixation device was first performed in a canine animal model by Synder et al. [17] in 1972. In 1977, Michielli and Miotti [18] used internal devices in lengthening of mandible in a canine animal model by gradual distraction.

McCarthy and colleagues [19] first used distraction osteogenesis in human mandible in 1992. Mandibular lengthening in four young patients and bilateral mandibular expansion in one patient were performed by gradual distraction. Since the first mention of distraction osteogenesis in the human mandible, it was recognized that the development of simple, multidirectional, miniaturized and buried devices would be necessary to broaden the application of distraction osteogenesis throughout the craniofacial skeleton [20].

4.2. Distraction histogenesis and phases

The gradual increase in soft tissue volume in response to the tension forces applied with bony distraction is called "distraction histogenesis". Conventional LeFort I osteotomy provides immediate bone advancement but, however, does not allow for compensatory growth of the soft tissues. The high rate of relapse after conventional maxillary advancement seems to be a result of scarring and memory of the soft tissues, though the soft tissue often contracts to its pre-operative state. On the other hand, DO creates a gradual increase in the amount of soft tissue by preventing its contraction [21].

In the distraction process, different biologic phenomena are produced and these can be summarized in three phases: **latency phase** is the period between the performance of osteotomy and the start of the traction, during which bone healing begins and soft callus (initial bone formation) is formed. The period is typically between 3–5 days, although in neonates and infants the latency period may be omitted or last only 24 hours. Waiting too long before distraction (beyond 10 to14 days) increases the risk of premature bone union; **distraction phase** is the period in which the process of distraction is activated to transport the bone fragment and the formation of new immature woven and parallel-fibered bone commences. The total time of the distraction phase is customized to the severity of the deformity. This phase usually lasts 1–2 weeks, and the traction modifies the normal development of the regeneration process. In contrast to the latency period, the rate and the rhythm (frequency) of distraction are important factors [22]. If lengthening of the osteotomy site occurs too slowly (<0.5 mm per day), premature bony union prevents lengthening to the desired dimension, whereas if the rate is too rapid (>2 mm per day), a fibrous nonunion will result. Therefore, most reports recommend a distraction rate of 1 mm per day. The ideal rhythm of DO is a continuous steady-state separation of the bone fragments [13–16]. However, this is not practical, and therefore, the recommended distraction frequency is 1 or 2 times daily [23–25]; and **consolidation phase** is the period that allows the maturation and corticalization of the regenerated bone and the surrounding soft tissues adapt to their new positions and lengths. In craniofacial bones, a 3–5 week phase is recommended for children and a 6–12 week phase for adults. In craniofacial skeleton the general rule is that the consolidation period should be at least twice the duration of the distraction phase [22, 26, 27]. The appearance of bone with identical characteristics to those of the initial bone may take more than a year [9].

4.3. Distraction osteogenesis in sagittal maxillary advancement

Maxillary surgical advancement is the most common surgical technique for correcting maxillary hypoplasia in patients with cleft lip and palate. An advancement of more than 10 mm in patients with no cleft and 6 mm in patients with cleft lip and palate is beyond the limit of conventional LeFort I advancement, and in such cases DO for advancement of the maxilla can be used [28–32].

The application of the force according to the center of resistance of the maxilla plays an important role in sagittal maxillary advancement. The mostly desired directions of the maxillary movements in DO are forward and downward. The center of the mass of the maxilla is considered to be located at the apex of the maxillary premolars. When the force is applied at the center of resistance of the maxilla, a straight anterior movement of the maxilla without any rotation is expected. If the same force is applied above, a clockwise rotation will be expected with a predictable increase in over bite and overjet negligible mandibular rotation. If the force is applied below, a counterclockwise rotation will be expected with a tendency of an anterior open bite [33].

External and internal distraction systems can be used for maxillary distraction osteogenesis [34].

4.3.1. Rigid external distraction osteogenesis

The rigid external distraction (RED) was developed by Polley and Figueroa [26, 35], and is composed by an external bow, which is fixed to the cranium screws, and by a custom-made intraoral splint cemented to the maxillary first molars. External traction hooks with eyelets are soldered to the splint, allowing the connection with the external device via surgical wires [36].

Advantages and disadvantages

RED devices have the ability to change the distractor vector during the distraction phase. Another advantage of this system is the ease of the installation and removal of the distractors. However, the main disadvantage is that the device is physically and socially inconvenient and uncomfortable for the patients [26, 35, 37, 38].

Technique and protocol

High-level complete LeFort I osteotomy is the most commonly performed osteotomy since tooth buds are located on a standard level of LeFort I osteotomy line in young patients [1, 36, 39–43]. Standard LeFort I and the 3-piece LeFort I osteotomies are also used with this protocol [7, 26, 35, 44, 45].

After a latency period of 4–7 days, initial activation of the RED device starts. The rate of distraction is 1 mm per day in two or three rhythms. The planned maxillary advancement is usually obtained in 2 to 3 weeks of active distraction. The duration of the activation varies according to the severity of the maxillary hypoplasia; therefore, many authors mention different protocols on this issue. Some activate the distractor until the proper overjet, overbite and stable posterior occlusion are achieved [39], some continued the activation until 5–8 mm of positive overjet is achieved [45], and some activate the distractor until the desired facial profile convexity, skeletal and dental relationships are achieved clinically [1, 7]. Long consolidation period of 8 to 12 weeks is generally accepted in UCLP patients to prevent the risk of possible skeletal relapse [1, 7, 43]. Radiographic bone healing and the presence of cortical outline should be checked using radiographs before removal of the distractors [43]. However, different consolidation period and retention period protocols exist. Nonunion of the external maxillary distraction after a consolidation period of 4–6 weeks was reported by He et al. [41] in 2010. The very first patients of them treated with external distraction had relapse after the early removal of the distractors, so they lengthened the consolidation time up to 12 weeks and had successful results without nonunion. After a consolidation period of 6–8 weeks, distractors and intraoral splints are removed and the maxillary retention by Class III intraoral elastics can be used [45]. Some radical rigid retention periods (consolidation period) such as 2–3 weeks were also mentioned in some studies [26, 39]. In these studies, after the removal of the RED devices, 4–8 weeks of face mask elastic traction at night time were utilized.

Skeletal changes (horizontal and vertical)

The sagittal maxillary advancement is measured as the forward movement of particular landmarks. Anterior maxillary movement (horizontal change in point A) varies between 8.03 to 13.4 mm [1, 26, 38–45].

For patients undergoing RED devices, the average increase in SNA angle is between 7.6 to 12.4 degrees [26, 38, 40, 42–45].

Clockwise rotation of the maxilla is one of the goals in most of the patients with unilateral cleft lip and palate due to the vertical maxillary growth deficiency. The vertical changes in point A are between −1.3 and −7 mm pointing an inferior movement [26, 43, 44]. Although there can be a positive downward displacement of the maxilla, an undesired counterclockwise rotation of the maxilla can be a result of inconvenient distraction force vector [1, 42]. Desired change in the palatal plane angle varies according to the application point of the distraction force. In patients without secondary alveolar bone graft, distraction force may also lead to a counter-clockwise rotation. This reversible undesired rotation of the maxilla can be corrected with the aid of intraoral elastics [1].

Dental changes

Dentoalveolar sagittal movement can be measured by the dental overjet and the displacement of the upper incisor tip. The increase of the overjet ranged from 12.7 to 15.8 mm, whereas the angular change of the upper incisor according to the palatal plane ranged from −1.2 to 3.6 degrees [7, 26, 42, 44].

Soft tissue changes

The main changes accompanying RED procedure are located in the upper lip and nasal region, with improved facial aesthetics. In these patients, the profile of the face changes from concave to convex. The increase in facial convexity angle is between 15.59 and 26.2 degrees [7, 26, 39, 43, 44].

4.3.2. Internal distraction osteogenesis

Internal miniature distractor was first reported by Cohen et al. [20] in 1997 on maxillary distraction in patients with CLP using an internal miniature distractor. This device produced no complications and permitted maxillary and midfacial advancement in patients with CLP and craniofacial syndromes.

Most surgeons accept that advancement of more than 6 mm in patients with CLP and more than 10 mm in non-cleft patients is beyond the present limit of one-stage maxillary advancement surgery using LeFort I osteotomy, and can only be achieved by distraction osteogenesis [29, 30].

There are many clinical research studies and case reports about sagittal maxillary advancement with DO. The biomechanical effects associated with this procedure still remain speculative. In

2011, we investigated the effects of DO in a patient with CLP using finite element analysis (FEM) and improved this preliminary study with another comparative study in 2014 [4, 46] (**Figures 5–8**). Three-dimensional (3D) finite element model (FEM) analysis is a helpful mathematical instrument for use in orthodontics and can determine the amount of stress, strain and displacement in the maxillofacial complex after different loading conditions of force.

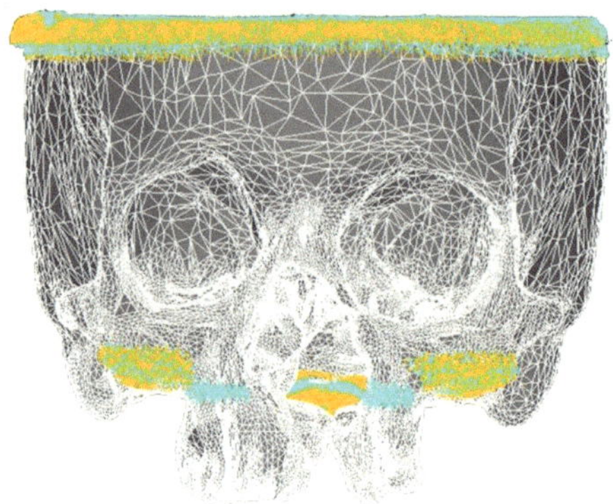

Figure 5. Three-dimensional finite element model of our patient with unilateral cleft lip and palate. Yellow colours represent the boundary conditions at the foramen magnum, upper side of the cranial vault and the zygomatic buttress, where the superior plates of the internal distractor are assumed to be placed.

The results of our study are similar to the clinical outcomes in some ways, and therefore may help surgeons and orthodontists to understand better the therapeutic effect of internal maxillary DO on the basal bones and sutures of the craniofacial system. The displacement distribution in the sagittal plane was asymmetric in the UCLP model rather than the non-cleft model. The non-cleft side of the UCLP FEM showed more anterior displacement than did the cleft side, which can result from the asymmetrical skeletal development of the anatomical structures.

The amount of transversal change at the lateral nasal walls was found to have expanded in both FEMs.

The maxillary rotation showed differences in both models. On the UCLP model, the maxilla rotated in a clockwise direction after maxillary advancement of 6 mm. On the cleft side, more inferior displacements were observed. In the control model, a counterclockwise rotation of the maxilla occurred. This can be the result of different placement of the anterior advancement vector in this finite element model.

Moreover, our results showed that the sagittal distraction forces produced not only advancement forces at the intermaxillary sutures but also higher stress values at the sutura nasomaxillaris, sutura frontonasalis and sutura zygomaticomaxillaris on the cleft side compared to the non-cleft side. In the non-cleft model, relatively high stress values were found at the sutura frontomaxillaris and sutura nasomaxillaris, similar to the findings on the non-cleft side of the UCLP FEM.

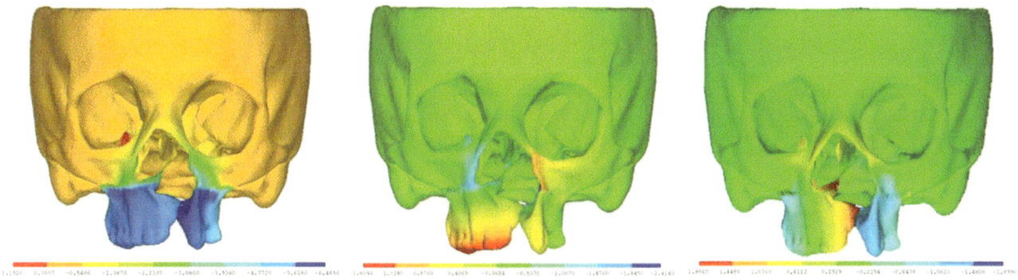

Figure 6. Displacement distribution in (a) sagittal, (b) transversal and (c) vertical planes after 6 mm of maxillary advancement for the UCLP model, respectively.

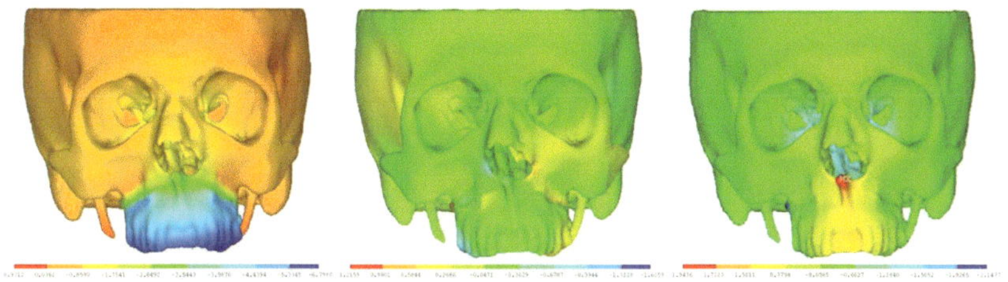

Figure 7. Displacement distribution in (a) sagittal, (b) transversal and (c) vertical planes after 6 mm of maxillary advancement for the non-cleft control model, respectively.

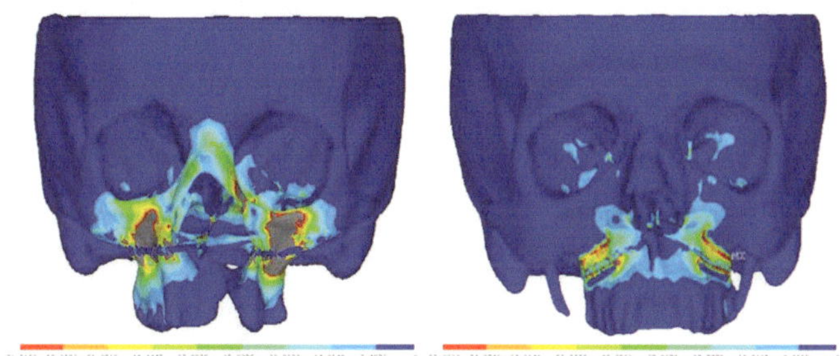

Figure 8. The magnitude and distribution of the von Mises stresses after 1 mm of maxillary advancement for the UCLP model and for the non-cleft control model, respectively.

Advantages and disadvantages

Internal distractors are socially and psychologically more tolerated than the external distractors [36, 47–49]. However, there are some disadvantages: (1) the difficulty of the position process, (2) the need for a second operation to remove the distractors, (3) the inability to change the distraction vector during the distraction phase (control of the maxillary segment can be achieved by intraoral elastics by which an adjustment in "molding the regenerate" bone corrects for an error in distraction direction or vector), (4) the difficulty in placement of the two parts of the distractors parallel to each other, (5) the limitation of the distraction length,

(6) the discomfort due to the stretch of the buccal tissues by the distractor's rods, (7) the need for pre-operative planning and/or stereolithographic modelling [34, 50–55].

Stereolithographic modelling

The desired vectors of the maxillary advancement are necessary and can be controlled via stereolithographic models. In patients with CLP, visualization of the bone thickness and decision of the bony cuts and distractor placements should be made on these models pre-operatively. However, in some countries there is an extra cost for stereolithographic modelling; therefore, pre-operative planning can also be simulated using specific computer software, which allows for three-dimensional craniofacial reconstruction from computed tomography scan images [51–54, 56] (**Figures 9–11**). Three-dimensional finite element model analysis is also a helpful mathematical instrument for use both in orthodontics and in orthopaedics, and can determine the amount of stress, strain and displacement in the maxillofacial complex [4, 57]. However, this technique cannot be used for all patients individually due to the long elapsed time for the analysis.

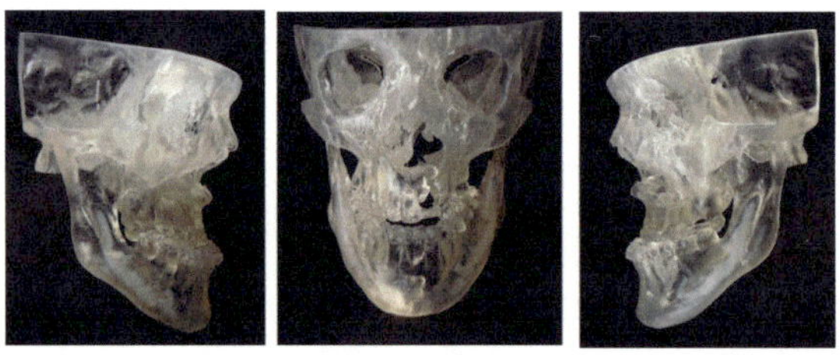

Figure 9. Stereolithographic model of our patient with UCLP.

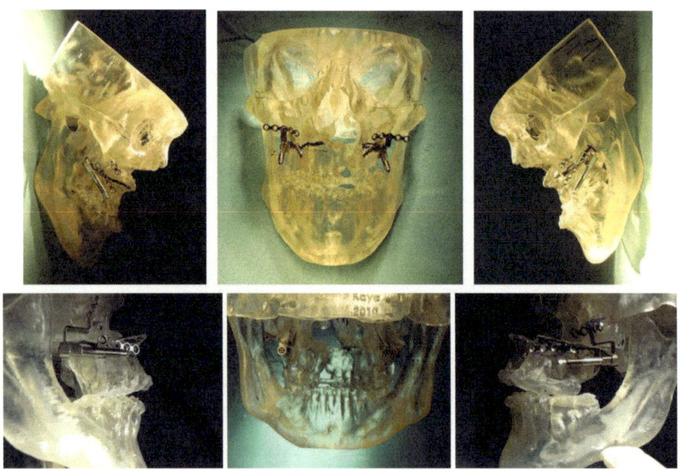

Figure 10. Demonstration of the surgery on the stereolithographic model, bending of the distractor plates during this section, and finally insertion of the bended distractor plates on the model.

http://dx.doi.org/10.5772/62545

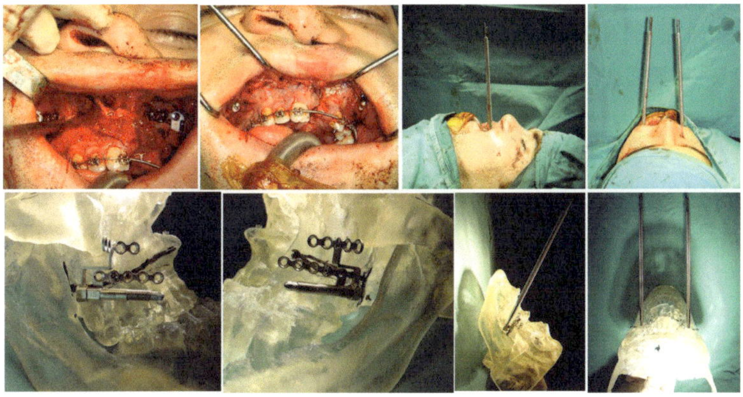

Figure 11. LeFort I osteotomy, and the checking for the parallelism of the inserted distractor plates using extension rods.

Technique and protocol

The need for the correction and severity of the maxillary deficiency is the key to choose the type of osteotomy. The maxillary osteotomies can be divided into three subgroups: (1) horizontal osteotomy, for anterior advancement of the maxilla, (2) oblique osteotomy, for forward and downward movement of the maxilla, (3) step osteotomy, for children in whom canine and premolar teeth buds are in a high position [51, 58]. The standard LeFort I osteotomy and down fracturing of the maxilla are the most commonly performed osteotomies since this technique is used in older patients than those treated with RED [51, 54, 59–61]. High LeFort I and the 2–3 piece LeFort I osteotomies (this can be performed after completion of distraction, at the time of device removal) are also used with this protocol [34, 54].

After the insertion of the internal bone-borne maxillary distractors, the screws were activated for a few millimeters or more to check the correctness of the maxillary movement and to overcome premature bony contacts during the activation process [4, 34, 60–62]. Mandibular osteotomies, if needed according to the skeletal diagnosis, can be performed in the same operation [59, 60, 62].

After the operation a latency period of 3–7 days, initial activation of the internal distraction device starts. The rate of distraction is 0.5 to 1 mm per day in one or two rhythms. Activation of the distractors can be performed by the patients themselves or by the patients' parents or relatives. The planned maxillary advancement is usually obtained in several days of active distraction. The duration of the activation phase depends on the severity of the maxillary deficiency. Activation of the distractors performed until the proper overjet, overbite and relative stable posterior and anterior occlusion (overcorrected Class I molar and incisal relationship) are achieved [4, 5, 36, 51, 54, 60–62].

In early post-operative period, many clinicians use orthodontic elastic traction to control the occlusion, to prevent posterior or anterior openbite and to guide the maxilla into position [34, 59–61].

Consolidation period of 8 to 12 weeks is generally accepted in UCLP patients to prevent the risk of possible skeletal relapse [32, 51, 54, 62]. During consolidation period, bone mineralization of the distraction zone and bone remodelling occur according to the Ilizarov's principles.

Skeletal changes (horizontal and vertical)

The horizontal maxillary advancement usually measured as the advancement of point A ranged from 5.7 to 34 mm [34, 54, 59, 61, 62]. The average increase in SNA angle is between 5.65 and 10.8 degrees [40, 54].

The vertical changes in point A are between −1.1 mm (meaning counterclockwise rotation of the maxilla) to 7 mm (meaning clockwise rotation of the maxilla) [34, 54, 61, 62].

The counterclockwise rotation of the maxilla can be a result of inconvenient distraction force vector and can be changed by the use of the orthodontic elastic traction that can be applied between upper and lower teeth [1, 4, 34, 42].

Dental changes

The increase of the overjet ranged from 6.59 to 13.66 mm [51, 61].

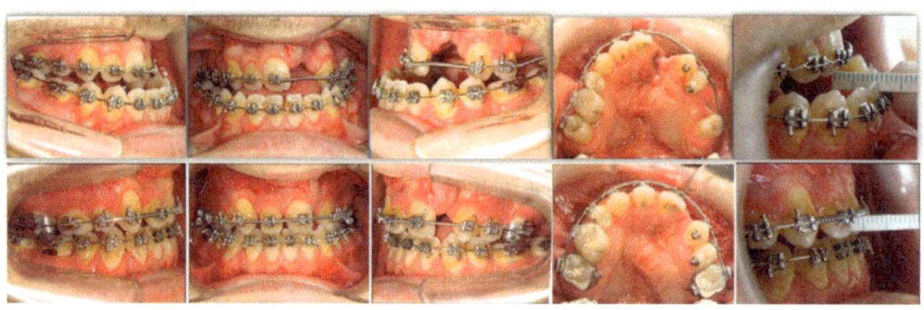

Figure 12. Intra-oral photographs of a 21-year-old boy affected by severe maxillary hypoplasia due to unilateral cleft lip and palate treated in our clinic before internal distraction and after consolidation period (after using orthodontic elastic traction and removal).

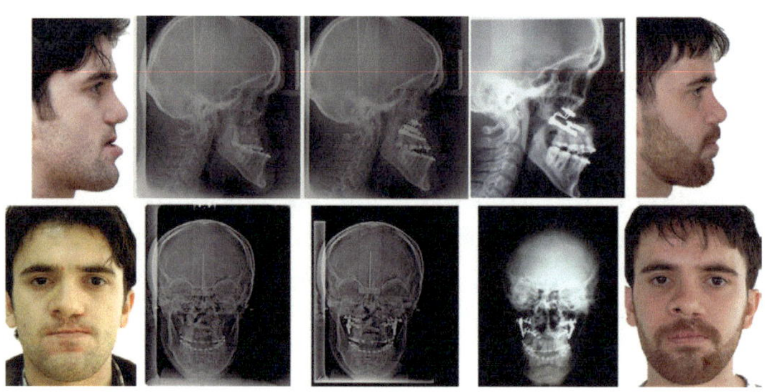

Figure 13. Pre-operative and post-operative extra-oral photographs and cephalometric films of the same patient.

http://dx.doi.org/10.5772/62545

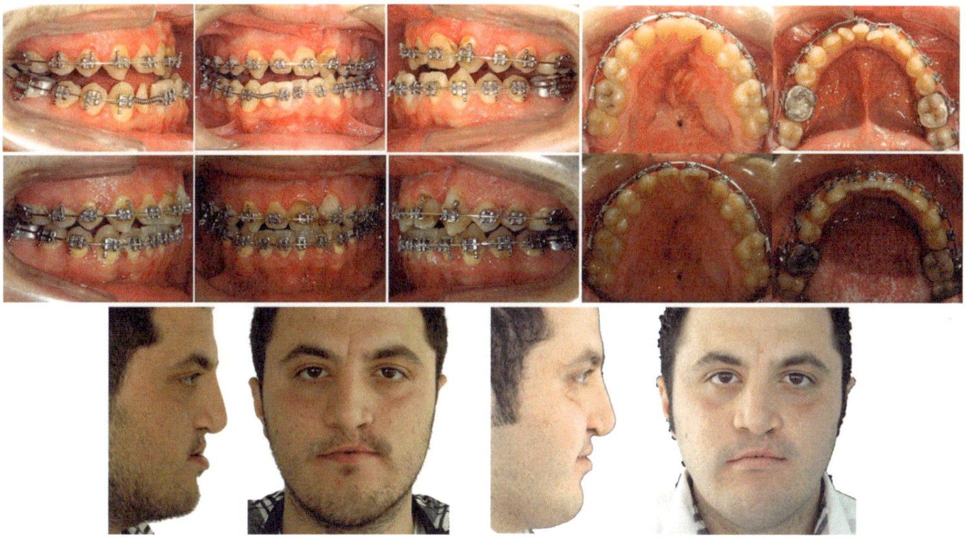

Figure 14. Intra-oral and extra-oral photographs of a 20-year-old boy affected by severe maxillary hypoplasia due to unilateral cleft lip and palate treated in our clinic before and after internal distraction osteogenesis.

5. Conclusion

The use of distraction osteogenesis was proved as a predictable method for major bone elongation with the generation of new bone in the distraction site. Newly formed bone can provide good support and thus contribute to stability. Many surgeons and orthodontists prefer sagittal maxillary distraction osteogenesis in maxillary deficiency, especially in patients with cleft lip and palate or in syndromic patients. Virtual surgical planning and/or stereolithographic modelling allow more predictable operation and distraction.

Sagittal distraction forces produce not only advancement forces at the intermaxillary sutures but also higher stress values at the sutura nasomaxillaris, sutura frontonasalis and sutura zygomaticomaxillaris on the cleft side of the patients with unilateral cleft lip and palate rather than the non-cleft side. Some patients feel pressure under the eyes, around the lateral nasal walls and generally throughout the face during and after the distractor activations. One should consider the consequences of the activation of the distractors under the light of these findings. Since the clinical effectiveness of the maxillary distraction osteogenesis, especially in patients with cleft lip and palate, is highly dependent on the presence of the scar tissue, it would be helpful to incorporate this soft tissue into future mathematical models.

For patients with mild to severe maxillofacial deficiencies, conventional one-step LeFort I maxillary advancement is out of limits, and advancement using distraction osteogenesis has been shown to be a stable, reliable treatment modality in such cases.

Author details

Sultan Olmez-Gurlen

Address all correspondence to: sultanolmez@gmail.com

Private Practitioner, Izmir, Turkey

References

[1] Aksu M, Saglam-Aydinatay B, Akcan CA, El H, Taner T, Kocadereli I, Tuncbilek G, Mavili ME Skeletal and dental stability after maxillary distraction with a rigid external device in adult cleft lip and palate patients. J Oral Maxillofac Surg. 2010;68:254-259.

[2] Ross RB Treatment variables affecting facial growth in complete unilateral cleft lip and palate. Cleft Palate J. 1987;24:5-77.

[3] Cheung LK, Chua HDP A meta-analysis of cleft maxillary osteotomy and distraction. Int J Oral Maxillofac Surg. 2006;35:14-24.

[4] Olmez S, Dogan S, Pekedis M, Yildiz H Biomechanical evaluation of sagittal maxillary internal distraction osteogenesis in unilateral cleft lip and palate patient and noncleft patients-a three dimensional finite element analysis. Angle Orthod. 2014;84:815-824.

[5] Austin SL, Mattick CR, Waterhouse PJ Distraction osteoegnesis versus orthognathic surgery for the treatment of maxillary hypoplasia in cleft lip and palate patients: a systematic review. Orthod Craniofac Res. 2015;18:96-108.

[6] Dogan S, Olmez S, Bilkay U, Aydinli E Treatment modalities of a unilateral cleft lip and palate patient from birth to adulthood-case report. Ortho Techniques. 2011;3(4):digital issue.

[7] Rachmiel A, Even-Almos M, Aizenbud D Treatment of maxillary cleft palate: distraction osteogenesis vs orthognathic surgery. Ann Maxillofac Surg. 2012;2(2):127-130.

[8] Constantino PD, Friedman CD Distraction osteogenesis: application for mandibular regrowth. Otolaryngol Clin North Am. 1991;24:1433-1442.

[9] Cohen SR, Rutrick RE, Burstein FD Distration osteogenesis of the human craniofacial skeleton: initial experience with new distraction system. J Craniofac Surg. 1995;6:368-374.

[10] Rachmiel A, Laufer D, Jackson IT, Lewinson D Midface membranous bone lengthening: a one year histological follow-up of distraction osteogenesis. Calcif Tissue Int. 1998;62:370-376.

[11] Rachmiel A, Rozen N, Peled M, Lewinson D Characterization of midface maxillary membranous bone formation during distraction osteogenesis. Plast Reconstr Surg. 2002;109:1611-1620.

[12] Codivilla A On the means of lengthening in the lower limbs, the muscles and tissues which are shortened through deformity. Clin Orthop Relat Res. 1994;301:4-9.

[13] Ilizarov GA Basic principles of transosseous compression and distraction osteosynthesis. Orthop Travmatol Protez. 1971;32:7-15.

[14] Ilizarov GA The principles of the Ilizarov method. Bull Hosp Jt Dis Orthop Inst. 1988;48:1-12.

[15] Ilizarov GA The tension-stress effect on the genesis and growth of tissues. Part I. The influence of stability of fixation and soft tissue preservation. Clin Orthop Relat Res. 1989a;238:249-281.

[16] Ilizarov GA The tension-stress effect on the genesis and growth of tissues. Part II. The influence of the rate and frequency of distraction. Clin Orthop Relat Res. 1989b; 239:263-285.

[17] SynderCC, Levine GA, Swanson HM, Browne EZ Jr Mandibular lengthening by gradual distraction. Preliminary report. Plas Reconstr Surg. 1973;51(5):506-508.

[18] Michielli S, Miotti B Lengthening of mandibular body by gradual surgical-orthodontic distraction. J Oral Surg. 1977;35(3):187-192.

[19] McCarthy JG, Schreiber J, Karp N, Thorne CH, Grayson BH Lengthening of the human mandible by gradual distraction. Plas Reconstr Surg. 1992;89(1):1-8.

[20] Cohen SR, Burstein FD, Stewart MB, Rathburn MA Maxillary-midface distraction in children with cleft lip and palate: a preliminary report. Plas Reconstr Surg. 1997;99(5): 1421-1428.

[21] Shah AR Distraction osteogenesis of the maxilla [Internet]. [Updated: December 15, 2014]. Available from: http://emedicine.medscape.com/article/844742-overview.

[22] Aronson J Experimental and clinical experience with distraction osteogenesis. Cleft Palate Craniofac. 1994;31:473-482.

[23] Guererero CA, Bell WH, Contasti GI Mandibular widening by intraoral distraction osteogenesis. Br J Oral Maxillofac Surg. 1997;35:383-392.

[24] Mommaerts MY Transpalatal distraction as a method of maxillary expansion. Br J Oral Maxillofac Surg. 1999;37(4):268-272.

[25] Bell WH, Gonzalez M, Samchukov ML Intraoral widening and lengthening of mandible in baboons by distraction osteogenesis. J Oral Maxillofac Surg. 1999;57(5):548-562.

[26] Polley JW, Figueroa AA Rigid external distraction: its application in cleft maxillary deformities. Plast Reconstr Surg. 1998;102:1360-1372.

[27] Shetye PR, Davidson EH, Sorkin M Evaluation of three surgical techniques for advancement of the midface in growing children with syndromic craniosyntosis. Plast Reconstr Surg. 2010;126(3):982-994.

[28] Saelen R, Tornes K, Halse A Stability after Le Fort I osteotomy in cleft lip and palate patients. Int J Adult Orthod Orthognath Surg. 1998;13:317-323.

[29] Molina F, Monasterio F, Aguliar M Maxillary distraction: aesthetic and functional benefits in cleft lip and palate and prognathic patients during mixed dentition. Plast Reconstr Surg. 1998;101:951-963.

[30] Costa F, Robiony M, Politi M Stability of Le Fort I osteotomy in maxillary advancement: review of the literature. Int J Adult Orthod Orthognath Surg. 1999;14:207-213.

[31] Yu H, Wang X, Fang B, Shen SG Comparative study of different osteotomy modalities in maxillary distraction osteogenesis for cleft lip and palate. J Oral Maxillofac Surg. 2012;70:2641-2647.

[32] Adolphs N, Ernst N, Menneking H, Hoffmeister B Significance of distraction osteogenesis of the craniomaxillofacial skeleton: A clinical review after 10 years of experience with the technique. J Craniomaxillofac Surg. 2014;42:966-975.

[33] Ahn JG, Figueroa AA, Braun S, et al. Biomechanical considerations in distraction of the osteotomized dentomaxillary complex. Am J Orthod Dentofacial Orthop. 1999;116:264-270.

[34] Tomita D, Omura S, Ozaki S, et al. Maxillary movement in distraction osteogenesis using internal devices in cleft palate patients. Cleft Palate Craniofac J. 2011;48(2): 161-166.

[35] Polley JW, Figueroa AA Management of severe maxillary deficiency in childhood and adolescence through distraction osteogenesis with an external, adjustable, rigid distraction device. J Craniofac Surg. 1997;8:181-185.

[36] Scolozzi P Distraction osteogenesis in the management of severe maxillary hypoplasia in cleft lip and palate patients. J Craniofac Surg. 2008;19(5):1199-1214.

[37] Figueroa AA, Polley JW, Ko EW Maxillary distraction for the management of cleft maxillary hypoplasia with a rigid external distraction system. Semin Orthod. 1999;5:46-51.

[38] Figueroa AA, Polley JW, Friede H, et al. Long-term skeletal stability after maxillary advancement with distraction osteogenesis using a rigid external distraction device in cleft maxillary deformities. Plast Reconstr Surg. 2004;114:1382-1392.

[39] Ko EWC, Figueroa AA, Polley JW Soft tissue profile changes after maxillary advancement with distraction osteogenesis by use of a rigid external distraction device: a 1 year follow-up. J Oral Maxillofac Surg. 2000;58:959-969.

[40] Rachmiel A, Aizenbud D, Peled M Distraction osteogenesis in maxillary deficiency using a rigid external distraction device. Plast Reconstr Surg. 2006;117:2399-2406.

[41] He D, Genecov DG, Barcelo R Nonunion of the external maxillary distraction in cleft lip and palate: analysis of possible reasons. J Oral Maxillofac Surg. 2010;68:2402-2411.

[42] Gürsoy S, Hukki J, Hurmerinta K Five-year follow-up of maxillary distraction osteogenesis on the dentofacial structures of children with cleft lip and palate. J Oral Maxillofac Surg. 2010;68:744-750.

[43] Dua G, Kumar AN, Roy ID, Roy SK Maxillary distraction osteogenesis in cleft lip and palate cases with midfacial hypoplasia using rigid external distractor: an alternative technique. J Craniofac Surg. 2014;25(3):746-751.

[44] Daimaruya T, Imai Y, Kochi S, Tachi M, Takano-Yamamoto T Midfacial changes through distraction osteogenesis using a rigid external distraction system with retention plates in cleft lip and palate patients. J Oral Maxillofac Surg. 2010;68:1480-1486.

[45] Rattan V, Jena AK, Singh SP, Utreja AK Maxillary distraction osteogenesis at Lefort I level induces bone apposition at infraorbital rim. Clin Oral Invest. 2014;18:1741-1748.

[46] Olmez S, Dogan S, Pekedis M, Yildiz H The evaluation of maxillary advancement technique using internal distraction osteogenesis in unilateral cleft lip and palate patient with finite element analysis. Journal of Biomechanics. 2011;44:e13-e14. DOI: 10.1016/j.jbiomech.2011.02.053.

[47] Gulsen, Ozmen S, Tuncer S, et al. Maxillary advancement with internal distraction device in cleft palate patients. J Craniofac Surg. 2007;18:177-185.

[48] Aikawa IS, Isomura ET, Namikawa M, Yatsuoka Y, Yamada C, Ymamoto T, Takigawa Y Breakage of internal maxillary distractor: considerable complication of axillary distraction osteogenesis. Oral Surg Oral Med Oral Pathol Oral Radiol Endod. 2008;106:e1-e7.

[49] Bevilacqua RG, Ritoli EL, Kang C, Mabry K, Castiglione CL Midmaxillary internal distraction osteogenesis: ideal surgery for the mature cleft patients. Plast Reconstr Surg. 2008;121:1768-1778.

[50] Nakagawa K, Ueki K, Takatsuka S, Marukawa K, Yamamoto E A device for determining the position of intraoral distractors for protracting the maxilla. J Craniomaxillofac Surg. 2003;31:234-237.

[51] Racmiel A, Aizenbud D, Peled M Long term results in maxillary deficiency using intraoral devices. Int J Oral Maxillofac Surg. 2005;34:473-479.

[52] Wang XX, Wang X, Yi B Internal midface distraction in correction of severe maxillary hypoplasia secondary to cleft lip and palate. Plast Reconstr Surg. 2005;116:51-60.

[53] Gateno J, Engel ER, Teichgraeber JF, et al. A new Le Fort I internal distraction device in the treatment of severe maxillary hypoplasia. J Oral Maxillofac Surg. 2005;63:148-154.

[54] Kumar A, Gabbay JS, Nikjoo R, et al. Improved outcomes in cleft patients with severe maxillary deficiency after Le Fort I internal distraction. Plast Reconstr Surg. 2006;117:1499-1509.

[55] Van Sickels JE, Madsen MJ, Cunningham LL Jr, Bird D The use of internal maxillary distraction for maxillary hypoplasia: a preliminary report. J Oral Maxillofac Surg. 2006;64:1715-1720.

[56] Olmez S Evaluation of maxillary distraction osteogenesis in patients with cleft lip and palate using finite element method [thesis]. Izmir-Turkey:2012.

[57] Ozan F, Yildiz H, Bora OA, et al. The effect of head trauma on fracture healing: biomechanical testing and finite element analysis. Acta Orthop Traumatol. 2010;44:313-321.

[58] Rachmiel S, Aizenbud D, Ardekian L, Peled M, Laufer D Surgically-assisted orthopedic protraction of the maxilla in cleft lip and palate patients. Int J Oral Maxillofac Surg. 1999;28:9-14.

[59] Cheung LK, Chua HDP, Hagg MB Ckeft maxillary distraction versus orthognathic surgery: clinical morbidities and surgical relapse. Plast Reconstr Surg. 2006;118:996-1008.

[60] Chua HDP, Whitehill TL, Samman N, Cheung LK Maxillary distraction versus orthognathic surgery in cleft lip and palate patients: effects on speech and velopharyngeal function. Int Journal Oral Maxillofac Surg. 2010a;39:633-640.

[61] Chua HDP, Cheung LK Soft tissue changes from maxillary distraction osteogenesis versus orthognathic surgery in patients with cleft lip and palate: a randomized controlled clinical trial. J Oral Maxillofac Surg. 2012;70:1648-1658.

[62] Chua HDP, Hagg MB, Cheung LK Cleft maxillary distraction versus orthognathic surgery- which one is more stable in 5 years? Oral Surg Oral Med Oral Pathol Oral Radiol Endod. 2010b;109:803-814.

Chapter 4

Sonographic Monitoring During Distraction Osteogenesis

Helder Groenwold Campos,
Bruna Olivotti Lahan Martins,
Daniel Miranda Ferreira and
Eduardo José Mariotoni Bronzatto

Additional information is available at the end of the chapter

http://dx.doi.org/10.5772/64112

Abstract

Distraction osteogenesis is a method of bone healing and regeneration widely used to correct bone malformations, shortenings, and other bone defects. Despite its benefits, it is a long-duration therapy with considerable physical and psychological morbidity. Treatment optimization is fundamental and monitoring techniques are being studied. This chapter discusses monitoring methods with a focus on ultrasound evaluation of distraction osteogenesis.

Keywords: sonographic monitoring, distraction osteogenesis, bone regeneration

1. Introduction

The distraction osteogenesis is a method of bone regeneration and fixation that was established by Ilizarov around the 1950s, causing revolution in the reconstruction and deformity correction surgeries [1]. The technique consists of a controlled bone fracture (osteotomy) and, after the formation of the soft callus (latency period), continuous traction of bone fragments in opposite directions, using an external fixator (lengthening phase), until the desired extension is reached, then fixing it until consolidation (neutral fixation/consolidation phase). This process does not use grafting and allows to cover extensive bone defects with newly formed bone (regenerated) or to remodel malformed structures. Nowadays it is applied in multiple orthopedic and maxillofacial surgeries. However, it is a long-duration therapy and the patient may remain in use of an external fixator for a period of up to 20 weeks.

The treatment duration generates great physical and psychological morbidity. Its importance was recognized by Ilizarov himself when he postulated: "keeping the apparatus for longer than necessary is as damaging as removing early" [2]. Therefore, the optimization of therapy is fundamental to reduce the complications and ensure its success. For that reason, the distraction osteogenesis monitoring must be realized. Several methods are available, with some being more suited to each phase. The histological characteristics of the regenerated tissue in each phase are fundamental for the comprehension of the monitoring methods, as we see later.

1.1. Latency period

Latency period consists in the physiological tissue repairing response initiated immediately after the osteotomy. The lesion unleashes an inflammatory reaction with clot formation

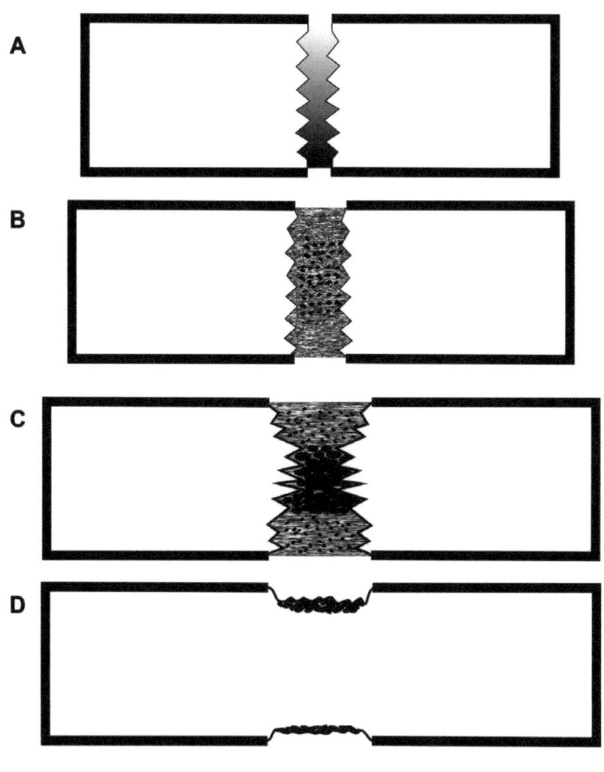

Figure 1. Distraction osteogenesis scheme. (A) Osteotomy, (B) gap increase with ossification centers (black dots), (C) progressive gap increase, confluence of ossification centers, and peripheral bone formation and (D) hard callous bridging the gap with mild corticalized margins and central invagination.

between and around the osteotomy segment and cytokine activation, growth factors, and mesenchymal cellular aggregation. A granulation tissue is formed, consisting of extracellular matrix rich in fibrin, collagen, neutrophils, fibroblasts, and cells with osteogenic potential [3]. This set is called soft callus (see **Figure 1**).

The goal of this phase is the formation and maturation of the soft callus, with sufficient neovascularization to stimulate ossification. Classically, its duration is established around 5–7 days. There is no need for monitoring in this phase.

1.2. Lengthening phase

After the latency phase, the distraction apparatus is activated and the soft callus is strained initiating several osteogenic processes. The straining produced in the longitudinal axis alters the cellular expression in the soft callus. At the gap center, high strain forces inhibit cellular differentiation and stimulate its proliferation. In the extremities, strain forces are milder, thus allowing cellular differentiation. Therefore, the callus center has high cellular density composed of precursor mesenchymal cells (fibroblasts and pre-osteoblasts), while the extremities are paucicellular and composed mostly of osteoblasts. Hence, the osteogenesis process occurs from the deeper region of the extremities toward the center and surface [3, 4].

The formation of bone tissue is modulated by the rate of distraction and its rhythm. The first is the total length gain in a day, which varies from 0.5 to 1.0 mm/day; the second refers to the number of daily activations to reach the desired length, varying from two to four activations per day. Excessive traction tends to stimulate the formation of cysts and fibrous tissue, reducing the resistance of the regenerated tissue; on the other hand, less traction leads to precocious consolidation, making it impossible to achieve the desired length [5].

1.3. Consolidation phase (neutral fixation)

Reaching the desired length, the external fixator is locked, fixing the bone extremities and ensuring proper support during the consolidation period. The apparatus must remain in position until the regenerated tissue is sufficiently consolidated to avoid complications such as deformations or post-distraction fractures. The duration of this period is usually defined as the number of the days of the lengthening phase multiplied by two (lengthening phase × 2). This rule, however, does not avoid the occurrence of complications, making other parameters of evaluation necessary.

2. Monitoring methods

Several complementary methods can be used to follow the evolution of the procedure, each one with advantages and disadvantages, depending on the phase of the process.

2.1. Ionizing radiation

X-ray, dual energy X-ray absorptiometry (DEXA) and computed tomography can be utilized for the evaluation of the bone callus. However, the necessity for a serialized evaluation, exposure to ionizing radiation, metallic artifacts susceptibility, and the high cost and more restricted availability of computed tomography and DEXA limit the utilization of these methods.

The X-ray is the most used, because it allows proper evaluation of the bone extremities and distraction distance (gap). Using the "three cortical rule," where the visualization of at least three corticals with 2 mm thickness on orthogonal views is necessary, the removal of the external fixator is indicated [6, 7]. Yet, it was observed that this method is subject to great observer variation, not being more accurate than random chance [8]. Other limitations are related to the initial stages where radiography is incapable of evaluating soft tissue.

Studies valued the role of DEXA in the evaluation of the regenerated tissue, from the lengthening stages until its attempt to objectively define the best moment to remove the external fixator. Some research parameters include the relation between the regenerated bone mineral density and contralateral limb, and also the percentage of the weekly increase of bone mineral density [9, 10]. Despite promising results, there is still no standardization of these parameters.

The quantitative computed tomography (QCT) sums the quantitative evaluation with high-resolution images of regenerating bones, presenting better correlation than the DEXA and allowing a global evaluation to the assistant doctor. However, high cost, little availability, and great exposure to radiation (more than the other methods) limit its application [1].

2.2. Ultrasonography

Recently, the role of ultrasonography in the monitoring and distraction has been target of several studies. Several characteristics make this a method of interest, as it does not use ionizing radiation, it is widespread, and it is not subject to artifacts related to external fixators. The top advantage is the possibility of characterization of soft tissue and precocious detection of complications like cysts and collections.

For the ultrasonographic evaluation, linear transducers for high resolution must be used (5–12 MHz). The osteotomy is evaluated with beams perpendicular to the bone corticals, longitudinally and transversely along the bone axis. In the initial evaluation, the ultrasonography identifies the osteotomy corticals as hyperechoic surfaces, with posterior acoustic shadow and acute margins. Between them is located the soft callus, defined as a hypoechoic area with great penetration of the ultrasonographic beam [11]. (see **Figure 1**)

In the first weeks, the appearance of echogenic outbreaks longitudinally oriented in the interior of the "gap" is noticed. In the cross-sectional assessment, there is a "cut wire" aspect. Between 2 and 4 weeks, the first individualized ossification center starts to be identified. Over time, there is an increase in number and size of those centers with the tendency to confluence on the longitudinal axis. Gradually, there is loss of penetration power in the callus and rounding of the edges of osteotomies. After 6–8 weeks, it is defined a cortical margin with mild central invagination and thickness markedly reduced in relation to the osteotomies corticals [12].

With the progression of the corticalization, the ultrasound beams are gradually more reflected, thus losing the correlation between the method and characterization of changes in the stiffness and strength of the regenerated tissue (attenuation × reflection) [13]. Eventually, the beams' reflection will be full, preventing the evaluation continuity with this method. Therefore, ultrasound assessment is limited in the final stages of consolidation and there are no studies in literature investigating its role establishing enough bone healing for the apparatus removal [1].

The ultrasound appearance during the entire process was compared with tissue density measurement with computerized tomography, evidencing an exponential increase in bone density through the consolidation time [14], but no objective ultrasound parameter was proposed as a follow-up measure. Ultrasound evaluation itself is mainly subjective and prone to multiple variables as transducer position and measurement site [15]. Troulis et al. proposed the use of through-transmission method, in which the beam penetration depth in the soft callus is used as the stiffness indicator. But in his work throught transmission was compared with the surgeon's intraoperative bone stiffness evaluation, which was also subjective [16]. The lack of objective parameters to assess bone mass index limits its application as a monitoring method.

Quantitative acoustic parameters (ultrasonometry) and its correlation with soft callus properties have been studied. Velocity propagation across the gap correlates with bone healing [17], while speed of sound, acoustic reflection, and attenuation correlate with trabecular bone mass index [18] and acoustic backscattering relates to trabecular microstructure [19]. Strong association between the penetration depth within the gap and maximum load and torsional stiffness of the consolidated callus has been shown. With noninvasive, radiation-free, objective data, follow-up protocols can be studied and early therapy modifications (distraction rate, medications) may optimize the distraction and consolidation processes.

3. Conclusion

The monitoring of the osteogenesis distraction is fundamental to avoid complications and reduce the time of use of the external fixator. Several methods are available, each one presenting advantages and disadvantages. The ultrasound seems like an excellent method in the initial evaluation of distraction; however, it is incapable of orienting objectively the moment of removal of the external fixator. The methods using ionizing radiation present several possibilities, but lack in objective and standard data limits its application. Considering these factors, a multimodal evaluation of the progression of the treatment, conciliating clinical expertise, and the rational use of the available complimentary exams for the optimization of the treatment must be used.

Author details

Helder Groenwold Campos, Bruna Olivotti Lahan Martins, Daniel Miranda Ferreira and Eduardo José Mariotoni Bronzatto*

*Address all correspondence to: edubronzatto@gmail.com

State University of Campinas – Unicamp, Campinas, Brazil

References

[1] O. M. Babatunde, A. T. Fragomen, and S. R. Rozbruch, "Noninvasive quantitative assessment of bone healing after distraction osteogenesis." *HSS J.*, vol. 6, no. 1, pp. 71–8, 2010.

[2] G. A. Ilizarov, "Clinical application of the tension-stress effect for limb lengthening." *Clin. Orthop. Relat. Res.*, vol. 250, pp. 8–26, Jan. 1990.

[3] L. R. Amir, V. Everts, and A. L. J. J. Bronckers, "Bone regeneration during distraction osteogenesis." *Odontology*, vol. 97, no. 2, pp. 63–75, 2009.

[4] T. Ol, O. D. P. Rool, D. G. D. Lul, Q. Jduzdo, and D. Q. G. Mlw, "The biology of distraction osteogenesis for correction of mandibular and craniomaxillofacial defects: a review." *Dent. Res. J.*, vol. Jan–Feb, no. 11(1), pp. 16–26, 2014.

[5] U. M. Djasim, E. B. Wolvius, J. A. Bos, H. W. van Neck, and K. G. van der Wal, "Continuous versus discontinuous distraction: evaluation of bone regenerate following various rhythms of distraction." *J. Oral Maxillofac. Surg.*, vol. 67, no. 4, pp. 818–26, 2009.

[6] D. L. Skaggs, A. I. Leet, M. D. Money, B. A. Shaw, J. M. Hale, and V. T. Tolo, "Secondary fractures associated with external fixation in pediatric femur fractures." *J. Pediatr. Orthop.*, vol. 19, no. 5, pp. 582–6, Jan. 1999.

[7] J. Fischgrund, D. Paley, and C. Suter, "Variables affecting time to bone healing during limb lengthening." *Clin. Orthop. Relat. Res.*, vol. 301, pp. 31–7, Apr. 1994.

[8] A. Anand, D. S. Feldman, R. J. Patel, W. B. Lehman, H. J. P. van Bosse, M. I. Badra, and D. A. Sala, "Interobserver and intraobserver reliability of radiographic evidence of bone healing at osteotomy sites." *J. Pediatr. Orthop. B*, vol. 15, no. 4, pp. 271–2, Jul. 2006.

[9] F. Chotel, P. Braillon, F. Sailhan, S. Gadeyne, J.-O. Gellon, G. Panczer, C. Pedrini, and J. Berard, "Bone stiffness in children: part II. Objectives criteria for children to assess healing during leg lengthening." *J. Pediatr. Orthop.*, vol. 28, no. 5, pp. 538–43, Jan. 2008.

[10] N. Saran and R. C. Hamdy, "DEXA as a predictor of fixator removal in distraction osteogenesis." *Clin. Orthop. Relat. Res.*, vol. 466, no. 12, pp. 2955–61, Dec. 2008.

[11] C. W. Hughes, R. W. Williams, M. Bradley, and G. H. Irvine, "Ultrasound monitoring of distraction osteogenesis." *Br. J. Oral Maxillofac. Surg.*, vol. 41, no. 4, pp. 256–8, 2003.

[12] A. Poposka, N. Atanasov, and R. Dzoleva-Tolevska, "Use of ultrasonography in evaluation of new bone formation in patients treated by the method of Ilizarov." vol. 208, pp. 199–208, 2012.

[13] K. S. Eyres, M. J. Bell, and J. A. Kanis, "Methods of assessing new bone formation during limb lengthening. Ultrasonography, dual energy X-ray absorptiometry and radiography compared." *J. Bone Joint Surg. Br.*, vol. 75, no. 3, pp. 358–64, May 1993.

[14] H. Selim, N. Elbargothy, Y. Nabil, and I. El-Hakim, "Evaluation of distracted mandibular bone using computed tomography scan and ultrasonography: technical note." *Dentomaxillofac. Radiol.*, vol. 38, no. 5, pp. 274–80, 2009.

[15] M. D. Markel and E. Y. Chao, "Noninvasive monitoring techniques for quantitative description of callus mineral content and mechanical properties." *Clin. Orthop. Relat. Res.*, vol. 293, pp. 37–45, Aug. 1993.

[16] M. J. Troulis, C. Coppe, M. J. O'Neill, and L. B. Kaban, "Ultrasound: Assessment of the distraction osteogenesis wound in patients undergoing mandibular lengthening." *J. Oral Maxillofac. Surg.*, vol. 61, no. 10, pp. 1144–9, 2003.

[17] C. B. Machado, W. C. de A. Pereira, M. Granke, M. Talmant, F. Padilla, and P. Laugier, "Experimental and simulation results on the effect of cortical bone mineralization in ultrasound axial transmission measurements: a model for fracture healing ultrasound monitoring." *Bone*, vol. 48, no. 5, pp. 1202–9, May 2011.

[18] M. A. Hakulinen, J. Töyräs, S. Saarakkala, J. Hirvonen, H. Kröger, and J. S. Jurvelin, "Ability of ultrasound backscattering to predict mechanical properties of bovine trabecular bone." *Ultrasound Med. Biol.*, vol. 30, no. 7, pp. 919–27, Jul. 2004.

[19] D. D. Deligianni and K. N. Apostolopoulos, "Characterization of dense bovine cancellous bone tissue microstructure by ultrasonic backscattering using weak scattering models." *J. Acoust. Soc. Am.*, vol. 122, no. 2, pp. 1180–90, Aug. 2007.

Chapter 5

A Strategy of Bone Regeneration for the Treatment of Idiopathic Femoral Head Necrosis

Tomoki Aoyama

Additional information is available at the end of the chapter

http://dx.doi.org/10.5772/62478

Abstract

Femoral head necrosis (FHN) is a difficult disease to treat. FHN results from an obstruction in the blood supply to the femoral head, which causes death of the bone-forming cells. For effective treatment of FHN, an osteogenic cell supply, revascularization, and provision of initial strength to resist collapse are needed. Evidence of favorable outcomes of cell transplantation therapy for the treatment of FHN is emerging. However, outcomes of treatment are influenced by the underlying FHN etiology and clinical stage. Therefore, understanding the epidemiology, clinical stage, and disease status of FHN is essential to inform treatment planning based on evidence. The aim of the chapter is to present and critically discuss the role of cell replacement therapy for the treatment of FHN based on clinical status.

Keywords: Femoral head necrosis, cell-based therapy, radiogenic stage, bone marrow, mesenchymal stromal cell

1. Epidemiology of osteonecrosis of the femoral head

Femoral head necrosis (FHN) is a painful disorder of the hip joint [1, 2]. Without treatment, more than 70% of clinically diagnosed cases of FHN proceed to collapse of the femoral head, requiring prosthetic joint replacement within 3–4 years after diagnosis [3, 4]. FHN typically occurs in adults, 30–40 years old, and is more prevalent in males than females, with evidence of bilateral involvement identified in 75% of cases [2]. The exact pathomechanism of FHN is not well understood. However, obstruction of blood supply caused by steroid use, alcoholism, sickle cell anemia, and femoral neck fracture are predisposing factors due to loss of osteogenic cells in the greater trochanteric region [1, 2].

In the natural history of FHN, 59% of cases progress to symptomatic disease and collapse of the femoral head [5]. The prognosis is different depending on the etiology. FHN resulting from sickle cell disease has the highest risk for progressing to collapse (73%), while 47% of cases due to excessive alcohol consumption are at risk of collapse and 46% of cases resulting from renal failure. The risk for collapse associated with corticosteroid use (26%) and for idiopathic FHN (38%) is comparable to the overall prevalence of collapse (38%). Cases of FHN associated with human immunodeficiency virus infection (15%) or systemic lupus erythematosus (7%) have a relatively lower risk for collapse, compared to the overall prevalence [5]. Therefore, understanding the etiologic factor of FHN is important for treatment planning.

Nonoperative treatment of FHN has been shown to have limited success in preventing disease progression [2]. Consequently, the use of joint preserving procedures has decreased in the United States, from being the treatment of choice in 25% of cases of FHN in 1992 compared to 12% of cases in 2008. Over the same period, total hip replacement for the management of FHN has increased from 75% in 1992 to 88% in 2008 [6].

2. Clinical stage assessed by radiographic image and prognosis

The clinical stages of FHN progression are classified based on radiographic examination, with magnetic resonance imaging (MRI) and bone scintigraphy used in the early stages. Although different radiographic classifications of clinical stage have been proposed, the underlying concept and indices of change are comparable between each classification [7–9]. The stage and classification, evaluated from plane, anterior–posterior, radiography images, are useful to understand the prognosis of FHN and to plan for treatment (**Table 1**). The classification of the Association Research Circulation Osseous (ARCO) Committee is the most widely used clinical grading classification for osteonecrosis of the femoral head (ONHF). The stages of FHN are defined as follows. Stage 1 is the identification of an osteonecrosis lesion by MRI and bone scintigraphy, with a marginal reaction emerging as a band of low signal intensity on T1-weighted images and a band of high signal intensity on T2-weighted images. Stage 2 is defined by radiographic appearance of demarcated regions of sclerosis and lucency. Blood vessels enter the necrotic zone as part of a repair process of bone resorption and formation, while toward the margin of the reactive interface, dead cancellous bone is invested by fibrous and lamellar tissues. In stage 3, resorption of bone causes fractures within the subchondral bone, with resulting segmental fractures identified on the radiographs by the 'crescent sign.' Stage 3 is subdivided into stage 3A, collapse of the femoral head <3 mm, and stage 3B, collapse of the femoral head ≥3 mm. In stage 4, osteoarthritic joint space narrowing, with osteophyte formation, is identified. According to Steinberg's classification, after stage 5, osteoarthritic changes are advanced.

The radiographic classification of the Specific Disease Investigation Committee (SDIC), under the auspices of the Japanese Ministry of Health, Labour and Welfare, defines the progression of FHN based on the extent of involvement of the weight-bearing surface of the femoral head (**Figure 1**) [9]. Plane, anterior–posterior radiographs are used to evaluate the necrotic area, and

http://dx.doi.org/10.5772/62478

the three types of lesions are defined as follows. The type A lesion occupies the medial one-third or less of the weight-bearing surface of the femoral head, while the type B lesion occupies the medial two-thirds or less of the weight-bearing surface. The type C lesion occupies more than two-thirds of the weight-bearing surface and is subdivided into C1 and C2 types: the C2 lesion extends laterally to the edge of the acetabulum, whereas the C1 lesion does not. Mont et al. [5] reported a risk for progression to collapse of 9% for type A lesions, 19% for type B lesions, and 59% for type C lesions. Nishii et al. [10] calculated an odds ratio (OR) for the incidence of collapse of the femoral head with type C lesions of 10.8 (95% confidence interval, 2.4–48.0), and an OR for progressive collapse of 26.0 (95% confidence interval, 1.9–358.5).

	Ficat	Steinberg	ARCO
Stage 1	Normal radiographs	Normal radiographs; abnormal bone scan and MRI	Normal radiographs; however, specific findings are observed on MRI, bone scintigraphy, or histology
Stage 2	Subchondral cyst formation and sclerosis	"Cystic" and sclerotic changes in femoral head	Demarcating sclerosis without collapse of the femoral head
Stage 3	Femoral head flattening, subchondral collapse, "crescent sign"	Subchondral collapse without femoral head flattening	Femoral head collapse, "crescent sign," no joint space narrowing
3A			Collapse <3 mm
3B			Collapse >3 mm
Stage 4	Osteoarthritic joint space narrowing, degenerative changes	Subchondral collapse, femoral head flattening, normal joint space	Osteoarthritic degenerative changes
Stage 5		Flattening, with joint space narrowing, acetabular changes, or both	
Stage 6		Advanced degenerative changes, secondary osteoarthritis	

Notes: ARCO, Association Research Circulation Osseous; MRI, magnetic resonance imaging.

Table 1. Clinical staging of osteonecrosis.

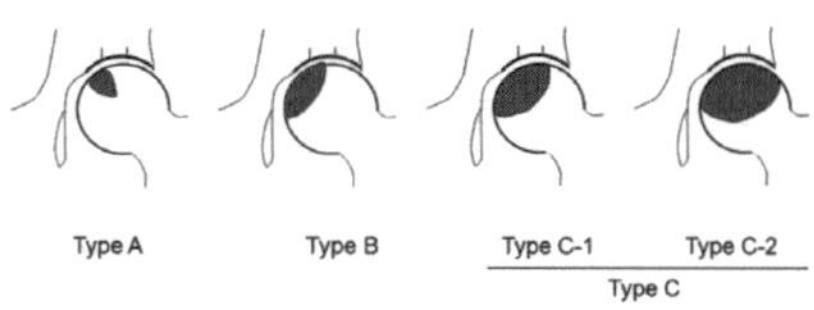

Figure 1 Radiographic classification of the Specific Disease Investigation Committee, under the auspices of the Japanese Ministry of Health, Labour and Welfare.

3. The treatment of FHN without cell-based therapy

Nonoperative treatment, which aims to offload forces exerted on the femoral head through limited weight bearing, activity modification, and physical therapy, has been shown to have limited success in preventing disease progression [2].

In the early stage of FHN (i.e., ARCO stage 1), intramedullary pressure is elevated and core decompression surgery is performed by drilling through the necrotic region, with a 6 or 8 mm short trephine drill, to reduce the pressure [7]. Core decompression treatment is more effective than conservative treatment [11], with clinically satisfactory results of core decompression obtained in 63.5% of cases of early FHN, compared to 22.7% with conservative treatment [12]. The clinical benefits of core decompression, however, have been questioned [13, 14]. Foremost, core decompression is not indicated for advanced stages of FHN. Mont et al. [15] reported satisfactory outcomes of core decompression of only 29% in patients with Steinberg stage 3 FHN, with 41% of patients in stage 3 and 92% in stage 4 requiring arthroplasty. In advanced stages of FHN, bone fragility is a more important consideration than elevated intrafemoral pressure.

Multiple microfractures of the subchondral bone are often present in advanced stages of FHN [16] and, therefore, reinforcing initial bone strength to prevent collapse of the femoral head is an important component of treatment at this stage. Vascularized bone grafts can offer reflux of blood flow and initial strength. Vascularized bone grafting is indicated for advanced stages of FHN [2, 17–19]. However, a radiographic study of outcomes after vascularized bone grafting by Ishizaka et al. [17] indicated continued progression of collapse in 50% of cases classified as Ficat stage 2 hips, and in 46% of cases classified as Ficat stage 3 hips. Therefore, vascularized bone grafting is not sufficient to prevent the collapse in cases of advanced FHN.

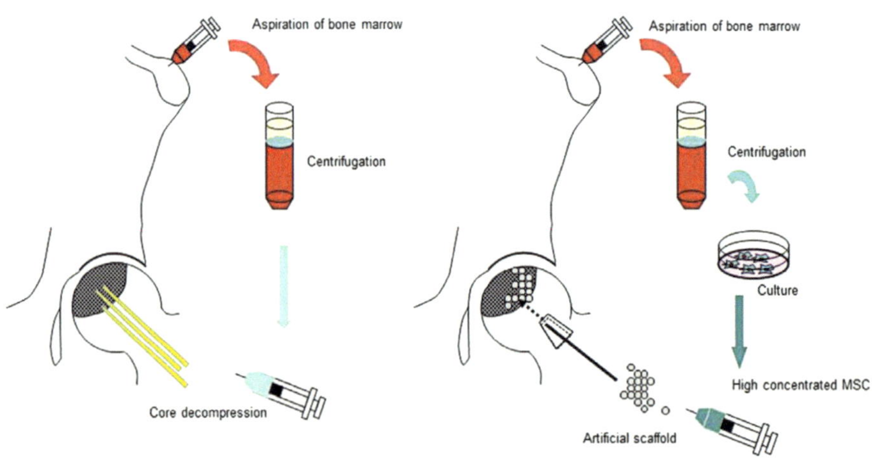

Figure 2 Cell-based therapy for osteonecrosis of the femoral head, combining concentrated bone marrow transplantation with core decompression is shown in the left panel. The right panel shows cultured mesenchymal stromal cell transplantation, combined with biomaterials, after removal of necrotic bone.

4. Concentrated bone marrow transplantation for the treatment of FHN

Core decompression offers not only a decrease in intramedullary pressure, but also a flow of living cells from regions surrounding the necrotic lesion. However, as FHN is not an isolated lesion of the femoral head, but rather involves the greater trochanteric area, the number of osteogenic cells throughout the trochanteric area is reduced [20, 21]. Hernigou et al. [22] and Gangji et al. [23] combined transplantation of concentrated autologous bone marrow from the iliac crest with core decompression with the aim of supplying osteoblastic cells. Gangji et al. [23] reported collapse of the femoral head to be significantly delayed with the use of concentrated bone marrow transplantation, compared with sole core decompression, when performed in the early stage of FHN (i.e., ARCO stage 1 or 2), with a collapse rate of 63% for the sole core decompression group, compared to 10% for the concentrated bone marrow transplantation group. Since the initial work of Hernigou et al. [22] and Gangji et al. [23], a number of studies have reported their outcomes of using concentrated autologous bone marrow transplantation in combination with core decompression [24–28], with relevant information from these studies reported in **Figure 2** and **Table 2**. Although clinically acceptable results for the combination of cell transplantation and core decompression were reported for patients classified in the early stages of FHN progression [23, 24], for patients with advanced stages of FHN, this combined treatment is not sufficient to prevent collapse of the femoral head [23–28]. The association between clinical stage of FHN and outcomes of the combined treatment was reported by Hernigou et al. [22], with 77% prevention of collapse for patients in stage 1 and 74% in stage 2, compared to 0% in stage 3 and 50% in stage 4. Therefore, additional treatment may be needed to enhance the positive effects of bone marrow transplantation. Martin et al. [29] used a combination of platelet rich plasma and bone marrow cells for transplantation after core decompression, with significant pain relief achieved in 86% of their cases, and with 79% of cases not progressing to collapse. Kang et al. [30] used a cancellous bone graft in combination with bone marrow transplantation after core decompression for both early and advanced stages of FHN, obtaining clinically successful outcomes in 80% of cases in stage 1, 65.7% in stage 2, 38.9% in stage 3, and 33.3% in stage 4.

Based on this evidence, it seems reasonable to suggest that for patients with the advanced stage of FHN (i.e., ARCO stage 3 or 4), providing initial strength to the femoral head is required to prevent further fracture and collapse. Bioactive scaffolding can provide the initial strength required. Yamasaki et al. [31] used interconnected porous calcium hydroxyapatite, in combination with concentrated bone marrow transplantation for patients with stages 1 and 2 FHN and advanced stage 3A. They reported no progression of the collapse in 56.7% of their case series, mild collapse of <2 mm in 33.3% and >2 mm of collapse in 10%. Liu et al. [32] used porous hydroxyapatite, with and without bone marrow transplantation, to treat patients in the precollapse stage of FHN progression (i.e., stage 2). They reported that 78.6% of their cases treated with the combination of porous hydroxyapatite and bone marrow transplantation did not progress to collapse, compared to 41.7% for patients treated only with bone marrow transplantation. A histological study by Arlot et al. [33], however, reported osteomalacia and osteoporosis to persist despite clinical improvement after treatment for FHN. Therefore, remodeling of the necrotic bone is difficult to achieve [34, 35]. To address this issue, Wang et al. [36] performed curettage of the necrotic bone, instead of core decompression, packing the free bone graft with concentrated bone marrow cells. Progression to collapse was prevented in 75% of their patients in stage 2 and 100% in stage 3.

Cell source	**Combined surgical technique**	**Radiographic stages (ARCO)**				
		Stage 1	**Stage 2**	**Stage 3**		**Stage 4**
				3A	**3B**	
Bone marrow cells	Core decompression	Gangji V (2004)				
		Wang BL (2010)				
		Chotivichit A (2012)				
		Mao Q (2013)				
		Ma Y (2014)				
		Tabatabaee RM (2015)				
		Hernigou P (2002)				
	Core decompression + bioderived material	Martin JR (2013)				
		Kang JS (2013)				
	Core decompression + bioactive scaffold	Yamasaki T (2010)				
			Liu Y (2013)			
	Curretage + bone graft		Wang T (2014)			
MSCs	Core decompression	Zhao D (2012)				
		Rastogi S (2013)				
		Persiani P (2015)				
	Curretage + bone graft + bioactive scaffold			Aoyama T (2014)		
						Kawate K (2006)

MSC, mesenchymal stem cell.

Table 2. Cell therapy according to the grade of osteonecrosis of the femoral head.

5. Mesenchymal stromal cell transplantation for the treatment of FHN

Reports of poor results using concentrated bone marrow transplantation combined with core decompression may reflect the low population of osteogenic cells in bone marrow of patients with FHN. Hernigou et al. [22] reported the osteogenic cell number to be low in patients with a history of steroid and alcohol use, as well as in patients who had undergone organ transplantation. Mesenchymal stromal cells (MSCs) may provide a solution to the problem of low osteogenic cell number.

MSCs hold promise for their use in regeneration of tissues of the musculoskeletal system [37]. MSCs are plastic dish-adherent cells that differentiate into osteogenic, chondrogenic, and adipogenic cell lineages, *in vitro* [38, 39]. The adherent cells can be easily proliferated, yielding a large number of cells [38]. The high proliferation nature of these cells in *in vitro* cultures could provide an effective compensation for low cell numbers [39]. MSCs can also differentiate into vascular endothelial cells [40]. This property to differentiate into vascular tissue would be useful to treat the avascular component of FHN. MSCs can be isolated from many tissues, including bone marrow, fat, and synovium [41]. The ideal source for MSC differentiation and proliferation remains controversial, with isolation of MSCs from bone marrow having been shown to be stable [42]. The technique to aspirate bone marrow is also well established [43] and relatively safe.

Zhao et al. [44] conducted a clinical trial on the use of MSCs for the treatment of FHN, with salient finding summarized in **Figure 2** and **Table 2**. Zhao et al. compared outcomes of transplanting cultured MSCs and bone marrow cells, in combination with core decompression, in patients with the early stage of FHN (i.e., ARCO stage 1 or 2). After 60-month follow-up, 4% of hip treated with MSCs progressed to collapse, compared to 23% of cases in the bone marrow treatment group. Rastogi et al. [45] also conducted a comparison of outcomes for treatment using cultured MSCs and bone marrow for transplantation in patients with the early (stages 1 and 2) and advanced (stage 3) stages of FHN. In contrast to Zhao et al., Rastogi et al. did not identify a significant difference in the rate of collapse between the two treatment groups, with a rate of collapse of 0% for both groups for stage 1 hips and 18% for stage 2 hips, and a rate of 20% for stage 3 hips for the MSC group, compared to 25% for the bone marrow group. Persiani et al. [46] reported that core decompression with MSCs transplantation was not a sufficient treatment for patients with advanced stages of FHN. Aoyama et al. [47] and Kawate et al. [48] performed curettage of the necrotic bone and packed beta-tricalcium phosphate with MSCs and a vascularized bone graft to treat patients with advanced stages of FHN. Aoyama et al. reported no progression to collapse for hips in stage 3A, while 50% of the hips in stage 3B progressed to collapse. In their 12-week follow-up, Kawate et al. did not report any progression to collapse of hips in stage 3 or 4 FHN.

6. The cell type used for the treatment of FHN

It is clear that transplantation of cells that can be differentiated to osteogenic cells is effective for the treatment of FHN. Preparation of concentrated bone marrow cells is easy, of low risk and of low cost. However, when the necrotic lesion is broad, preparation of a large number of cells is needed [49]. The condition of the host tissue influences the number and quality of osteogenic cells harvested [49]. Therefore, it is a great benefit that MSCs can be differentiated into both osteogenic and vascular endothelial cells [40]. The cytokine and paracrine effect of MSCs is important in yielding a large number of differentiated MSC cell lineages *in vitro* [50, 51]. However, the differentiation property of MSCs is highly influenced by the conditions of the host, such as age, disease, medication, etc. [52]. Peripheral CD34-positive MSCs may be another source for the treatment of FHN. They have the potential to differentiate into osteogenic and vascular endothelial cells and are easily prepared by *in vivo* induction of granulocyte colony-stimulating factors [53]. Despite the different possible sources of MSCs, remodeling of the osteonecrotic bone is an issue that remains to be solved. In healthy bone tissue, the balance between bone formation and bone resorption is under precise regulation [54]. In contrast, in pathological conditions, such as osteoporosis, prolonged fracture repair, and osteonecrosis, there is a dysregulation of the balance between osteoclast and osteoblast activity [35, 54]. In FHN, both living osteoclast and osteoblast cells are reduced in number. Therefore, pathogenic tissue, such as necrotic bone, should be removed as a component of treatment to facilitate bone remodeling. MSCs have the ability not only to differentiate into osteogenic cells, but they can also stimulate the osteoclastogenesis [55–57]. Therefore, the cytokine effect of MSCs induces a healthy remodeling regulation.

7. Biomaterials

Implantation of biomaterial is useful to provide initial strength to avoid collapse of the femoral head. Recent development of biomaterials aims to implement osteoinduction and osteoconduction ability in biomaterials themselves [58, 59]. Tantalum rods have high volumetric porosity, providing excellent osteoconductive properties, while their elastic modulus is similar to that of bone, providing exceptional biocompatibility [60]. In their case series of 50 hips treated with tantalum rods, Veillette et al. [61] reported a conversion rate to total hip arthroplasty in only 15.5% of their cases. Miao et al. [62] compared tantalum rod implantation to core decompression in patients with the early stage FHN (i.e., Steinberg stage 1 or 2) hips. After treatment, clinical score on radiographic assessment was improved in both the treatment groups. Pakos et al. [63] used tantalum rods with bone marrow and autologous bone grafting to treat patients with Steinberg stage 2 or stage 3 FHN. Five years after treatment, only 3% of hips in stage 2 and 15% in stage 3 were converted to total hip replacement.

Other biodegradable materials have also been used. Nano-hydroxyapatite/polyamide (n-HA/PA) 66 rods were used for the treatment of FHN [61, 64]. In their case series of 84 FHN cases, Yang et al. [64] allocated patients to two treatment groups, the first combining core decompression in combination with insertion of a n-HA/PA 66 rod and the second combining core decompression with an autologous cancellous bone graft. In the n-HA/PA 66 rod group, 21.1% of hips progressed to collapse of the femoral head, compared to 45.7% in the bone grafting group. A distinct advantage of biomaterials is their ability to change their form to easily fill cavities of different shapes. The clinical benefits of different biomaterials in the treatment of hips with FHN have been reported: Yamasaki et al. [31] used rod type porous hydroxyapatite; Liu et al. [32] used composite filler; and Aoyama et al. [47] and Kawate et al. [48] used porous beta-tricalcium phosphate granules in combination with cultured MSCs. Although there is evidence of satisfactory clinical outcomes using biomaterials, when these materials are used in combination with cell transplantation, the balance between the timing of degradation and osteogenesis is an important factor influencing outcome. Specifically, the activity of osteoclasts has been shown to be influenced by the type of biomaterial [65]. In the presence of biomaterials that facilitate early resorption of bone, compared to bone formation, the biomaterial does not have sufficient strength to protect against collapse. Therefore, the combination between biomaterial and cell type needs to be carefully examined.

8. Growth factors

Growth factors, such as transforming growth factor-β1, platelet-derived growth factor, vascular endothelial growth factors, fibroblast growth factor-2 (FGF-2), and bone morphogenetic protein (BMP) treatment, aim to promote revascularization and bone formation in hips with FHN [66]. Samara et al. [67] reported a lower expression of BMP-2 and BMP-6 in the femoral head of patients with FHN, compared to healthy controls. Therefore, supplying the lacking growth factor may be a reasonable adjunct treatment option. Lieberman et al. [68] used BMP-2 replacement in combination with allogenic fibula transplantation, reporting a radiographic progression of FHN in 17.6% of hips in Ficat stages 2 and 3. Sun et al. [69] compared the outcomes of recombinant BMP-2 treatment in combination with artificial bone implantation to implantation of artificial bone alone. The radiographic survival rate of the femoral head for hips in the BMP-2 treatment group was 100.0% for ARCO stage 2b hips, 84.2% for ARCO stage 2C hips, and 30.0% for ARCO stage 3 hips. By comparison, in the control group treated by implantation alone, the survival rate was 100.0% for ARCO stage 2b, 76.5% for ARCO stage 2C, and 37.5% for ARCO stage 3. Sun et al. concluded that BMP-2 was effective for selected patients. Papanagiotou et al. [70] used BMP-7 in combination with autologous, nonvascularized fibular grafting for hips in Steinberg stage 2 or stage 3. Over a 4-year follow-up, 29% of hips progressed to collapse and required total hip replacement. Papanagiotou et al. did report that BMP-7 in combination with autologous, nonvascularized, fibular grafting, is effective for shortening operative time and the postoperative rehabilitation period. Kuroda et al. [71] used recombinant FGF-2 impregnated with gelatin hydrogel for minimally invasive surgical treatment of patients in early stages of FHN. In their case series, 10% of hips progressed to collapse 1-year posttreatment, with improvement in radiographic clinical score in all other cases. Results of these preliminary studies provide evidence of the safety and feasibility of treatment using growth factors. Abe et al. [72] also reported elevation in levels of interleukin-6 and tumor necrosis factor-α in the joint fluid of hip in advanced stages of FHN. Therefore, modulation of cytokine activity, in combination with growth factors, may be an effective treatment strategy. Therefore, although there is currently no clinical report combining cell-based therapy and growth factor treatment, this combination holds promise for treatment of FHN and should be evaluated in future studies.

9. Conclusion

For an effective treatment of FHN, an osteogenic cell supply, revascularization, and providing initial strength to resist collapse are needed. The combination of cell-based therapy, growth factor, and biomaterial may effectively meet these requirements [73]. The development of new procedures is required, with treatment being according to the pathology and clinical status being extremely important considerations.

Acknowledgements

This work was supported by JSPS KAKENHI Grant Number 26282154.

Author details

Tomoki Aoyama

Address all correspondence to: blue@hs.med.kyoto-u.ac.jp

Human Health Sciences, Graduate School of Medicine, Kyoto University, Kyoto, Japan

References

[1] Mankin HJ. Nontraumatic necrosis of bone (osteonecrosis). N Engl J Med. 1992;326(22): 1473–1479. DOI: 10.1056/NEJM199205283262206.

[2] Kaushik AP, Das A, Cui Q. Osteonecrosis of the femoral head: an update in year 2012. World J Orthop. 2012;3(5):49–57. DOI: 10.5312/wjo.v3.i5.49.

[3] Steinberg ME. Osteonecrosis of the hip: summary and conclusions. Semin Arthroplasty. 1991;2(3):241–249. DOI: 10.1097/B TO.0b013e31816b476e.

[4] Steinberg ME, Steinberg DR. Classification systems for osteonecrosis: an overview. Orthop Clin North Am. 2004;35(3):273–283. DOI: http://dx.doi.org/10.1016/j.ocl. 2004.02.005.

[5] Mont MA, Zywiel MG, Marker DR, McGrath MS, Delanois RE. The natural history of untreated asymptomatic osteonecrosis of the femoral head: a systematic literature review. J Bone Joint Surg Am. 2010;92(12):2165–2170. DOI: 10.2106/JBJS.I.00575.

[6] Johnson AJ, Mont MA, Tsao AK, Jones LC. Treatment of femoral head osteonecrosis in the United States: 16-year analysis of the Nationwide Inpatient Sample. Clin Orthop Relat Res. 2014;472(2):617–623. DOI: 10.1007/s11999-013-3220-3.

[7] Ficat RP. Idiopathic bone necrosis of the femoral head. Early diagnosis and treatment. J Bone Joint Surg Br. 1985;67(1):3–9.

[8] Steinberg ME. Classification of avascular necrosis: a comparative study. Acta Orthop Belg. 1999;65(Suppl 1):45–46.

[9] Sugano N, Atsumi T, Ohzono K, Kubo T, Hotokebuchi T, Takaoka K. The 2001 revised criteria for diagnosis, classification, and staging of idiopathic osteonecrosis of the femoral head. J Orthop Sci. 2002;7(5):601–605. DOI: 10.1007/s007760200108.

[10] Nishii T, Sugano N, Ohzono K, Sakai T, Haraguchi K, Yoshikawa H. Progression and cessation of collapse in osteonecrosis of the femoral head. Clin Orthop Relat Res 2002;400:149–157. DOI: 10.1097/00003086-200207000-00019.

[11] Stulberg BN, Davis AW, Bauer TW, Levine M, Easley K. Osteonecrosis of the femoral head. A prospective randomized treatment protocol. Clin Orthop Relat Res. 1991;268:140–151. DOI:10.1016/j.injury.2013.09.014.

[12] Mont MA, Carbone JJ, Fairbank AC. Core decompression versus nonoperative management for osteonecrosis of the hip. Clin Orthop Relat Res 1996;324:169–178. DOI: 10.1097/00003086-199603000-00020.

[13] Rajagopal M, Balch Samora J, Ellis TJ. Efficacy of core decompression as treatment for osteonecrosis of the hip: a systematic review. Hip Int. 2012;22(5):489–493. DOI: 10.5301/HIP.2012.9748.

[14] Neumayr LD, Aguilar C, Earles AN, Jergesen HE, Haberkern CM, Kammen BF, Nancarrow PA, Padua E, Milet M, Stulberg BN, Williams RA, Orringer EP, Graber N, Robertson SM, VichinskyEP; National Osteonecrosis Trial in Sickle Cell Anemia Study Group. Physical therapy alone compared with core decompression and physical therapy for femoral head osteonecrosis in sickle cell disease. Results of a multicenter study at a mean of three years after treatment. J Bone Joint Surg Am. 2006;88(12):2573–2582. DOI: http://dx.doi.org/10.2106/JBJS.E.01454.

[15] Mont MA, Jones LC, Pacheco I, Hungerford DS. Radiographic predictors of outcome of core decompression for hips with osteonecrosis stage III. Clin Orthop Relat Res 1998;354:159–168. DOI: 10.1097/00003086-199809000-00019.

[16] Meier R, Kraus TM, Schaeffeler C, Torka S, Schlitter AM, Specht K, Haller B, Waldt S, Rechl H, Rummeny EJ, Woertler K. Bone marrow oedema on MR imaging indicates ARCO stage 3 disease in patients with AVN of the femoral head. Eur Radiol. 2014;24(9):2271–2278. DOI: 10.1007/s00330-014-3216-8.

[17] Ishizaka M, Sofue M, Dohmae Y, Endo N, Takahashi HE. Vascularized iliac bone graft for avascular necrosis of the femoral head. Clin Orthop Relat Res 1997;337:140–148.

[18] AldridgeJM3rd, Urbaniak JR. Vascularized fibular grafting for osteonecrosis of the femoral head with unusual indications. Clin Orthop Relat Res. 2008;466(5):1117–1124. DOI: 10.1007/s11999-008-0201-z.

[19] Korompilias AV, Lykissas MG, Beris AE, Urbaniak JR, Soucacos PN. Vascularised fibular graft in the management of femoral head osteonecrosis: twenty years later. J Bone Joint Surg Br. 2009;91(3):287–293. DOI: 10.1302/0301-620X.91B3.21846.

[20] Gangji V, Hauzeur JP, Schoutens A, Hinsenkamp M, Appelboom T, Egrise D. Abnormalities in the replicative capacity of osteoblastic cells in the proximal femur of patients with osteonecrosis of the femoral head. J Rheumatol. 2003;30(2):348–351. DOI: 10.1016/j.bone.2014.04.034.

[21] Hernigou P, Beaujean F, Lambotte JC. Decrease in the mesenchymal stem-cell pool in the proximal femur in corticosteroid-induced osteonecrosis. J Bone Joint Surg Br. 1999;81(2):349–355. DOI: 10.1302/0301-620X.81B2.8818.

[22] Hernigou P, Beaujean F. Treatment of osteonecrosis with autologous bone marrow grafting. Clin Orthop Relat Res 2002;405:14–23. DOI: 10.4103/0019-5413.45322.

[23] Gangji V, Hauzeur JP, Matos C, De Maertelaer V, Toungouz M, Lambermont M. Treatment of osteonecrosis of the femoral head with implantation of autologous bone-marrow cells. A pilot study. J Bone Joint Surg Am. 2004;86-A(6):1153–1160.

[24] Wang BL, Sun W, Shi ZC, Zhang NF, Yue DB, Guo WS, Xu SQ, Lou JN, Li ZR. Treatment of nontraumatic osteonecrosis of the femoral head with the implantation of core decompression and concentrated autologous bone marrow containing mononuclear cells. Arch Orthop Trauma Surg. 2010;130(7):859–865. DOI: 10.1016/j.bone.2011.07.032.

[25] Chotivichit A, Korwutthikulrangsri E, Pornrattanamaneewong C, Achawakulthep C. Core decompression with bone marrow injection for the treatment of femoral head osteonecrosis. J Med Assoc Thai. 2014;97(Suppl 9):S139-S143.

[26] Mao Q, Jin H, Liao F, Xiao L, Chen D, Tong P. The efficacy of targeted intraarterial delivery of concentrated autologous bone marrow containing mononuclear cells in the treatment of osteonecrosis of the femoral head: a five year follow-up study. Bone. 2013;57(2):509–516. DOI: 10.1016/j.bone.2013.08.022.

[27] Ma Y, Wang T, Liao J, Gu H, Lin X, Jiang Q, Bulsara MK, Zheng M, Zheng Q. Efficacy of autologous bone marrow buffy coat grafting combined with core decompression in patients with avascular necrosis of femoral head: a prospective, double-blinded, randomized, controlled study. Stem Cell Res Ther. 2014;5(5):115. DOI: 10.1186/scrt505.

[28] Tabatabaee RM, Saberi S, Parvizi J, Mortazavi SM, Farzan M. Combining concentrated autologous bone marrow stem cells injection with core decompression improves outcome for patients with early-stage osteonecrosis of the femoral head: a comparative study. J Arthroplasty. 2015;30(9 Suppl):11–15. DOI: 10.1016/j.arth.2015.06.022.

[29] Martin JR, Houdek MT, Sierra RJ. Use of concentrated bone marrow aspirate and platelet rich plasma during minimally invasive decompression of the femoral head in the treatment of osteonecrosis. Croat Med J. 2013;54(3):219–224. DOI: 10.3325/cmj.2013.54.219.

[30] Kang JS, Moon KH, Kim BS, Kwon DG, Shin SH, Shin BK, Ryu DJ. Clinical results of auto-iliac cancellous bone grafts combined with implantation of autologous bone marrow cells for osteonecrosis of the femoral head: a minimum 5-year follow-up. Yonsei Med J. 2013;54(2):510–515. DOI: 10.3349/ymj.2013.54.2.510.

[31] Yamasaki T, Yasunaga Y, Ishikawa M, Hamaki T, Ochi M. Bone-marrow-derived mononuclear cells with a porous hydroxyapatite scaffold for the treatment of osteo-

necrosis of the femoral head: a preliminary study. J Bone Joint Surg Br. 2010;92(3):337–341. DOI: 10.1302/0301-620X.92B3.22483.

[32] Liu Y, Liu S, Su X. Core decompression and implantation of bone marrow mononuclear cells with porous hydroxylapatite composite filler for the treatment of osteonecrosis of the femoral head. Arch Orthop Trauma Surg. 2013;133(1):125–133. DOI: 10.1007/s00402-012-1623-3.

[33] Arlot ME, Bonjean M, Chavassieux PM, Meunier PJ. Bone histology in adults with aseptic necrosis. Histomorphometric evaluation of iliac biopsies in seventy-seven patients. J Bone Joint Surg Am. 1983;65(9):1319–1327.

[34] Gangji V, Hauzeur JP. Cellular-based therapy for osteonecrosis. Orthop Clin North Am. 2009;40(2):213–221.

[35] Chim SM, Tickner J, Chow ST, Kuek V, Guo B, Zhang G, Rosen V, Erber W, Xu J. Angiogenic factors in bone local environment. Cytokine Growth Factor Rev. 2013;24(3): 297–310. DOI: 10.1016/j.cytogfr.2013.03.008.

[36] Wang T, Wang W, Yin ZS. Treatment of osteonecrosis of the femoral head with thorough debridement, bone grafting and bone-marrow mononuclear cells implantation. Eur J Orthop Surg Traumatol. 2014;24(2):197–202. DOI: 10.1007/s00590-012-1161-2.

[37] Steinert AF, Rackwitz L, Gilbert F, Nöth U, Tuan RS. Concise review: the clinical application of mesenchymal stem cells for musculoskeletal regeneration: current status and perspectives. Stem Cells Transl Med. 2012;1(3):237–247. DOI: 10.5966/sctm.2011-0036.

[38] Pittenger MF, Mackay AM, Beck SC, Jaiswal RK, Douglas R, Mosca JD, Moorman MA, Simonetti DW, Craig S, Marshak DR. Multilineage potential of adult human mesenchymal stem cells. Science. 1999;284(5411):143–147. DOI: 10.1126/science.284.5411.143.

[39] Dominici M, Le Blanc K, Mueller I, Slaper-Cortenbach I, Marini F, Krause D, Deans R, Keating A, Prockop Dj, Horwitz E. Minimal criteria for defining multipotent mesenchymal stromal cells. The International Society for Cellular Therapy position statement. Cytotherapy. 2006;8(4):315–317. DOI: 10.1080/14653240600855905.

[40] Aoyama T, Toguchida J. Isolation of bone marrow stromal cells from bone marrow by using a filtering device (Method). Stem Cells and Cancer Stem Cells. Vol. 2; Netherlands: Springer; 2012. p.3-12. DOI: 10.1007/978-94-007-2016-9_1.

[41] Sun Q, Zhang Z, Sun Z. The potential and challenges of using stem cells for cardiovascular repair and regeneration. Genes Dis. 2014;1(1):113–119. DOI: 10.1016/j.gendis.2014.07.003.

[42] Mohal JS, Tailor HD, Khan WS. Sources of adult mesenchymal stem cells and their applicability for musculoskeletal applications. Curr Stem Cell Res Ther. 2012;7(2):103–109. DOI: 10.2174/157488812799219027.

[43] Hernigou J, Alves A, Homma Y, Guissou I, Hernigou P. Anatomy of the ilium for bone marrow aspiration: map of sectors and implication for safe trocar placement. Int Orthop. 2014;38(12):2585–2590. DOI: 10.1007/s00264-014-2353-7.

[44] Zhao D, Cui D, Wang B, Tian F, Guo L, Yang L, Liu B, Yu X. Treatment of early stage osteonecrosis of the femoral head with autologous implantation of bone marrow-derived and cultured mesenchymal stem cells. Bone. 2012;50(1):325–330. DOI: 10.1016/j.bone.2011.11.002.

[45] Rastogi S, Sankineani SR, Nag HL, Mohanty S, Shivanand G, Marimuthu K, Kumar R, Rijal L. Intralesional autologous mesenchymal stem cells in management of osteonecrosis of femur: a preliminary study. Musculoskelet Surg. 2013;97(3):223–228. DOI: 10.1007/s12306-013-0273-0.

[46] Persiani P, De Cristo C, Graci J, Noia G, GurzìM, Villani C. Stage-related results in treatment of hip osteonecrosis with core-decompression and autologous mesenchymal stem cells. Acta Orthop Belg. 2015;81(3):406–412.

[47] Aoyama T, Goto K, Kakinoki R, Ikeguchi R, Ueda M, Kasai Y, Maekawa T, Tada H, Teramukai S, Nakamura T, Toguchida J. An exploratory clinical trial for idiopathic osteonecrosis of femoral head by cultured autologous multipotent mesenchymal stromal cells augmented with vascularized bone grafts. Tissue Eng Part B Rev. 2014;20(4):233–242. DOI: 10.1089/ten.teb.2014.0090.

[48] Kawate K, Yajima H, Ohgushi H, Kotobuki N, Sugimoto K, Ohmura T, Kobata Y, Shigematsu K, Kawamura K, Tamai K, Takakura Y. Tissue-engineered approach for the treatment of steroid-induced osteonecrosis of the femoral head: transplantation of autologous mesenchymal stem cells cultured with beta-tricalcium phosphate ceramics and free vascularized fibula. Artif Organs. 2006;30(12):960–962. DOI: 10.1111/j.1525-1594.2006.00333.x.

[49] Hernigou P, Poignard A, Zilber S, Rouard H. Cell therapy of hip osteonecrosis with autologous bone marrow grafting. Indian J Orthop. 2009;43(1):40–45. DOI: 10.4103/0019-5413.45322.

[50] Salem HK, Thiemermann C. Mesenchymal stromal cells: current understanding and clinical status. Stem Cells. 2010;28(3):585–596. DOI: 10.1002/stem.269.

[51] Liang X, Ding Y, Zhang Y, Tse HF, Lian Q. Paracrine mechanisms of mesenchymal stem cell-based therapy: current status and perspectives. Cell Transplant. 2014;23(9):1045–1059. DOI: 10.3727/096368913X667709.

[52] Schimke MM, Marozin S, Lepperdinger G. Patient-specific age: the other side of the coin in advanced mesenchymal stem cell therapy. Front Physiol. 2015;6:362. DOI: 10.3389/fphys.2015.00362.

[53] Kuroda R, Matsumoto T, Kawakami Y, Fukui T, Mifune Y, Kurosaka M. Clinical impact of circulating CD34-positive cells on bone regeneration and healing. Tissue Eng Part B Rev. 2014;20(3):190–199. DOI: 10.1089/ten.

[54] Xiao W, Li S, Pacios S, Wang Y, Graves DT. Bone remodeling under pathological conditions. Front Oral Biol. 2015;18:17–27. DOI: 10.1159/000351896.

[55] Ikeguchi R, Kakinoki R, Aoyama T, Shibata KR, Otsuka S, Fukiage K, Nishijo K, Ishibe T, Shima Y, Otsuki B, Azuma T, Tsutsumi S, Nakayama T, Otsuka T, Nakamura T, Toguchida J. Regeneration of osteonecrosis of canine scapho-lunate using bone marrow stromal cells: possible therapeutic approach for Kienböck disease. Cell Transplant. 2006;15(5):411–422. DOI: 10.3727/000000007783465190.

[56] Bielby R, Jones E, McGonagle D. The role of mesenchymal stem cells in maintenance and repair of bone. Injury. 2007;38(Suppl 1):S26-S32. DOI: 10.1016/j.injury.2007.02.007.

[57] Crane JL, Cao X. Bone marrow mesenchymal stem cells and TGF-β signaling in bone remodeling. J Clin Invest. 2014;124(2):466–472. DOI: 10.1172/JCI70050.

[58] Kokubo T, Yamaguchi S. Growth of novel ceramic layers on metals via chemical and heat treatments for inducing various biological functions. Front Bioeng Biotechnol. 2015;3:176. DOI: 10.3389/fbioe.2015.00176.

[59] García-Gareta E, Coathup MJ, Blunn GW. Osteoinduction of bone grafting materials for bone repair and regeneration. Bone. 2015;81:112–121. DOI: 10.1016/j.bone. 2015.07.007.

[60] Bobyn JD, Poggie RA, Krygier JJ, Lewallen DG, Hanssen AD, Lewis RJ, Unger AS, O'Keefe TJ, Christie MJ, Nasser S, Wood JE, Stulberg SD, Tanzer M. Clinical validation of a structural porous tantalum biomaterial for adult reconstruction. J Bone Joint Surg Am. 2004;86-A(Suppl 2):123–129. DOI: 10.1038/srep02243.

[61] Veillette CJ, Mehdian H, Schemitsch EH, McKee MD. Survivorship analysis and radiographic outcome following tantalum rod insertion for osteonecrosis of the femoral head. J Bone Joint Surg Am. 2006;88(Suppl 3):48–55. DOI: 10.1016/j.injury.2014.11.016.

[62] Miao H, Ye D, Liang W, Yao Y. Effect of osteonecrosis intervention rod versus core decompression using multiple small drill holes on early stages of necrosis of the femoral head: a prospective study on a series of 60 patients with a minimum 1-year-follow-up. Open Orthop J. 2015;9:179–184. DOI: 10.2174/1874325001509010179.

[63] Pakos EE, Megas P, Paschos NK, Syggelos SA, Kouzelis A, Georgiadis G, Xenakis TA. Modified porous tantalum rod technique for the treatment of femoral head osteonecrosis. World J Orthop. 2015;6(10):829–837. DOI: 10.5312/wjo.v6.i10.829.

[64] Yang P, Bian C, Huang X, Shi A, Wang C, Wang K. Core decompression in combination with nano-hydroxyapatite/polyamide 66 rod for the treatment of osteonecrosis of the femoral head. Arch Orthop Trauma Surg. 2014;134(1):103–112. DOI: 10.1007/ s00402-013-1885-4.

[65] Detsch R, Boccaccini AR. The role of osteoclasts in bone tissue engineering. J Tissue Eng Regen Med. 2015;9(10):1133–1149. DOI: 10.1002/term.1851.

[66] Rackwitz L, Eden L, Reppenhagen S, Reichert JC, Jakob F, Walles H, Pullig O, Tuan RS, Rudert M, Nöth U. Stem cell- and growth factor-based regenerative therapies for avascular necrosis of the femoral head. Stem Cell Res Ther. 2012;3(1):7. DOI: 10.1186/scrt98.

[67] Samara S, Dailiana Z, Varitimidis S, Chassanidis C, Koromila T, Malizos KN, Kollia P. Bone morphogenetic proteins (BMPs) expression in the femoral heads of patients with avascular necrosis. Mol Biol Rep. 2013;40(7):4465–4472. DOI: 10.1007/s11033-013-2538-y.

[68] Lieberman JR, Conduah A, Urist MR. Treatment of osteonecrosis of the femoral head with core decompression and human bone morphogenetic protein. Clin Orthop Relat Res. 2004;429:139–145. DOI: 10.1097/01.blo.0000150312.53937.6f.

[69] Sun W, Li Z, Gao F, Shi Z, Zhang Q, Guo W. Recombinant human bone morphogenetic protein-2 in debridement and impacted bone graft for the treatment of femoral head osteonecrosis. PLoS One. 2014;9(6):e100424. DOI: 10.1371/journal.pone.0100424. eCollection 2014.

[70] Papanagiotou M, Malizos KN, Vlychou M, Dailiana ZH. Autologous (non-vascularised) fibular grafting with recombinant bone morphogenetic protein-7 for the treatment of femoral head osteonecrosis: preliminary report. Bone Joint J. 2014;96-B(1):31–35. DOI: 10.1302/0301-620X.96B1.32773.

[71] Kuroda Y, Asada R, So K, Yonezawa A, Nankaku M, Mukai K, Ito-Ihara T, Tada H, Yamamoto M, Murayama T, Morita S, Tabata Y, Yokode M, Shimizu A, Matsuda S, Akiyama H. A pilot study of regenerative therapy using controlled release of recombinant human fibroblast growth factor for patients with pre-collapse osteonecrosis of the femoral head. Int Orthop. Dec 29, 2015. [Epub ahead of print]. DOI: 10.1007/s00264-015-3083-1.

[72] Abe H, Sakai T, Ando W, Takao M, Nishii T, Nakamura N, Hamasaki T, Yoshikawa H, Sugano N. Synovial joint fluid cytokine levels in hip disease. Rheumatology (Oxford). 2014;53(1):165–172. DOI: 10.1093/rheumatology/ket334.

[73] Sun H, Yang HL. Calcium phosphate scaffolds combined with bone morphogenetic proteins or mesenchymal stem cells in bone tissue engineering. Chin Med J (Engl). 2015;128(8):1121–1127. DOI: 10.4103/0366-6999.155121.

Chapter 6

Treatment of Non-Union and Bone Loss of Tibial Pilon

Giorgio Maria Calori, Massimiliano Colombo,
Emilio Mazza, Miguel Simon Bucci, Piero Fadigati,
Alessandra Ines Maria Colombo and
Simone Mazzola

Additional information is available at the end of the chapter

http://dx.doi.org/10.5772/62664

Abstract

Non-union is a fracture with no healing potential without a further surgical procedure. Diagnosis of non-union can be done in case of healing failure from 6 to 9 months after the first fracture. We consider appropriate to keep the attention of the reader on the relevance that more frequent traumatic mechanisms have in relationship with evolution and eventual failure of healing processes. In literature, non-union mean rate for tibial pilon fractures is around 5% independently from the synthesis technique used; as main causes we can recognize a significant fracture's comminution ad eventual bone loss, vascular damage, and local infection. Risk factors can be divided into two big groups: factors proper of the patient at the moment of injury (age, diseases, drugs, smoke, etc.) and characteristics of the trauma itself (comminution and dislocation of fragments, involvement of soft tissues, topography, distance between fragments). Tibial pilon fractures are mainly caused by high-energy trauma. This kind of dynamic determines not only more serious damage to the bone, but often cause damage of the surrounding tissues. Following important lesions of the periosteum and of the vascular network and after a suboptimal synthesis caused by comminution and dislocation of fragments is frequent with the evolution toward a bad bone healing process. Bone healing was, in the last 50 years, argument of intense research activity. The incidence of non-union is growing steadily, although principles and materials of synthesys are well standardized. Recently it has been codified the "diamond concept," which clarified different appliances mechanical and biological, these distinguished between cells, scaffolds, and growth factors. Under the mechanical profile, it must be restored the spectrum of stability that consider the set of bone and synthesis implanted. The spectrum of stability interprets Wolf's law providing indications on the need to modulate the rigidity of the synthesis in reason of the level of instability of the pseudoarthrosis itself. During the years several kinds of non-union classifications have been proposed. The most widespread until now is the one proposed by

Weber–Cech in 1976, which distinguishes vital forms (hypertrophic and oligotrophic) from non-vital forms (atrophic). In 2007 a new score classification system has been processed, which is the "Non-Union Scoring System (NUSS)," which divides patients in four big groups by score awarded based on the real non-healing risk. The NUSS represents an innovative approach to the problem because it understand the multifactorial reasons of failure, explains why in a variable percentage of cases (depending from de district affected), the healing is not obtained, even with a correct treatment and above all make possible the drafting of a therapeutic choice algorithm. Biotechnologies at our disposal are synthetic growth factors, the autologous growth factors and platelet-rich plasma, mesenchymal stem cells, and scaffolds or bone substitute. The biologic chamber represent the ideal site for bone regeneration; it is a bio-reactor in which are present all those elements at the base of the concept of diamond. The chamber needs to be aseptic, vital, mechanically stable, and sealed but selectively permeable. Thanks to the use of megaprosthesis not only in oncologic orthopaedics, but also it is now possible to avoid the amputation or long and often inconclusive treatment of lengthening or ankle arthrodesis. The new frontier in treatment of non-unions will be genetic therapy, that is, the possibility to transport to the patient those genes that con drive to the formation of good bone callus and his maturation toward strong bone.

Keywords: Tibial pilon, tibial plafond, non-union, biological chamber, biotechnologies, NUSS, megaprosthesis, stem cells, growth factor, diamond concept

1. Definition

Non-union is a fracture with no healing potential without a further surgical procedure. Diagnosis of non-union can be done in case of healing failure from 6 to 9 months after the first fracture. Time is variable between fracture types, at the level of the tibial pilon diagnosis can be done only 9 months after trauma. Between long bones, tibia is the most frequently involved by this complication.

We consider appropriate to keep the attention of the reader on the relevance that more frequent traumatic mechanism have in relationship with evolution and eventual failure of healing processes.

As known, tibial plafond fractures are mainly caused by axial overload more than torsional forces, that are, responsible more frequently of malleolus fractures.

The mechanism of axial overload presupposes a major transfer of energy which leads to a more rapid deformation of the bone tissue until resistance limit is reached. The energy released at the broken point to soft tissues surrounding causes characteristics soft tissues lesions, which are present in those kinds of fractures and make the healing more complex: associated fractures, dislocation of the astragalus; vascular and nervous lesions; muscle and skin lesions with comparison of enlarged edema.

2. Incidence

The tibial pilon non-union incidence in the literature ranges between 2 [1] and 18% for Ruedi and Ovadia [2], and those results have been confirmed even by McFerran [3].

Studies of Havet in 2006 and Bacon and Wang in 2010 [4–6] report similar statistic data from which result in similar non-union rate independently from the kind of ostheosynthesis used.

After those premises and therapeutic compromises sometimes adopted in treatment of the tibial pilon fractures, it is easy to understand the data present in literature for which non-union mean rate is around 5% independently from the technique used, recognizing as main causes a significant fracture's comminution ad eventual bone loss, vascular damage, and local infection [4–7].

3. Risk factor

At this moment, we are able to classify risk factors, related to the establishment of non-union, in two big groups: factors proper of the patient at the moment of injury and characteristics of the trauma itself.

Between general risk factors, we can found advanced age (especially in female population penalized by hormonal imbalances resulting from the menopause); non-compensated diabetes (besides the well-known vascular and nervous disorders, it was observed a decrease in the formation of collagen and cells involved in bone callus formation and maturation); osteoporosis; muscle atrophy; lifestyle (food, smoke, alcohol); drugs as NSAD, often prescribed against pain after surgery (the reason of their bad influence on healing time is to be found in decreased macrophagic activity and prostaglandin synthesis induced by COX 1 and 2 inhibition) [8].

Local risk factors, that are inherent to the trauma itself, include

- High-energy trauma (very frequent in tibial pilon fracture) in which occurs a greater comminution and dislocation of fragments and a greater involvement of soft tissues and vascular system, with heavy impact on blood support at the fracture's site. Experimental studies have demonstrated as the physiological healing process is guided, with a peak 2 weeks after the trauma, by blood supply from the cortical bone. As a consequence, a wide lesion of soft tissues and large hematoma, narrowing blood support to the cortex itself, reduce the inflow of nutrients and osteogenic cell to the fracture site, condition that determine an increased risk of necrosis and delayed healing, with possible evolution toward atrophic pseudoarthrosis [9].
- Topography: metaphyseal and diaphyseal fractures have different healing time and a different incidence of non-union, due to the bone callus synthesis process that involve mainly spongy bone, highly vascularized, and with a faster regenerative kinetics [10].
- Interfragmentary distance: an excessive distance between bone fragments, or the presence of a third fragment, induces to the onset of non-union [11]. In this situation, a correct

anatomic reduction of fragments with the intent to preserve vascularization is a positive prognostic factor.

Tibial pilon fractures are mainly caused by high-energy trauma. This kind of dynamic determines not only more serious damage to the bone, but often cause damage of the surrounding tissues.

Following important lesions of the periosteum and of the vascular network and after a suboptimal synthesis caused by comminution and dislocation of fragments is frequent with the evolution toward a bad bone healing process.

After the end of the 1980s, thanks to statistic analysis proposed by authors as McFerran [3] and Dillin [12] and, more recently Piper et al. [13], it was possible to clarify the importance of risk factors that affect the prognosis of tibial pilon fractures.

Distal tibia is characterized by a relatively poor vascularization and skin coverage. These structures, when seriously damaged from the mechanism of injury, penalize the healing of fractures.

There are several factors to whom was charged complicity in the development of such an eventuality; among the most important, we find:

- A residual bone loss after the reduction of the fracture;
- The precariousness of the metaphyseal vascularization;
- A loss of skin coverage after injury;
- An inadequate mounting in case of external fixation synthesis;
- A wide deperiostization during synthesis with plate and screws.

Its, however, not negligible the eventuality that fractures of patients treated correctly, and with low-risk rate, could evolve toward non-union.

It seems that the population of patients affected by non-union is somehow selected toward those patients that present a higher risk of this complication. For this reason, it seems even more important to analyze and classify these patients to define better surgical program and even in some way to clarify the risk of treatment failure.

Is not a rare observation that some subject, unfortunately few in number, even if treated not correctly shows "miraculous healing." Instead, is greater the number of patients that, although treated in a good way, under go several in effective surgical procedures.

4. Bone healing

Bone healing was, in the last 50 years, argument of intense research activity. The number of non-union is constantly growing although principles and material of synthesis are standardized. This observation finds an explanation in increase of life expectancy, in a population of female and "young" senior addicted to activities at risk of injuries and in survival to car crash deadly until few years ago. But does not clarify the feedback of those cases which, even after good cares, does not undergo to healing.

It can be reasonably supposed that the improvement of cares offered to the injured patient has in some way modified the population of patients with non-union.

In the past surgical errors, lack of knowledge of biomechanical principles that guide a good synthesis and low-quality materials created cases of non-union that need only a more correct treatment.

Recently is been codified the "diamond concept" that clarified different appliances mechanical and biological, these distinguished between cells, scaffolds, and growth factors [14].

Under the mechanical profile, it must be restored the spectrum of stability that consider the set of bone and synthesis implanted. The spectrum of stability interprets Wolf's law providing indications on the need to modulate the rigidity of the synthesis in reason of the level of instability of the pseudoarthrosis itself [15].

5. Non-union classification

To be able to encode treatment's guidelines, we must first proceed to a correct nosological assessment of the problem. During the years, it has been proposed several kinds of non-union classifications.

The most widespread until now is the one proposed by Weber–Cech in 1976, which distinguishes vital forms, hypertrophic, and oligotrophic, or rather with possible biologic response, from non-vital forms or rather non-reactive atrophic kind, frequently accompanied by osteonecrosis, and even by bone loss [16].

This classification is based on a descriptive radiological analysis of the kind of non-union evaluating only the bone, we think that a more complete classification, even from a prognostic point of view, should take into account even the quality of soft tissues and the general conditions of the patient (comorbidity, lifestyle, drugs, genetic diseases).

For this reason in 2007 have been identified through the study of international literature all possible risk factors in the healing of fractures [8].

After has been processed a score classification system, the "Non-Union Scoring System (NUSS)" [17] with double finality: not to detect a "radiographic case" but a "patient" and then detect, in relationship with the real non-healing risk, those cases in which is necessary, not only a correct surgical treatment, but even a right biotechnological approach. The NUSS represents an innovative approach to the problem because it understand the multifactorial reasons of failure, explains why in a variable percentage of cases (depending from de district affected) the healing is not obtained, even with a correct treatment and above all make possible the drafting of a therapeutic choice algorithm [18, 19].

6. The NUSS

In the new NUSS classification of 2008 are considered all the variables and all risk factors, giving to anyone a score based on clinical experience and scientific evidences and defining so a treatment guideline depending from the final score [17].

The final score, obtained by the sum of the individual score, allows to compare different patients with different non-union, making them objectively comparable according to a principle of complexity.

Atrophic forms of non-union can have better prognosis and greater chance of healing than oligotrophic reactive forms, in patients affected by impaired general health condition, as in example a non-compensated diabetes.

7. The variables considered are as follows:

- The bone (quality, kind of fracture, number of previous surgical procedures, and their invasiveness, non-union classification according to Weber–Cech, adequate first surgical procedure in order to mechanical stability, bone gap, alignment);
- Soft tissues (tissues conditions, vascurarization and possible surgical procedures on soft tissues and skin coverage);
- The patient (ASA score—American Society of Anesthesiologists—diabetes, laboratorys exams, infective condition, drugs, and smoke).

First group, score from 0 to 25, made mainly as mechanical problem, the treatment indicated is the fracture stabilization, optimizing or changing the synthesis system.

Second group, score from 26 to 50, made the problem as both mechanical and biologic, the treatment needs correction of the synthesis and biologic stimulation of the fracture site, obtained with the help of physical means (magnetic electro-pulsated fields, extracorporeal shock wave) or with the application of biotechnologies in monotherapy [20–22].

Third group with score from 51 to 75. Is a complex problem characterized by high gravity of both biological and mechanical conditions? It is almost always required the resection of the non-union site, and then, is present a bone loss that have to be restored. Next to bone transport techniques with external fixator and tibiotarsal joint arthrodesis at the docking point, there is indication to autologous bone transplant and biotechnologies (cells, scaffolds, and growth factors) applied in polytherapy according to the principles of the "Biological Chamber" [23–25] [case 1].

http://dx.doi.org/10.5772/62664

Fourth group with score from 76 to 100. Are non-union of such gravity to be assimilated to an almost unsolvable problem and so can require a limb amputation or the implant of megaprothesis [case 2].

There are no doubt that the third group non-union (51–75 points) are the more difficult to treat and often are those recalcitrant forms that come to experts after too many surgical procedures without outcome.

In this group, we think is appropriate the application of biotechnologies in order to avoid unnecessary use of economic resources.

8. Biotechnology

Biotechnology at our disposition are synthetic growth factors (GFs) as human bone morphogenetic recombinant proteins (rh-BMPs), autologous growth factors (AGFs) contained in platelet-enriched plasma (PRP), mesenchymal stem cells (MSCs), and scaffolds or bone substitutes.

- Growth factors (GFs)

  Since the second half of 1990s, it has been demonstrated that some growth factors act as powerful stimulators of the in vitro osteoblastic proliferation and of the in vivo bone healing, such as to turn out really useful in aiding the healing process if correctly applied at the site of the lesion [26]. Thanks to the evolution of the tissue engineering, it is been possible to produce the single growth factors with the recombinant-DNA technique, particularly the rh-BMPs. Although they have been identified at least 40 different rh-BMPs, a clear clinical demonstration of the osteoinductive potential is available only for the rh-BMP-7, also known as osteogenic protein-1 (OP-1), and for the rh-BMP-2 [27], belonging to the transforming growth factors family (TGF-β), whose receptors are expressed on chondrocytes and osteoblasts [28]. The osteoinduction phenomenon is characterized by the transformation of the perivascular mesenchymal cells in bone progenitor cells that can regenerate bone tissue. The recombinant human osteogenic protein-1 (rh-OP-1), also known as rh-BMP-7 (eptodermina-α), conveyed by type-I collagen, has been the first to be approved in the world to treat non-union of long bones and in the USA as "humanitarian device exemption" (HDE) in the treatment of spinal non-union. It allows, also, the regeneration from vascularized bone and of healthy bone surrounding toward the inside deficient area. Thanks to several preclinical and clinical studies, the efficacy of the use of rh-BMP-7 has been demonstrated reporting in some studies success percentage between 85 and 89%; at the same time, it has been found a real decrease of complications linked to the use of autologous bone, considered even at this time the "gold standard" [29–38].

- Autologous growth factors (AGFs) and platelet-rich plasma (PRP)

  The PRP is the most advanced product of the "blood management." It is a biologically active concentrate of mediators extracted from patient's plasma and is a source of non-specific autologuos growth factors [platelet-derived growth factor (PDGF), TGF-β1-β2, insulin-like growth factor type 1-2 (IGF1-2) and vascular endothelial growth factor (VEGF)] able to stimulate bone, cartilage, and soft tissues healing processes on the site of use. It is characterized by an elevate concentration of trombocytes able to degranulate releasing several growth factors and cytokines that can induce osteogenesis and angiogenesis with a chemotactic and mitogenic mechanism [39]. It can be obtained from autologous or heterologous blood. Depending from the procedure used to treat the withdrawal can be obtained final platelet concentration from 4 to 8 times higher from the initial situation. In a randomized study of 2007 on 60 long-bones non-union has been demonstrated a minor healing capabilities by the PRP (63.8%) both in comparison with BMP-7 than to the autograft [30].

The AGFs contained in the PRP, as clarified by preclinical and clinical data, are promoters of the cellular division (mitogenesis) nonspecific for the bone cells, unable to promote the differentiation of the mesenchymal cells and to induce the formation of new bone tissue. They seem to be not useful when used alone or in association with scaffold in treatment of tibial pilon non-union.

- Mesenchymal stromal cells (MSCs)

Studies based on cellular therapies are concentrated on a rare non-hematopoietic cells population, the MSCs, which are present in patient's bone marrow and can be increased in colture in an undifferentiated state [40, 41]. In addition to their pluripotent properties, the MSCs are considered osteogenic progenitor cells with demonstrated ability to repair bone defects [42]. Their concentration at bone marrow level, however, can result not ever elevated [43, 44]. The influence of this factor seems to be fundamental to the aim to obtain the healing, and there are clinical evidences that a better prognosis is obtained with a progenitor cells concentration >1500/cm^3. Recently, new techniques have become available to obviate to this problem, between these patient's bone marrow aspirate permit the mesenchymal stem cells concentration directly in the operatory room. Those new methods have demonstrated two big advantages: a reduction in costs respect to the in vitro expansion of the MSCs and a drastic decrease of the donor site morbidity compared to the traditional collection in open surgery of the iliac crest [44, 45]. The clinical use of the MSCs, especially if associated with the BMPs, it has proven effective determining the non-union healing [46].

- Scaffold

The osteoconduction mediated by the scaffold is determined by the chemical–physical characteristics of the substratum act to favor the adhesion and the growth of the cells on the surface. The mechanical characteristics of the bone graft, and their resistance to the compression and torsion, are influenced from their shape (massive, cortical splint, spongious block, morcellized), from the withdrawal modality, processing, conservation, and from the kind of synthesis meaning used.

The synthesis substitutes used are mineral structures similar to human bone kind. They have only osteoconductive power. Between synthesis substitutes you can find calcium phosphate as hydroxyapatite, coralline hydroxyapatite (absorbable), tricalcium phosphate (TCP, absorbable), and biphasic calcium phosphate (BCP = HA + TCP). For small defects, the hydroxyapatite is good filler ad favorite, thanks to their osteoconductive properties, the progressive revascularization and reossification of the treated area. All materials available have some limit. Ceramic, particularly, presents three important disadvantages: the difficulty to remain in place, the long time needed to absorption, and the complete substitution with neoformed bone and the impossibility to fill important bone gap.

The allogenic transplant from bone bank and heterologous animal origin (porcine, bovine, or equine) have demonstrate osteoconductive power but not osteoinductive. They need, then, to be revascularization and repopulated from the outside, needing a surrounding enabling environment. Con be used as filler (morcellized/granules) or as mechanical support (wedges, blocks, splints) [47, 48].

9. Biological chamber and polytherapy

The biological chamber is a concept that represents the ideal site in which to brought out the bone regeneration processes. Is a natural bio-reactor within which are present all the elements at the base of the diamond concept. It is even, physically, the site of non-union or of bone loss specially prepared from the surgeon with the aim to create the best condition for the regeneration. The chamber has to be aseptic, mechanically stable, and sealed in a selectively permeable way [25].

To use the chamber is necessary to remove completely the pathologic non-union tissue, removing all external bodies and meaning of synthesis. Is important to remove in a complete way all the necrotic tissue up to a bleeding bone resection that means vitality. The non-union tissue can be assimilated to a "meta-traumatic tumor" and as such, it must be removed entirely. In case of non-union or septic bone loss is important to do cultural withdrawal with the aim to identify the pathogen responsible of sepsis and perform targeted antibiotic therapy. Over the removal of the infected bone tissue is important to do a debridement and an accurate toilette of the soft tissues.

In septic cases is always preferable to do a two times treatment, then, once performed the removal of the pathologic tissue need to be implanted a cement spacer usually two antibiotics added (the choice of the active principle has to be done on the base of the antibiogram, when available) able to sterilize the site and create a reactive pseudo synovial membrane (described by Masquelet) extremely useful in the second reconstructive time [49].

In non-septic cases you can run a single surgical time reconstruction. Once created the biological chamber is then possible to insert within it polytherapy, or rather the simultaneous application of the three elements at the base of the diamond concept (growth factors, mesenchymal stem cells, and scaffolds). The fourth element, that is mechanical stability, will be provided by ostheosynthesis meaning (angular stability plates).

Case 1 (**Figures 1–4**)

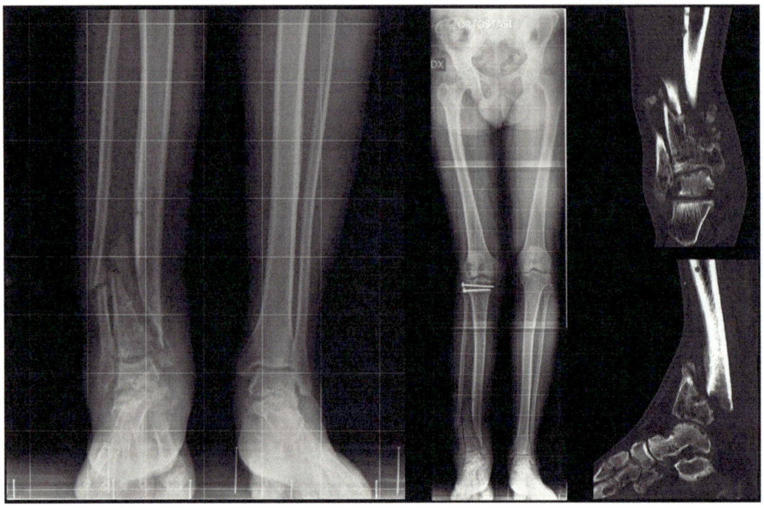

Figure 1. Clinical case 1—Man, 49 years, initial trauma following a motorcycle accident in which suffered exposed tibial pilon fracture, four ineffective treatments previously, comes to our attention (see X-rays and TC images) with a picture of septic non-union with serious bone loss and varus deformity, NUSS: 56 points.

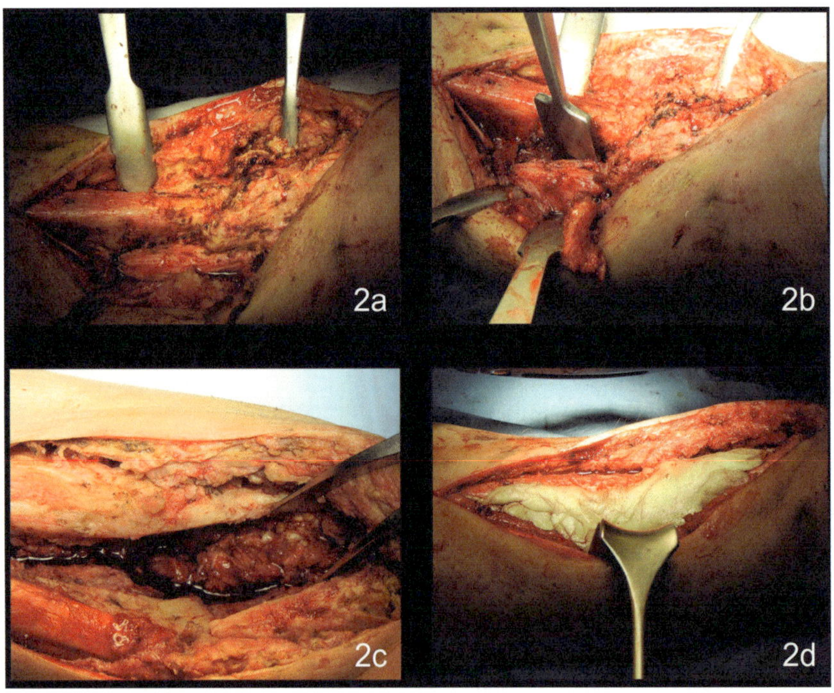

Figure 2. Intraoperative pictures that evidence: non-union site (a). Osteotomy with cruentation and removal of the pathologic tissue saving the joint surface came to healing after all previous treatments (b). The creation of the "biological chamber" (c). The implantation of antibiotic cement added with gentamicin and clindamycin (d).

http://dx.doi.org/10.5772/62664

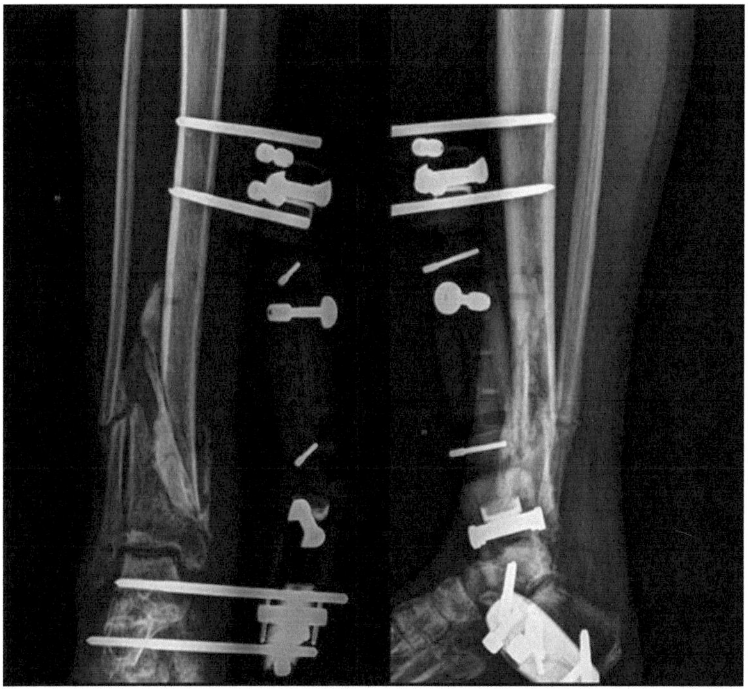

Figure 3. Radiographic post-op images that evidence the stabilization with external fixation, the positioning of the cement spacer and the deformity correction.

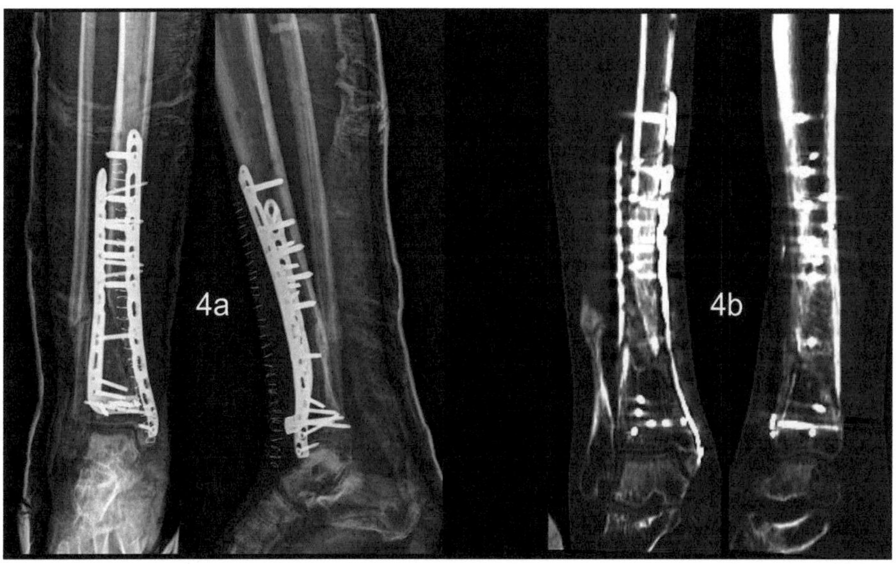

Figure 4. X-rays post-op images after the second reconstructive surgery performed by grafting biotechnologies in polytherapy and stabilization with double angular stability plate (a). CT control after 9 months (b).

10. Megaprosthesis

The development of megaprosthesis in serious segmental bon defects happened thanks to the biomedical application of the metallurgic industry on the field of surgical oncology. The development of new prosthesis for large resections offered important opportunities to oncologic orthopaedic surgeons for the substitution of skeletal segment, as long bones of the upper and lower limbs and near joints.

Our experience in treatment of non-union and serious bone loss led us, sometimes, to confront with the reality of some failure, after futile attempts to reconstruct the bone, eve with the use of advanced technologies as biotechnologies in monotherapy or polytherapy. In case of patients with a NUSS score of 76–100, the severity of the lesions and the clinical conditions usually makes sure that the surgical options of arthrodesis and amputation are implemented. In front of these drastic situations, radiologic and clinic, and to patients that have no intention to consider the amputation as a solution of their problem, we decided to apply the principles of the oncologic surgery, trying to remedy at their extreme cases with a solution of massive prosthetic [50, 51].

Actually in commerce you can find modular prosthetic system able to replace the entire femur including hip and knee joints up to the distal third of the tibia.

This surgical instrument presents peculiar characteristics:

- Custom-made realized on radiologic images,
- Stabilized with a tibial stem and a talocalcaneal stem locked with a screw,
- It allows to be stretched according to the necessity on the way to restore the correct length of the lower limbs,
- It offers the possibility to be resurfaced by silver in septic cases, exploiting the bacteriostatic action of this element.

Thanks to these new implants are now possible to avoid the amputation or long and often inconclusive treatments of lengthening and arthrodesis of the ankle with external fixators. Those patients, being part of the fourth NUSS category, cannot have benefit nor from the application of biotechnologies because the real possibilities of regeneration of the subject are too compromised. Therefore in those patients, we think more opportune to do a substitution treatment that can give back the function to the patient rapidly rather than follow again useful reconstruction attempts. More studies will be carried out to value the efficacy and the longevity of those new instruments.

Case 2 (**Figures 5–7**)

http://dx.doi.org/10.5772/62664

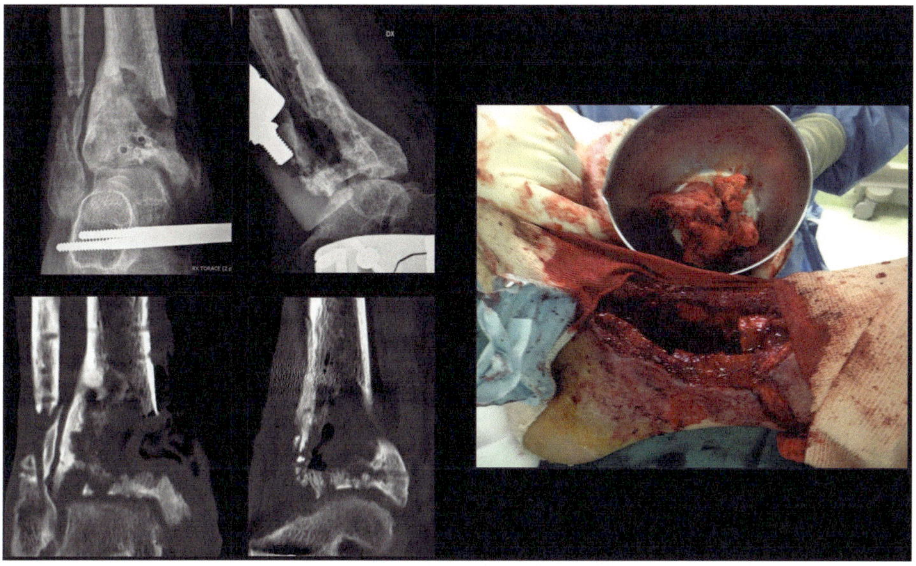

Figure 5. Clinical case 2—man, 46 years, initial injury following an accident on work in which suffered of comminuted tibial pilon fracture treated with synthesis with plate and complicated by septic condition. Comes to our attention with bone defect of the tibial distal epiphysis and severe bone loss with bone exposition and deep sepsis after the removal of the synthesis means and stabilization with external fixation. NUSS: 78 points. On the left X-rays and CT images, on the right intraoperative picture after the resection of the distal tibia, evident the severe skin loss that has been treated by covering flap.

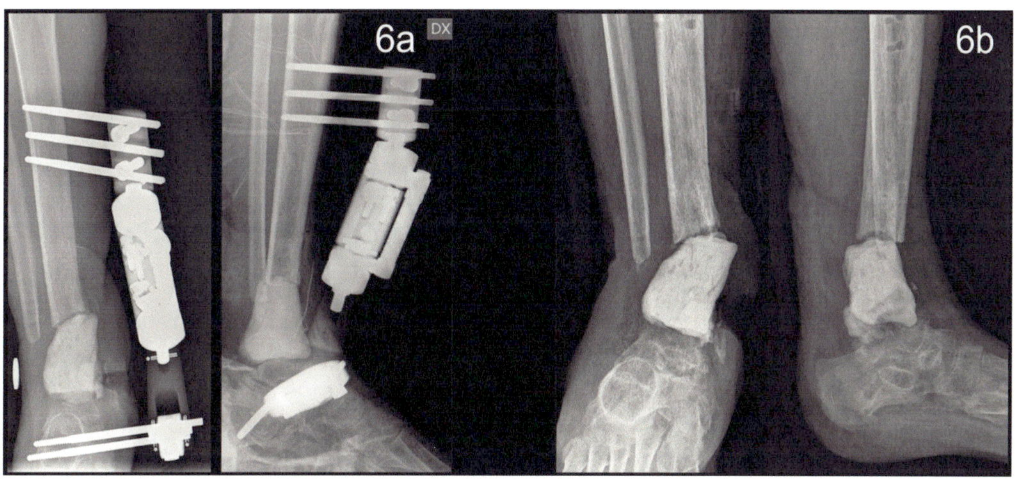

Figure 6. X-rays post-op images that evidence the stabilization with external fixator and positioning of antibiotic cement spacer with gentamicin and clindamycin (a), and after 3 months, resolved the septic condition, after the removal of the external fixator (b).

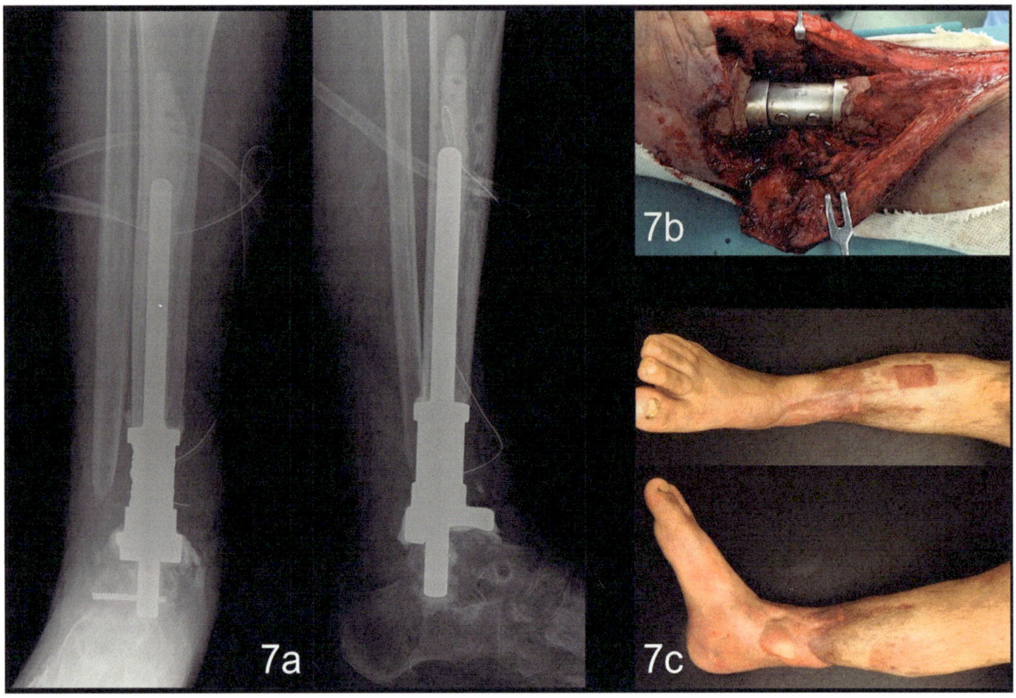

Figure 7. X-rays post-op images (a) after the implant of arthrodesing megaprosthesis of the distal leg (b) and clinical pictures (c) of the operated limb and of the skin condition.

11. Conclusions and future perspectives

The objective difficulty of those specific cases, evidenced or classified correctly by an elevated NUSS, cannot be representative in cases in which, in front of presumable mechanic necessities and correct surgical treatment, presents real biological difficulties.

This biologic difficulty is presumable to be searched in genetic expression [52, 53] but is difficult to assess in her real essential components and even more in the single clinical case.

The even more depth study of those which are the causes that can induce to non-union is today more important than ever. The new frontier will be the gene therapy or rather the possibility to transport inside the patient those genes acted to determine the succession of events that conduce to the formation of a bone callus and his maturation to strong bone.

Several studies, on animals, evidence today show that the gene therapy is viable both with the use of carrier virus [54, 55], both with the use of other non-viral carrier as for example particular pulsed electric fields (DNA electroporation) [56]. These therapies are still futuristic realities and provide an ulterior wide preclinic and clinic evaluation. A lot of road has been done until today on the ground of knowledge and of clinic treatment of non-union, and we think that in

http://dx.doi.org/10.5772/62664

the near future there will be understanding of how the non-union pathology could be by herself a pathology on a vulnerable patient.

In these patients in which the regeneration possibilities are compromised, a valid solution is offered from the biological chamber and from the new mega prosthetic implants that can avoid the amputation and restoring the function to the patient.

Is today recognized the importance of a global and polyspecialists approach in the treatment of non-union and of large bone loss of the tibial pilon? Recent studies costs–benefits on the choice of the most appropriate treatment have demonstrate that the probabilities of a better outcome offered by multidisciplinary approach with biotechnology have a fewer impact on the sanitary economy compared to that expected for long-time care in case of repeated features [57].

It is therefore our opinion that the use of secure and trusted traditional techniques must be accompanied by the best is offered today by new technologies both on the respect of the quality of patient's life, both keeping in mind of the economic feasibility.

Author details

Giorgio Maria Calori*, Massimiliano Colombo, Emilio Mazza, Miguel Simon Bucci, Piero Fadigati, Alessandra Ines Maria Colombo and Simone Mazzola

*Address all correspondence to: gmc@studiocalori.it

Orthopaedic and Trauma Reparative Surgery Department, Gaetano Pini Institute, University of Milan, Italy

References

[1] Heim U: Fractures du pilon tibial. Cahiers d'enseignement de la SOFCOT: Conférences d'enseignement. 35–51, 1997

[2] Ruedi TP, Allgower M: The operative treatment of intra-articular fractures of the lower end of the tibia. Clin Orthop 138: 105–110, 1979

[3] McFerran MA, Smith SW, Boulas HJ, et al.: Complications encountered in the treatment of pilon fractures. J Orthop Trauma 6: 195–200, 1992

[4] Bacon S, Smith WR, Morgan SJ, et al.: A retrospective analysis of HYPERLINK "http://www.ncbi.nlm.nih.gov/pubmed/18241864"comminutedHYPERLINK "http://www.ncbi.nlm.nih.gov/pubmed/18241864" intra-HYPERLINK "http://www.ncbi.nlm.nih.gov/pubmed/18241864"articularHYPERLINK "http://www.ncbi.nlm.nih.gov/pubmed/18241864" fractures of the HYPERLINK "http://

www.ncbi.nlm.nih.gov/pubmed/18241864"tibialHYPERLINK "http://www.ncbi.nlm.nih.gov/pubmed/18241864" plafond: Open reduction and internal fixation versus external HYPERLINK "http://www.ncbi.nlm.nih.gov/pubmed/18241864"IlizarovHYPERLINK "http://www.ncbi.nlm.nih.gov/pubmed/18241864" fixation. Injury 39(2):196–202, 2008

[5] Havet E, Alovor G, Gabrion A, et al.: Résultat thérapeutiques à long terme des fracture du pilon tibial: à propos de 50 fractures à 7 ans de recul minimum. Revue de Chirurgie Orthopédique 89:97, 2003 (suppl.).

[6] Wang C, Li Y, Huang L, et al.: Comparison of two-staged ORIF and limited internal fixation with external HYPERLINK "http://www.ncbi.nlm.nih.gov/pubmed/20182880"fixatorHYPERLINK "http://www.ncbi.nlm.nih.gov/pubmed/20182880" for closed HYPERLINK "http://www.ncbi.nlm.nih.gov/pubmed/20182880"tibialHYPERLINK "http://www.ncbi.nlm.nih.gov/pubmed/20182880" plafond fractures. Arch Orthop Trauma Surg 130(10):1289–1297, 2010

[7] Calori, G.M., Tagliabue, L., Mazza, E., de Bellis, U., Pierannunzii, L., Marelli, B.M., Colombo, M., Albisetti, W: Tibial pilon fractures: Which method of treatment? Injury 41:1183–1190, 2010

[8] Calori GM, Albisetti W, Agus A, et al.: Risk factors contributing to fracture non-unions. Injury 38(suppl. 2):11–18, 2009

[9] Dickinson K, Katzman S, Delgado E, et al.: Delayed union and non-unions of open tibial fractures: Correlation with arteriography results. Clin Orthop 302:189–193, 1994

[10] Calori GM, Albisetti W, Mazza E, et al.: Long bone nonunions and defects. G.I.O.T. 36:183–189, 2010

[11] Claes L, Augat P, Suger G, Wilke HJ: Influence of size and stability of the osteotomy gap on the success of fracture healing. J Orthop Res 15:577–584, 1997

[12] Dillin L, Slabaugh P: Delayed wound healing, infection, and non-union following open reduction and internal fixation of tibial plafond fractures. J Trauma 26:1116–1192, 1986

[13] Piper KJ, Won HY, Ellis AM: Hybrid external fixation in complex tibial plateau and plafond fractures: An Australian audit of outcomes. Injury 36:178–184, 2004

[14] Giannoudis PV, Einhorn TA, Marsh D: Fracture healing: the diamond concept. Injury 38(Suppl. 4):S3–S6, 2007

[15] Wolff J: Das Gesetz der Transformation der Knochen. Berlin: Hirschwald, 1982. (Transl. The Law of Bone Remodelling. Berlin: Springer, 1986)

[16] Weber BG, Cech O: Pseudarthrosis. Bern, Hans Huber, 1976

[17] Calori GM, Phillips M, Jeetle S, et al.: Classification of non-union: Need for a new scoring system? Injury 39(Suppl.):S59–S63, 2008

http://dx.doi.org/10.5772/62664

[18] Abumunaser LA, Al-Sayyad MJ: Evaluation of the Calori, et al.: Nonunion scoring system in a retrospective case series. Orthopedics 34(5):359, 2011

[19] Calori GM, Colombo M, Mazza EL, Mazzola S, Malagoli E, Marelli N, Corradi A: Validation of the Non-Union Scoring System in 300 long bone non-unions. Injury 45 Suppl 6:S93–S71, Dec2014

[20] Jingushi S, Mizuno K, Matsushita T, et al.: Low-intensity pulsed ultrasound treatment for postoperative delayed union or non-union of long bone fractures. J Orthop Sci 12:35–41, 2007

[21] Bara T, Synder M: Nine-years experience with the use of shock waves for treatment of bone union disturbances. Ortop Traumatol Rehabil 9:254–258, 2007

[22] Calori GM, Colombo M, Mazza E, Ripamonti C, Mazzola S, Marelli N, Mineo GV: Monotherapy vs polytherapy in the treatment of forearm non unions and bone defects. Injury 44(suppl. 1):S63–S69, 2013

[23] Calori GM, Mazza E, Colombo M, Ripamonti C, Tagliabue L: Treatment of long bone non unions with polytherapy: Indications and clinical results. Injury 42(6):587–590, 2011

[24] Calori GM, Colombo M, Ripamonti C, Bucci M, Fadigati P, Mazza E, Mulas S, Tagliabue L: Polytherapy in bone regeneration: Clinical applications and preliminary considerations. Int J Immunopathol Pharmacol 24(1 Suppl. 2), 85–89, 2011

[25] Calori G.M., Giannoudis P: Enhancement of fracture healing with the diamond concept: The role of the biological chamber. Injury 42:1191–1193, 2011

[26] Wozney JM: The bone morphogenetic protein family and osteogenesis. Mol Reprod Devel 32:160–167, 1992

[27] Lieberman JR, Daluiski A, Einhorn TA: The role of growth factors in the repair of bone. J Bone Joint Surg Am 84-A:1032–1044, 2002

[28] Celeste AJ, Iannazzi JA, Taylor RC, et al.: Identification of transforming growth factor family members present in bone inductive protein purified from bovine bone. Proc Natl Acad Sci USA 87:9843–9847, 1990

[29] Burkus JK, Sandhu HS, Gornet MF, et al.: Use of rhBMP-2 in combination with structural cortical allografts: Clinical and radiographic outcomes in anterior lumbar spinal surgery. J Bone Joint Surg Am 87:1205–1212, 2005

[30] Calori GM, Tagliabue L, Gala L, et al.: Application of rhBMP-7 and platelet-rich plasma in the treatment of long bone non-unions: A prospective randomized clinical study on 120 patients. Injury 39:1391–1402, 2008

[31] Govender S, Csimma C, Genant HK, et al.: Recombinant human bone morphogenetic protein-2 for treatment of open tibial fractures: A prospective, controlled, randomized study of our hundred and fifty patients. J Bone Joint Surg Am 84A:2123–2134, 2002

[32] Kanakaris NK, Calori GM, Verdonk R, et al.: Application of BMP-7 to tibial non-unions: A 3-year multicenter experience. Injury 39(S2):S83–S90, 2008

[33] Kanakaris NK, Lasanianos N, Calori GM: Application of bone morphogenetic proteins to femoral non-unions: A 4-year multicentre experience. Injury 40(S3):S54–S60, 2009

[34] Kanakaris N.K, Mallina R, Calori GM, Kontakis G, Giannoudis PV: Use of bone morphogenetic proteins in arthrodesis: Clinical results. Injury, Int J Care Injured 40(S3):S62–S66, 2009

[35] Dimitriou R, Dahabreh Z, Katsoulis E, et al.: Application of recombinant BMP-7 on persistent upper and lower limb non-unions. Injury 36S:S51–S59, 2005

[36] Dinopoulos H, Giannoudis PV: (iv) The use of bone morphogenetic proteins (BMPs) in long-bone non-unions. Curr Orthop 21:268–279, 2007

[37] Friedlaender GE, Perry CR, Cole JD, et al.: Osteogenic protein-1 (BMP-7) in the treatment of tibial nonunions. J Bone Joint Surg Am 83(Suppl. 1):S151–S158, 2001

[38] Zimmermann G, Wagner C, Schmeckenbecher K, et al.: Treatment of tibial shaft non-unions: Bone morphogenetic proteins versus autologous bone graft. Injury 40(Suppl. 3):S50–S53, 2009

[39] Slater M, Patava J, Kingham K, et al.: Involvement of platelets in stimulating osteogenic activity. J Orthop Res 3:655–659, 1995

[40] Pountos I, Corscadden D, Emery P, et al.: Mesenchymal stem cell tissue engineering: Techniques for isolation, expansion and application. Injury 38(Suppl.):S23–S33, 2007

[41] Kadiyala S, Jaiswal N, Bruder SP: Culture-expanded, bone marrow-derived mesenchymal stem cells can regenerate a criticalsized segmental bone defect. Tissue Eng 3:173–185, 1997

[42] Connolly JF: Clinical use of marrow osteoprogenitor cells to stimulate osteogenesis. Clin Orthop Relat Res 355(Suppl.):S257–66, 1998

[43] Hamanishi C, Yoshii T, Totani Y, et al.: Bone mineral density of lengthened rabbit tibia is enhanced by transplantation of fresh autologous bone marrow cells. Clin Orthop 303:250–255, 1994

[44] Weiner BK, Walker M: Efficacy of autologous growth factors in lumbar intertransverse fusions. Spine 28:1968–1971, 2003

[45] Hernigou P, Poiguard A, Beaujean F, et al.: Percutaneous autologous bone marrow grafting for non-unions. Influence of the number and concentration of progenitor cells. J Bone Joint Surg Am 87:1430–1437, 2005

[46] Saito A, Suzuki Y, Ogata SI, et al.: Accelerated bone repair with the use of a synthetic BMP-2-derived peptide and bone-marrow stromal cells. J Biomed Mater Res 72:77–82, 2005

[47] De Long WG, Einhorn TA, Koval K, et al.: Bone grafts and bone graft substitutes in orthopaedic trauma surgery. A critical analysis. J Bone Joint Surg Am 89:649–658, 2007

[48] Calori GM, Mazza E, Colombo M, Ripamonti C: The use of bone graft substitutes in large bone defects: Any specific needs? Injury 42:S56–S63, 2011

[49] Masquelet AC, Fitoussi F, Be′ gue′ T, Muller GP: Reconstruction of long bones induced membrane and spongy autograft. Ann Chir Plast Esthet 45:346–353, 2000

[50] Calori GM, Colombo M, Ripamonti C, Malagoli E, Mazza E, Fadigati P, Bucci M: Megaprosthesis in large bone defects: Opportunity or chimaera? Injury, Int J Care Injured 45:388–393, 2013

[51] Calori GM, Colombo M, Malagoli E, Mazzola S, Bucci M, Mazza E: Megaprosthesis in post-traumatic and periprosthetic large bone defects: Issues to consider. Injury 45 Suppl. 6:S105–S110, Dec 2014

[52] Zimmermann G, Schmeckenbecher KHK, Boeuf S, et al.: Differential gene expression analysis in fracture callus of patients with regular and failed bone healing. Injury, Int J Care Injured 43:347–356, 2012

[53] Dimitrioua R, Kanakaris N, Soucacos PN, et al.: Genetic predisposition to non-union: Evidence today. Injury, Int J Care Injured 44(S1):S50–S53, 2013

[54] Evans CH: Gene delivery to bone. Adv Drug Deliv Rev 64:1331–1340, 2012

[55] Ashman O, Phillips AM: Treatment of non-unions with bone defects: Which option and why? Injury, Int J Care Injured 44(S1):S43–S45, 2013

[56] Kimelman-Bleich N, Pelled G, Zilberman Y, et al.: Targeted gene-and-host progenitor cell therapy for nonunion bone fracture repair. Mol Ther 19:53–59, 2011

[57] Calori GM Capanna R, Colombo M, De Biase P, O'Sullivan Carol, Cartareggia V, Conti C: Cost-effectiveness of tibial non unions treatment: A comparison between rhBMP-7 and autologous bone graft in two Italian centres. Injury, Int J Care Injured 44:1871–1879, 2013

Section 2

Basic Science and Research

Chapter 7

Nature-Inspired Nanotechnology and Smart Magnetic Activation: Two Groundbreaking Approaches Toward a New Generation of Biomaterials for Hard Tissue Regeneration

Simone Sprio, Monica Sandri, Michele Iafisco,
Silvia Panseri, Monica Montesi, Andrea Ruffini,
Alessio Adamiano, Alberto Ballardini and
Anna Tampieri

Additional information is available at the end of the chapter

http://dx.doi.org/10.5772/63229

Abstract

Today, as the need of new regenerative solutions is steadily increasing, the demand for new bio-devices with smart functionality is pushing material scientists to develop new synthesis concepts. Indeed, the conventional approaches for biomaterials fail when it comes to generate nano-biocomposites with designed biomimetic composition and hierarchically organized architecture mimicking biologically relevant tissue features. In this respect, an emerging concept in material science is to draw inspiration from natural processes and products, which we may consider as the most advanced examples of smart nanotechnology. Natural processes of supramolecular assembly and mineralization of organic macromolecules, known as biomineralization, generate complex hybrid 3D constructs that are the basis of skeletons, exoskeletons, nacre and shells. On the other hand, natural structures such as woods and plants exhibit multi-scale hierarchic organization that is the source of smart and anisotropic mechanical properties associated with high porosity and lightness. The association of nature-inspired nano-technological products with smart functionalization can provide new advanced solutions to critical and still unmet clinical needs. In this respect, magnetic activation of biomaterials by the use of a recently developed biocompatible, resorbable magnetic apatite promises to represent a new safe and effective switching tool, enabling personalized applications in regenerative medicine and theranostics that so far were not feasible, due to the cytotoxicity of the currently used magnetic materials.

Keywords: bone regeneration, bioinspired materials, biomineralization, biomorphic transformation, magnetic activation

1. Introduction

Materials science today is experiencing a paradigmatic change in the development of new smart devices for biomedical applications. Particularly, the regeneration of hard tissues (i.e. bone, cartilage, tooth) is one of the most demanding issues in medicine and requires smart devices showing high mimicry of the host tissues and ability to instruct and drive progenitor cells to activate the regenerative cascade. Therefore, among the various approaches pursued so far for the synthesis of bone biomaterials, wide consensus is now consolidated around the concept of "*biomimetics*". Such a definition indicates the ability of a synthetic material to closely reproduce the chemical composition, physical properties, and architecture of native tissues, with the purpose to create 3-D environments able to deliver signals stimulating cell chemotaxis and specific differentiation of autologous stem cells [1]. In this way, the main concept is that bone regeneration can be greatly aided by the fact that, by implantation of a biomimetic scaffold, the patient body acts as a natural bioreactor guiding proper tissue regeneration without the need of complicated tissue engineering procedures or of the use of biological factors, thus improving the safety of clinical approaches.

In this respect the chapter highlights some emerging concepts related to the development of bio-inspired materials addressed to hard tissue regeneration. In particular, the focus is on assembling/mineralization techniques that reproduce the cascade of phenomena acting in the formation of hybrid nanocomposites such as bone and shells, that can generate hybrid fibrous structures with excellent regenerative ability. This process, pinning on the exchange of information stored in the structure of natural polymers, is characterized by great versatility that enable the synthesis of smart multifunctional scaffolds for regeneration of tissue complexes such as joints and periodontium.

On the other side, the chapter is focused on the emerging concept of biomorphic transformations by which natural structures with hierarchic architecture are converted into apatitic biomaterials with unpreceded bioactivity and structure, by multi-step chemical processes. In fact, as the process bases on heterogeneous reactions at the interface between a solid template and a gaseous phase, the obtained scaffolds result well consolidated without the need of sintering treatments and exhibit enhanced mechanical properties, due to the hierarchical architecture, thus being very promising for regeneration of load-bearing bones such as those of the limbs. Finally, the chapter highlights the recent development of an iron-substituted hydroxyapatite (HA) nanophase that, thanks to its excellent biocompatibility and intrinsic magnetic properties, demonstrated ability to be activated by remote magnetic signalling, thus representing a new switching tool for the development of a multifunctional platform generating smart bio-devices for various applications in regenerative medicine and theranostics. This new material, overcoming the limitations of toxic iron oxide nanoparticles currently used in nanomedicine, is very promising for the future establishment of new and more effective and personalized approaches for bone regeneration and cancer therapies. Moreover, the possibility of boosting bone regeneration by magnetic stimulation in patients with reduced endogenous potential is a key issue, in consideration of the progressive ageing of the population for which more effective and personalized regenerative therapies will be increasingly demanded in the incoming decades.

2. Bio-inspired synthesis processes: hybrid biomimetic scaffolds through biomineralization

In the last decade *bio-nanocomposites* emerged as a new class of materials including a natural polymer (biopolymer) in combination with an inorganic phase, rather than using synthetic polymers. Indeed the need of biomimetic materials and the limitations of the current fabrication methods are increasingly stimulating material scientists to explore this new class of compounds, thus benefitting of the presence of a polymer matrix that can be subjected to physiological, cell-mediated resorption in vivo, rather than to processes of chemical dissolution. In fact, the chemical leaching of polymeric scaffolds is one of the possible cause of failure in vivo, as the dissolution process can be too fast with respect to the new bone formation process, and also, the degradation products of many polymers can result in harmful effects, jeopardizing the regenerative cascade so that fibrous scars may form, rather than healthy, organized bone tissue. The inspiration for the design and development of bio-nanocomposites takes place from living organisms that are able to produce natural nanocomposites showing an amazing hierarchical arrangement of their organic and inorganic components from the nano to the macro scale (**Figure 1**).

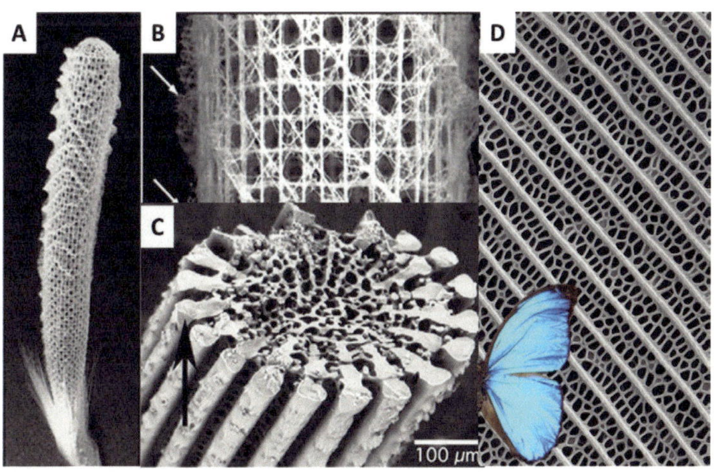

Figure 1. Natural bio-nanocomposites.

These outstanding architectures are the key of the insuperable performance of natural structures, particularly by a mechanic perspective: nacre, shells, bones, ligaments, tooth enamel, and dentine are just some examples of hierarchical, hybrid bio-nanocomposites found in nature. The mechanism at the basis of this outstanding structural arrangement is the establishment of hybrid building blocks formed upon heterogeneous nucleation of inorganic nanophases (such as carbonates and apatites) onto natural polymers, driven by several control mechanisms acting at the molecular scale [2]. In particular, during new bone formation, type I collagen, extruded by fibroblast cells, acts as a template for the nucleation of the mineral phase through a hierarchical assembly of collagen molecules into fibrils and ever thicker fibres, whereas HA nano-nuclei nucleate onto specific positively charged sites located in the collagen molecules. This process is governed by several control mechanisms inherent in the molecular structure of collagen that guide the formation of new bone at all scale sizes: a) the chemical interaction of HA with collagen prevents the crystallization and growth of the mineral phase, which results in a nearly amorphous material characterized by an apatite-like lattice; b) the growth of mineral nuclei is controlled by the organic matrix, so that the size of the nuclei are constrained up to few nanometers; c) the topotactic interaction induces specific crystal orientation of the mineral phase growing on the collagen fibers and evolving into lamellae; d) finally, lamellae are organized through different hierarchical levels to form the structure of the macroscopic bone [3–8]. The use of scaffolds able to guide cells to the re-growth of new bone tissue is an approach now considered as necessary for bone regeneration. Native extra-cellular matrix contains multiple signals whose presentation follows precise spatial and temporal patterns. In designing scaffolds for hard tissue regeneration, such signals must be reproduced so as to give chemical, physical, structural, and morphological information to cells and compel them to express specific phenotypes. Besides, ideal scaffolds guiding tissue regeneration should also have adequate properties with respect to degradation, cell binding, cellular uptake, non-immunogenicity, and mechanical performance. In particular, the essential characteristics of regenerative bone scaffolds are: surface activity enabling the establishment of a tight interface between the scaffold and the new tissue; osteoconductivity i.e. the ability to function as a template for 3D cell colonization; appropriate degradation profile without host tissue responses such as inflammation or fibrous encapsulation of the implant [9].

The reproduction of the bone biomineralization process in laboratory enabled the synthesis of hybrid HA/collagen composites reproducing most of the relevant features of newly formed bone and osteochondral tissues [10, 11]. Type I collagen extracted by equine tendon and dispersed into acetic acid in the form of nanofibrils can be subjected to controlled assembly in aqueous environment by pH variation, simultaneously to the mineralization with apatite nanophases where the content of foreign ions can be tailored to reach bio-competent compositions. In fact, the maintenance of a disordered crystal structure allows the entrapment of ions naturally present in the physiological environment (i.e. Mg^{2+}, CO_3^{2-}, Sr^{2+}, Na^+, K^+, SiO_4^{4-}) into the structure of the mineral phase. The molecular habitus of type I collagen acts as a 3D substrate for heterogeneous nucleation of the mineral phase but also as a constraint for the growth and long-range ordering of the mineral crystals (**Figure 2**).

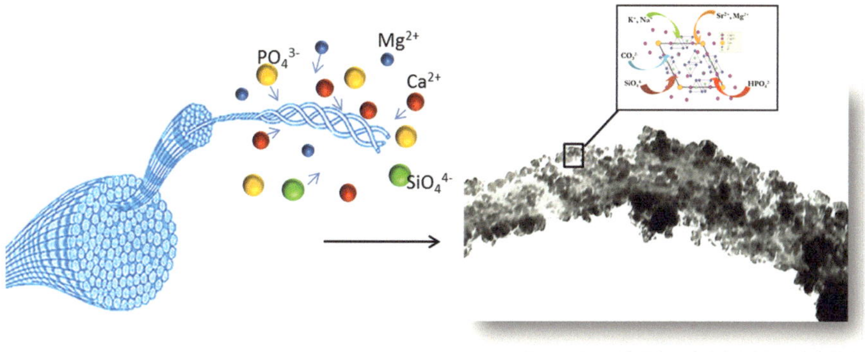

Figure 2. Scheme of collagen assembling and mineralization.

By this process CO_3^{2-} ions can be introduced to preferably occupy the phosphate site of the HA lattice (B type position) [4], thus providing the mineral phase with enhanced activity for cell adhesion and resorbability. Carbonate ions are abundant in young and newly formed bone tissue, and decrease in mature bone, thus evidencing their role in bone development. Among the foreign ions present in biologic apatite, Mg^{2+} have the marked property of increasing the nucleation kinetics of HA on collagen fibres but, in the meantime, hampering crystal growth, thus generating nano-size HA nuclei, strongly enhancing the bioavailability of the mineral phase. In fact, magnesium is found in much higher concentrations in young and newly formed mineralized tissues and is considered today as a fundamental element governing the first stages of bone formation [12]. Silicon is a minor element, essential for healthy skeletal development in higher biological organisms [6, 13], in particular for its role in the formation of crosslinks between collagen and proteoglycans [14], that provide stabilization of the new bone matrix and prevent enzymatic degradation.

The bone-like features of HA/Collagen hybrid composites reflect in bio-resorbability at physiological pH and high surface activity, particularly referred to the crystal size (i.e. ranging from 30–50 nm long, 15–30 nm wide, and 2–10 nm thick) [7, 8, 15–17] and to the specific orientation of the apatite nuclei, in respect to the long axis of collagen. The preferential growth of apatite nuclei along the *c* axis, as induced by the presence of particular functional chemical groups on the surface of the organic template, affects the surface polarity of the final hybrid composites, and consequently protein adhesion and cell attachment. The hierarchical assembly of these nano-size building blocks into macroscopic objects occurs upon supramolecular arrangement of collagen fibrils into thicker fibres, thus resulting into a final hybrid composite where, on a macroscopic scale, the mineral phase assumes a complex and hierarchical architecture, strictly dependent on the combination of the various above-described phenomena, which hierarchically occur on different dimensional scales in correspondence with the sites of heterogeneous nucleation.

The HA/Col composites assume a fibrous structure as well as high and interconnected porosity, the amount and morphology of which can be tailored by customized freeze drying processes (**Figure 3**).

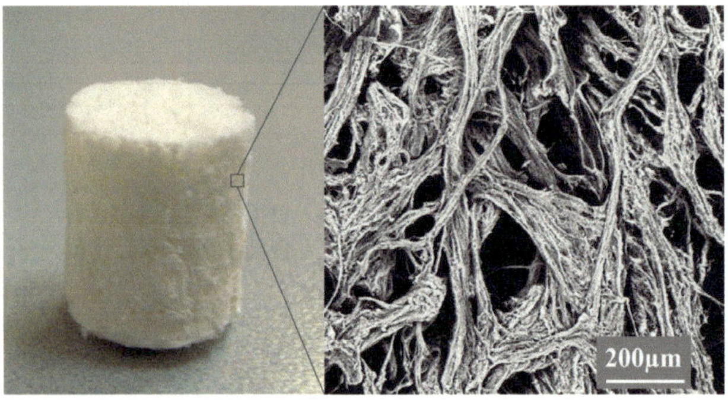

Figure 3. Bio-hybrid HA/Collagen composites.

The final dried scaffolds exhibit high activity towards cells; therefore they can be easily resorbed in vivo whereas new tissue forms. However, to limit the enzymatic degradation possibly preventing successful cell colonization and integration, cross-linking methods can be applied by using physical or chemical approaches addressing specific links among functional groups of collagen, thus enabling fibre bridging and tailored stability against resorption.

The in-lab reproduction of the phenomena occurring in biological processes can be considered as a conceptually new approach for nanotechnology and may pave the way to the development of new devices with outstanding properties. On the basis of the recognition of the different requirements to regenerate cartilaginous and bony part, such processes can be directed to graded scaffolds reproducing different histological areas in the osteochondral tissue by simply varying the degree of mineralization and the alignment of collagen fibres [11]. Therefore, hydrogels with designed features can be engineered into three-layered devices reproducing the sub-chondral bone (mineralization = 60-70 wt%), mineralized cartilage (mineralization = 30-40 wt%), and the hyaline cartilage (mineralization = 0 wt%) (**Figure 4**).

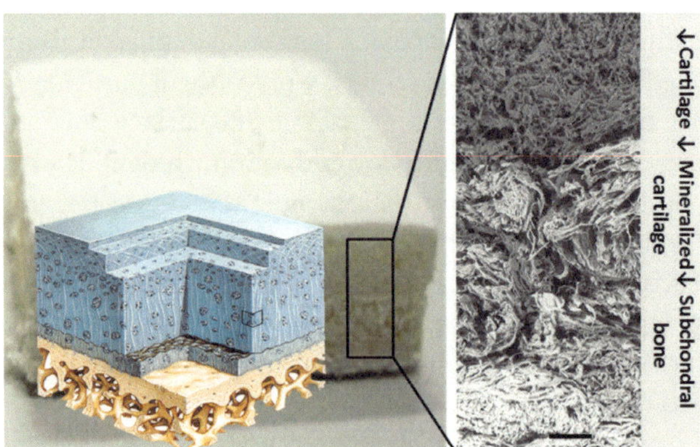

Figure 4. Scheme of osteochondral scaffolds.

In particular, the collagen-like layer, based on collagen and added with hyaluronic acid to create microstructural features improving the hydrophilic behaviour of the construct, reproduces some cartilaginous environmental cues such as the formation of a columnar-like structure converging towards the external surface where it forms horizontal flat ribbons, resembling the morphology of the *lamina splendens* [10, 11].

Such composites have demonstrated enhanced cell proliferation with very spread cell morphology, as well as high osteoinductivity and regenerative potential. The HA/collagen graded composites differentially support cartilage and bone tissue formation in the different histological layers, as demonstrated by comparative *in vivo* study carried out on adult sheep, where HA/collagen graded composites have been implanted on femoral condyles [18]. In particular, histological evaluation showed the formation of new hyaline-like tissue and good integration of scaffolds with host cartilage, with a strong proteoglycan staining and columnar rearrangement of chondrocytes, and an underlying well-ordered sub-chondral trabecular bone.

In this section it has been discussed that biologic processes pin on information exchanged at the molecular scale and on environmental boundary conditions that guide the process towards the establishment of 3-D hybrid composites with defined characteristics. This implies that bio-inspired syntheses are flexible processes that can be directed to fabricate specific devices *on demand*. In this respect, hybrid HA/Col composites can be developed to assume specific 3D morphologies, thus mimicking human multifunctional tissues such as periodontal regions. Indeed, human tooth is a tissue complex formed by the periodontium, in turn including alveolar bone and cementum, linked together by the periodontal ligament firmly bound to the root, and the dentin, a highly mineralized collagen matrix with tubular organization that is protected by the enamel (**Figure 5**).

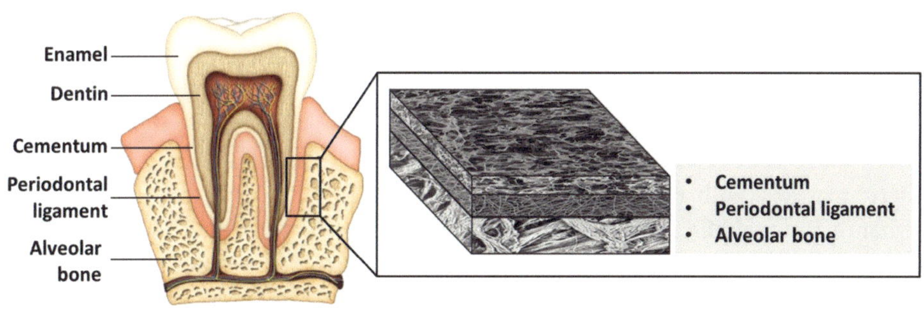

Figure 5. Scheme of dental tissues.

All the components of tooth form upon biologic phenomena close to those leading to formation of bone and cartilage [19]. The relevant differences are related to the mineralization extent of the different tissues (i.e. alveolar bone ~70 wt%, cementum ~50 wt%, dentine ~75 wt%, enamel ~98%), the degree of aggregation of collagen fibres, and the structural organization. Therefore, bio-inspired in-lab mineralization can be directed to develop new biomimetic scaffolds mimicking the different parts of the tooth by varying the concentration of calcium and phosphate ions with respect to collagen thus achieving the desired mineralization extent. Then, oriented channel-like porosity mimicking the tubular organization of dentine can be obtained by ionotropic gelation techniques applied to the as-synthesized hydrogels (**Figure 6**).

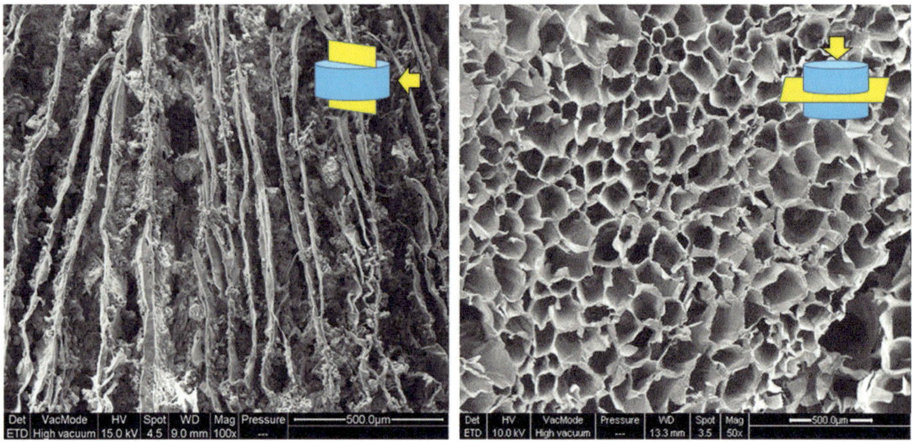

Figure 6. Dentin-like scaffolds.

Preliminary research shows that the application of bio-inspired synthesis techniques can enable the development of new implantable devices for the complete regeneration of dental tissues. This is a major and highly demanding clinical need and a target of high impact for materials science and medicine.

In perspective, the in-lab biomineralization process may be in principle translated to wider applications, possibly extending the range of natural polymers that can be combined to form composite matrices activating self-assembly and mineralization with specific inorganic phases. Non-mineralized constructs can be used as scaffolds for soft tissues and organs, where the biologic and mechanical performance can be tailored by combining various raw materials such as gelatin, nanocellulose, chitosan, alginate, and fibroin characterized by different hydrophilic behaviour and stiffness. On the other hand, the simultaneous mineralization of composite polymeric matrices with nano-apatites can generate scaffolds with improved mechanical performance, thus enabling wider applications in bone surgery, particularly referred to load-bearing applications where the soft nature of hybrid scaffolds does not allow to withstand strong biomechanical loads in the early stages of new bone formation.

3. Nature-derived biomaterials: biomorphic bone scaffolds with hierarchic architecture

The regeneration of load-bearing bone parts is still a high demanding challenge. Particularly, therapies to solve serious diseases involving the limbs, due to trauma or tissue degeneration, are today restricted to reconstructive approaches based on multiple surgery and the use of metallic parts that often give rise to secondary effects such as infections, pseudoarthrosis, and non-unions which can also lead to the complete loss of the limb functionality and also to amputation [20–22]. The incidence of such events is great and steadily increasing globally due to the modern lifestyle and also to the progressive ageing of the population, thus leading to high disability with huge impact on the healthcare costs and the patient's life.

Today the use of grafts to assist the regeneration of long segmental bones is considered as a promising approach, with different alternatives including autologous vascularized bone grafts, homologous bone graft, heterologous bone graft (xenograft), or prostheses, each one of them dealing with both specific advantages and drawbacks, such as: donor site morbidity and limited available amount, possible immune response and viral transmission, possible animal-derived pathogen transmission and risk of immunogenic rejection, high invasiveness and surgery-related systemic risks, long recovery time and need of prostheses revision [23–27].

Due to these very serious drawbacks, the use of synthetic bone substitutes with osteogenic and osteoconductive ability may offer clear benefits compared to natural bone grafts. Adequate osteogenic ability is required to stimulate the formation of new bone by exhibiting highly exposed active surfaces, favouring cell adhesion and proliferation. Also, osteoconductivity enables the penetration of the scaffold by cells which is a key aspect to achieve early osseointegration in turn enabling adequate stability of the bone/implant construct and the possibility for the patient to stimulate bone regeneration by progressively increasing loading [28, 29]. Adequate osteoconductivity is provided by the presence of open and interconnected porosity in the bone scaffold, in association with high surface affinity with bone cells. However, most of the bio-devices today developed exhibits tortuous porosity that hampers the development of extensive angiogenesis and penetration of blood vessels in the inner parts of the scaffold; in consequence, even though a good surface integration occurred, bone penetration is limited thus penalizing the stability of the bone/implant construct and the mechanical performance. [30–32].

HA, and particularly ion-doped apatites are the golden materials for bone scaffolding. However, the feasibility of synthesizing large porous HA bodies with high bioactivity, osteoconductivity, and mechanical strength is hampered by the need of thermal consolidation that destroys the bioactivity features of HA, that means: segregation of the foreign ions outside the HA lattice, thermally-induced grain growth with strong reduction of the specific surface area and reduction of the hydrophilic character and surface reactivity. Moreover, the weak mechanical properties of HA make it difficult to develop large scaffolds with high porosity extent. However, it can be envisaged that early and extensive penetration of new bone into the scaffold pores may significantly enhance the strength of the bone/biomaterial construct and enable mechanical loading. This process may lead to the complete recovery of limb functionality by progressive and assisted stimulation of the implanted part [32].

Since the unique biomechanical properties of bone mainly depend on its hierarchically organized structure ranging from the molecular to the nano-, micro-, and macro-scales, only scaffolds endowed with a 3D structure capable of exhibiting complex biomechanical performances may activate mechano-transduction processes in a biological-like fashion and yield regeneration of well-organized bone [33–39].

In consideration to the limits imposed by the ceramic technology (particularly by means of the existing forming techniques and the sintering), new manufacturing approaches are required for synthesis of scaffolds with adequate requisites for regeneration of long segmental bones. In this respect, the complex structural organization exhibited by living beings such as woods and plants is an interesting source of inspiration for material scientists towards the generation of smart devices with strongly improved performances. Indeed, these structures possess a hierarchic organization on multiple size scales that provide high strength and lightness (**Figure 7**).

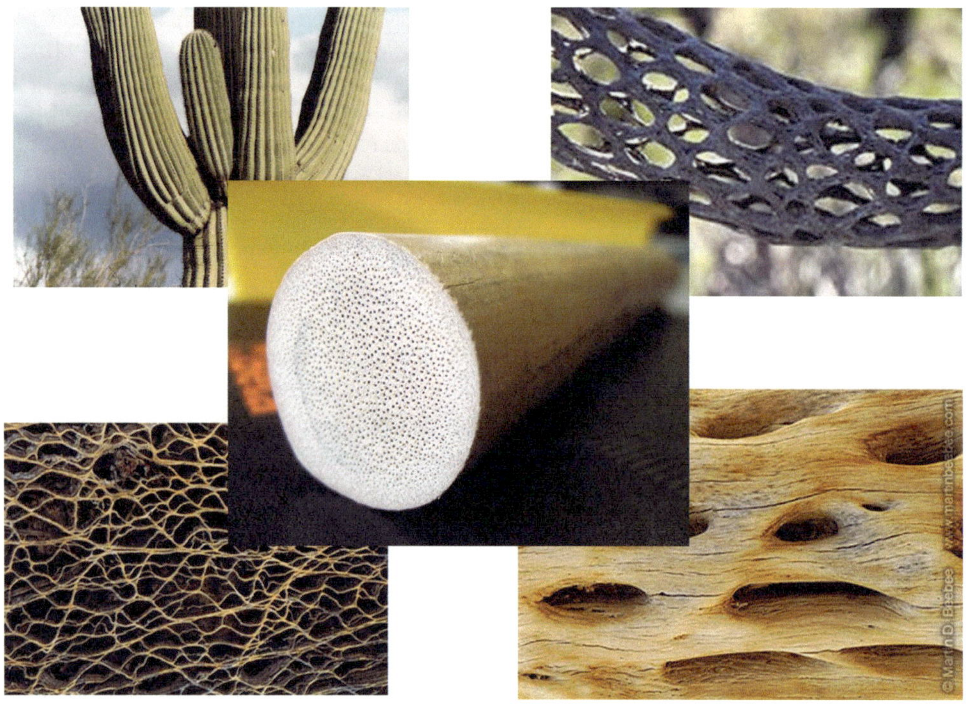

Figure 7. Structure of various woods and plants.

Among these, ligneous structures endowed with open porosity and suitable interconnection enabling extensive permeability to cells and fluids, as well as, at the same time, with adequate anisotropic mechanical behaviour, may be investigated as templates to develop new porous scaffolds with bone-like structural features [40–42].

Porous woods like pine and rattan were recently transformed into HA scaffolds with hierarchic organization, by a multi-step biomorphic transformation process (**Figure 8**) enabling precise control of phase composition and crystal ordering, as well as of the microstructure, since the different reactions occurred between a gas and the solid template at a molecular level, where calcium, oxygen, carbonate, and phosphate ions were progressively added, while building the HA molecules [43].

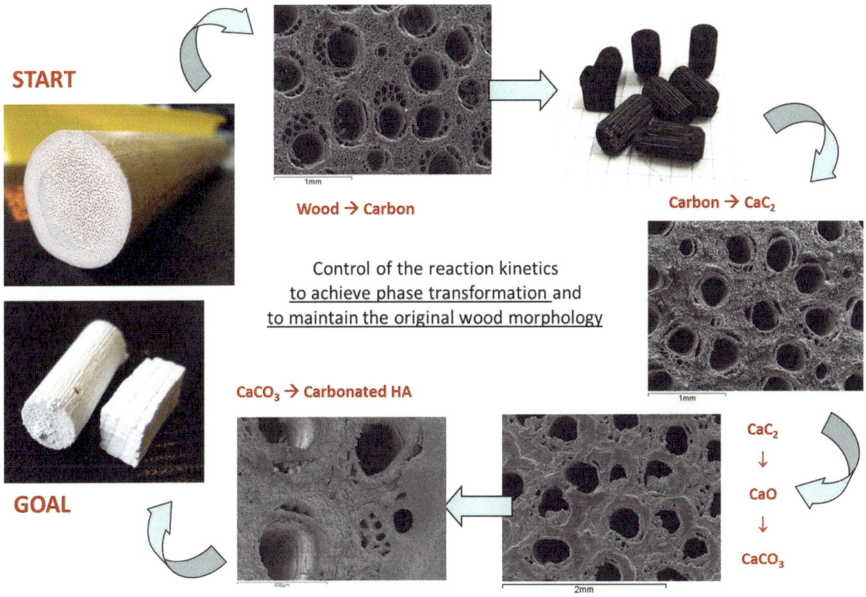

Figure 8. Biomorphic transformation process generating hydroxyapatite scaffolds.

By this process, it was possible to incorporate foreign ions, such as carbonate, in the final consolidated apatite scaffold [43] and to control the chemico-physical features related to the scaffold bioactivity and resorbability, such as the Ca/P ratio and the extent of crystal ordering of the HA phase. Among the existing ligneous sources rattan possesses a structure particularly suitable for bone scaffolding, i.e. a channel-like porosity very close to the Haversian structure with wide pores having diameter adequate for enhanced cell hosting and 3D colonization (**Figure 9**), thus being very promising for the activation of extensive vascularization throughout large volumes.

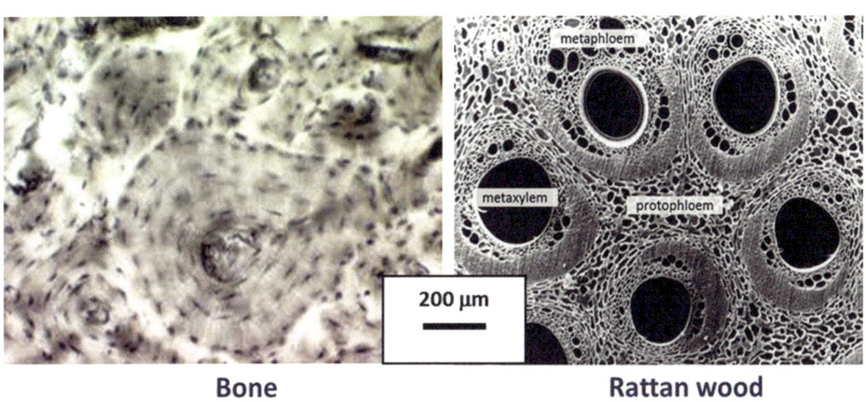

Figure 9. Bone mimicry of rattan wood.

Moreover, the endowment of the bone scaffolds with the channel-like structure of rattan resulted into anisotropic mechanical properties with values in the range of the trabecular bone, that reflect the complex bone response to directional loading. Preliminary biologic tests reported an outstanding affinity with cells, with complete coverage of the scaffolds by well spread cells (i.e. MG63 osteoblast-like cells) after 1 week and enhanced osteogenic ability compared to sintered HA scaffolds (**Figure 10**). Also, preliminary in vivo tests reported extensive bone formation and colonization in femoral bone defects, also showing good morphological organization after one month from implantation [20].

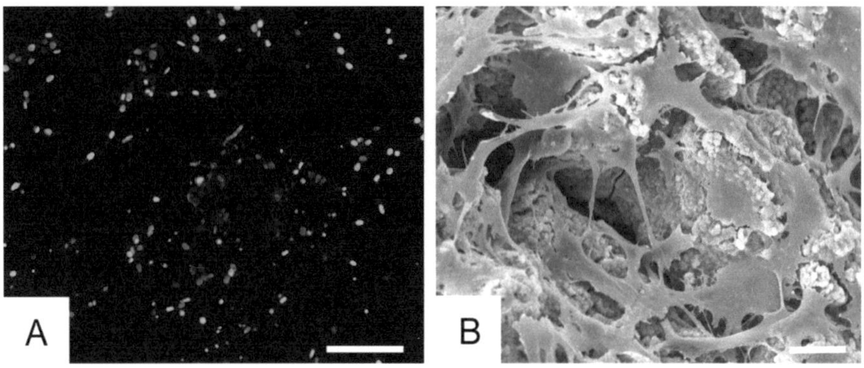

Figure 10. MG63 cells morphology in contact with wood-derived HA scaffold.

The first results obtained with this new type of bone scaffolds are very promising for further development and application into more clinically-relevant models, for assessing the feasibility of regenerating long segmental bone parts. In this respect the exploitation of natural sources as models for generation of new hierarchically organized scaffolds can be considered as a completely new synthesis approach that may open to still unexplored applications in the incoming years.

4. Biocompatible magnetic materials: a new smart, multifunctional tool in nanomedicine

The use of biomimetic scaffolds can be an effective approach for bone tissue regeneration, however the patients' metabolism plays an important role in the regulation of the kinetics and extent of new bone formation. Indeed, metabolic diseases, as well as degenerative conditions induced by aging, can seriously penalize new bone formation and fracture healing. In consideration of the ever increasing ageing of the world population, the occurrence of degenerative diseases is expected to steadily rise in the next decades, thus new therapeutic approaches are strongly required to boost and assist tissue regeneration in patients with reduced endogenous regenerative potential. Tissue engineering approaches and the use of drug delivery systems able to deliver growth factors are two main approaches for enhancing tissue regeneration. Particularly, a great effort is being dedicated to the development of scaffolds with the ability of controlled biochemical stimulation that should be delivered in temporo-spatially defined fashion [44].

In this respect, recent advances in material science suggest that the use of weak magnetic fields is appealing as remote signalling for non-invasive controlling and *on demand* activation of biomedical devices in vivo [1]. The use of magnetic materials in nanomedicine is thus raising a steadily growing interest, as they can open to new personalized applications including cancer therapy by hyperthermia, magnetic resonance imaging, and other diagnostic approaches based on the guiding of such particles to specific targeted areas in vivo and their use as nano-probes [45–52]. A serious drawback in the use of magnetic materials in nanomedicine is their long term cytotoxicity [53, 54]. Intense effort is therefore dedicated to engineering SPIONs (i.e. superparamagnetic iron oxide nanoparticles) with surface treatments to achieve enhanced biocompatibility and affinity with cells [55–57]. A significant advance can be the development of magnetic materials with intrinsic biocompatibility and resorbability. In this respect, it has been shown that the doping of the apatite lattice with Fe^{2+}/Fe^{3+} ions in specific calcium sites yields a new phase with intrinsic paramagnetic behaviour (FeHA) [58]. By virtue of its chemical composition very close to the one of mineral bone, FeHA is characterised by excellent bio-compatibility, as also confirmed by in vitro studies revealing that FeHA nanoparticles do not reduce cell viability and at the same time enhance cell proliferation compared to undoped HA particles [59]. Moreover, a pilot animal study of bone repair (a rabbit critical bone defect model) demonstrated the in vivo biocompatibility and biodegradability of FeHA [59]. The achievement of biocompatible nano-biomaterials with magnetic properties opens new perspectives in regenerative medicine. Particularly, the development of bone scaffolds with the ability of remote magnetic activation is now an emerging concept in regenerative medicine [60], since it has been demonstrated that weak magnetic or pulsed electromagnetic fields are effective in promoting bone fracture healing, spinal fusion, and bone ingrowth in various animal models [61–65]. However, the incorporation of FeHA phase into ceramic bone scaffolds is made difficult by the need of consolidating green ceramic bodies by high temperature treatments provoking lattice destabilization and loss of magnetic properties [59]. In this respect FeHA can also be synthesized by suitable modification of the biomineralization process to induce heterogeneous nucleation of FeHA nanophase on Type I collagen [66]. This method yielded biomimetic hybrid scaffolds with paramagnetic ability and mineralization extent that could be tailored from cartilage to bone-like level. The presence of a mineral phase with bone-like features and ability to be activated by remote magnetic signal make this new biomaterial very promising to boost regeneration of extended bone and osteochondral regions, even in patients with reduced endogenous regenerative potential [67–70].

Besides, the use of biocompatible magnetic materials can open to further, different approaches for enhanced bone regeneration. It is accepted that a key limiting factor in the regeneration of extended bone defects is the inability of cells to self-propagate in the inner part of the scaffold and to establish new bone and vascular tissue [20]. Recent progresses show that it is possible to locally guide the migration of magnetic nanoparticles and nanoparticle-labelled cells through the use of an externally applied magnetic field gradient [71]. In this respect FeHA nanoparticles can be easily incorporated into cells by endocytosis, thus obtaining "magnetic cells" without negatively affecting cell behavior (e.g. proliferation, morphology, differentiation). Through the application of an external magnetic field of low intensity, these cells can be guided within a scaffold, in order to have faster and more selective seeding for tissue engineering application (**Figure 11**).

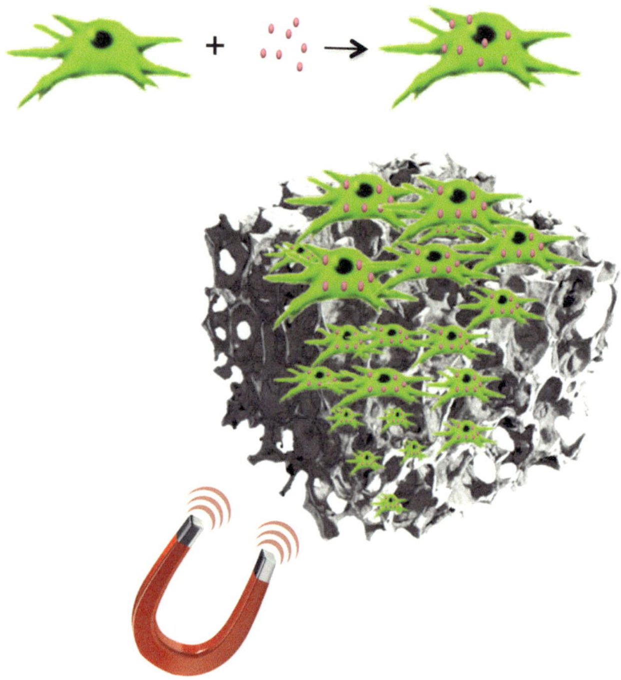

Figure 11. Scheme of magnetic guiding enabling enhanced scaffold colonization.

Biocompatible magnetic media can also be associated to polymeric or hybrid carriers to achieve new smart drug delivery systems with the ability of magnetic activation [72–77].

Hollow micro- and nano-spheres with controlled size and magnetization level, made of polycaprolacton coated with adequate amounts of FeHA displayed dose-dependent biocompatibility towards bone marrow mesenchymal stem cells, thus highlighting the positive effect of the mineralization extent on cell behaviour [78–80]. These carriers could be developed as magnetically-responsive drug delivery systems with activation and delivery kinetics modulated by phenomena of magnetoshaking or hyperthermia [81]. To explore these new approaches for controlled drug delivery, careful investigation is needed to investigate the most suitable conditions, by means of intensity and frequency of alternated magnetic fields that shall provide the energy needed for the release of the linked bioactive molecules. Therefore, in the incoming years further development of this approach may represent a new tool enabling the release of different chemical species under defined temporo-spatial patterns, thus opening to more advanced and personalized therapies.

5. Conclusions and future perspectives

The incoming decades will experience a growing role of smart biomaterials in therapies for bone regeneration. In this respect, a significant effort to develop nature-inspired synthesis approaches will generate new scaffolds endowed with high mimicry of host tissues and smart functions that will greatly improve the existing therapies and, might also generate new ones that were prevented so far by the inadequateness of the existing biomaterials. On the basis of some existing examples of nature-inspired biomaterials showing effective regenerative ability, and on the increasing effort of material scientists in the synthesis of biomimetic devices, it can be envisaged that significant advances will be reached in the next decade. In this respect, new emerging concepts of fabrication, such as biomineralization or biomorphic transformation, will overcome the limitations of current manufacturing techniques that, particularly in the case of ceramics, are not able to provide highly organized structures with details defined at the micron size. In this respect, due to the innumerable examples of natural structures exhibiting smart properties that are not achievable by conventional fabrication approaches, there are virtually no limits to the potential applications of biomorphic materials in various high-impact fields other than the biomedical one. Besides, the attainment of smart functionalization is another key topic that is engaging a significant part of the biomaterials researchers, particularly due to the increasing need to overcome the systemic drug administration and to provide more effectiveness and targeting to the existing therapies. In this respect, as safety, effectiveness, and targeting are key objectives for real applicability in nanomedicine, the use of magnetic stimulation can be considered as a promising concept that is raising ever increasing interest among scientists and will probably experience extended diffusion in the incoming years.

Acknowledgements

The research leading to these results has received funding from the European Union 7th Framework Programme under Grant agreement no. 310637 (SMILEY), the PNR-CNR Aging Program 2012–2014 and the Flagship project Nanomax (PNR-CNR 2011–2013).

Author details

Simone Sprio*, Monica Sandri, Michele Iafisco, Silvia Panseri, Monica Montesi, Andrea Ruffini, Alessio Adamiano, Alberto Ballardini and Anna Tampieri

*Address all correspondence to: simone.sprio@istec.cnr.it

Institute of Science and Technology for Ceramics, National Research Council, Faenza, Italy

References

[1] Tampieri A, Sprio S, Sandri M, Valentini F. Mimicking natural bio-mineralization processes: A new tool for osteo-chondral scaffold development. Trends in Biotech. 2011; 29(10): 526–535. DOI: 10.1016/j.tibtech.2011.04.011.

[2] Mann S. Bio-Mineralization: Principles and Concepts in Bioinorganic Materials Chemistry. Oxford University Press, Great Clarendon Street, Oxford , U.K. 2001. ISBN: 0198508824.

[3] LeGeros RZ. Calcium phosphate in oral biology and medicine. Karger, Basel, Switzerland; 1991. DOI: 10.1159/000419232.

[4] Boskey AL. Mineralization, structure and function of bone. In: Seibel MJ, Robins SP, Bilezikian JP, editors. Dynamics of Bone and Cartilage Metabolism: Principles and Clinical Applications. Academic Press, Theobald's road, London, U.K. 2006. pp. 201–212. ISBN: 9780120885626.

[5] Bigi A, Foresti E, Gregorini R, Ripamonti A, Roveri N, Shah JS. The role of magnesium on the structure of biological apatite. Calcif Tissue Int. 1992; 50: 439–444. DOI: 10.1007/BF00296775.

[6] Matsko NB, Žnidaršič N, Letofsky-Papst I, Dittrich M, Grogger W, Štrus J, Hofer F. Silicon: The key element in early stages of biocalcification. J Struct Biol. 2011; 174: 180–186. DOI: 10.1016/j.jsb.2010.09.025.

[7] Lowenstam HA, Weiner S. On Bio-Mineralization. Oxford University Press, Great Clarendon Street, Oxford , U.K. 1989. ISBN: 9780195049770.

[8] Jackson SA, Cartwright AG, Lewis D. The morphology of bone-mineral crystals. Calcif Tissue Res 1978; 25(1): 217–222. DOI: 10.1007/BF02010772.

[9] Wagoner Johnson AJ, Herschler BA. A review of the mechanical behavior of CaP and CaP/polymer composites for applications in bone replacement and repair. Acta Biomater. 2011; 7(1): 16–30. DOI: 10.1016/j.actbio.2010.07.012.

[10] Tampieri A, Celotti G, Landi E, Sandri M, Roveri N, Falini G. Biologically inspired synthesis of bone like composite: Self-assembled collagen fibers/hydroxyapatite nanocrystals. J Biomed Mater Res. 2003; 67A: 618–625.

[11] Tampieri A, Sandri M, Landi E, Pressato D, Francioli S, Quarto R, Martin I. Design of graded biomimetic osteochondral composite scaffolds. Biomaterials. 2008; 29(26): 3539–3546. DOI: 10.1016/j.biomaterials.2008.05.008.

[12] Bigi A, Foresti E, Gregorini R, Ripamonti A, Roveri N, Shah JS. The role of magnesium on the structure of biological apatite. Calcif Tissue Int. 1992; 50: 439–444. DOI: 10.1007/BF00296775.

[13] Pietak AM, Reid JW, Stott MJ, Sayer M. Silicon substitution in the calcium phosphate bioceramics. Biomaterials. 2007; 28: 4023–4032. DOI: 10.1016/j.biomaterials.2007.05.003.

[14] Schwarz K. A bound form of Si in glycosaminoglycans and polyuronides. Proc Nat Acad Sci USA. 1973; 70: 1608–1612. DOI: 10.1073/*pnas*.70.5.1608.

[15] Eppell SJ, Tong WD, Katz JL, Kuhn L, Glimcher MJ. Shape and size of isolated bone mineralites measured using atomic force microscopy. J Orthop Res. 2001; 19: 1027–1034.

[16] Weiner S, Price PA. Disaggregation of bone into crystals. Calcif Tissue Int. 1986; 39: 365–375.

[17] Traub W, Arad T, Weiner S. Three-dimensional ordered distribution of crystals in turkey tendon collagen fibers. Proc Natl Acad Sci 1989; 86: 9822–9826.

[18] Kon E, Delcogliano M, Filardo G, Fini M, Giavaresi G, Francioli S, Martin I, Pressato D, Arcangeli E, Quarto R, Sandri M, Marcacci M. Orderly osteochondral regeneration in a sheep model using a novel nano-composite multilayered biomaterial. J Orthop Res. 2010; 28: 116–124. DOI: 10.1002/jor.20958.

[19] Linde A, Goldberg M. Dentinogenesis. Crit Rev Oral Biol Med. 1993; 4(5): 679–728. DOI: 10.1007/s00418-009-0556-6.

[20] Sprio S, Sandri M, Iafisco M, Panseri S, Filardo G, Kon E, Marcacci M, Tampieri A. Composite biomedical foams for engineering bone tissue. In: Netti PA, editor. Biomedical Foams for Tissue Engineering Applications. Cambridge (UK): Woodhead Publishing Limited; 2014. pp. 249–280. ISBN: 9780857096968.

[21] Giannoudis PV, Atkins R. Management of long-bone non-unions. Injury. 2007; 38(Suppl. 2): S1–S2. DOI: 10.1016/j.injury.2011.03.036.

[22] Kanakaris NK, Giannoudis PV. The health economics of the treatment of long-bone non-unions. Injury. 2007; 38(Suppl. 2): S77. DOI: 10.1016/S0020-1383(07)80012-X.

[23] Stevenson S. The immune response to osteochondral allografts in dogs. J Bone Joint Surg Am. 1987; 69(4): 573–582. DOI: 10.1007/s11999-008-0444-8.

[24] Lord CF, Gebhardt MC, Tomford WW, Mankin HJ. Infection in bone allografts. Incidence, nature, and treatment. J Bone Joint Surg Am. 1988; 70(3): 369–376.

[25] Mankin HJ, Gebhardt MC, Tomford WW. The use of frozen cadaveric allografts in the management of patients with bone tumors of the extremities. Orthop Clin North Am. 1987; 18(2): 275–289.

[26] Alman BA, De Bari A, Krajbich JI. Massive allografts in the treatment of osteosarcoma and Ewing sarcoma in children and adolescents. J Bone Joint Surg Am 1995; 77(1): 54–64. DOI: 10.1007/s11999-010-1362-0.

[27] Berrey BH Jr, Lord CF, Gebhardt MC, Mankin HJ. Fractures of allografts. Frequency, treatment, and end-results. J Bone Joint Surg Am. 1990; 72(6): 825–833.

[28] Daculsi G. Biphasic calcium phosphate concept applied to artificial bone, implant coating and injectable bone substitute. Biomaterials. 1998; 19: 1473–1478. DOI: 10.1016/S0142-9612(98)00061-1.

[29] Kessler S, Mayr-Wohlfart U, Ignatius A, Puhl W, Claes L, Günther KP. The impact of bone morphogenetic protein-2 (BMP-2), vascular endothelial growth factor (VEGF) and basic fibroblast growth factor (b-FGF) on the osteointegration, the degradation and biomechanical properties of a synthetic bone substitute. Z Orthop. 2003; 141: 472–480. DOI: 10.1055/s-2003-41569.

[30] Conor TB, O'Kelly KU. Fabrication and characterization of a porous multidomain hydroxyapatite scaffold for bone tissue engineering investigations. J Biomed Mater Res Part B: Appl Biomater. 2010; 93B: 459–467. DOI: 10.1002/jbm.b.31603.

[31] Babis GC, Soucacos PN. Bone scaffolds: The role of mechanical stability and instrumentation. Int J Care Injured. 2005; 36S: S38–S44. DOI: 10.1016/j.injury.2005.10.009.

[32] Sprio S, Ruffini A, Valentini F, D'Alessandro T, Sandri M, Panseri S, Tampieri A. Biomimesis and biomorphic transformations: New concepts applied to bone regeneration. J Biotechnol. 2011; 156(4): 347–355. DOI: 10.1016/j.jbiotec.2011.07.034.

[33] Ingber DE. The architecture of life. Sci Am. 1998; 278(1): 48–57.

[34] Li J, Han D, Zhao Y-P. Kinetic behaviour of the cells touching substrate: The interfacial stiffness guides cell spreading. Sci Rep. 2014; 4: 3910. DOI: 10.1038/srep03910.

[35] Cameron AR, Frith JE, Cooper-White JJ. The influence of substrate creep on mesenchymal stem cell behaviour and phenotype. Biomaterials. 2011; 32(26): 5979–5993. DOI: 10.1016/*j.biomaterials*.2011.04.003.

[36] Wells RG. The role of matrix stiffness in regulating cell behavior. Hepatol. 2008; 47: 1394–1400. DOI: 10.1002/hep.22193.

[37] Pavalko FM, Norvell SM, Burr DB, Turner CH, Duncan RL, Bidwell JP. A model for mechanotransduction in bone cells: The load-bearing mechanosomes. J Cell Biochem. 2003; 88: 104–112. DOI: 10.1002/jcb.10284.

[38] Sikavitsas VI. Biomaterials and bone mechanotransduction. Biomaterials. 2001; 22: 2581–2593. DOI: 10.1016/S0142-9612(01)00002-3.

[39] Bilezikian JP, Raisz LG, Rodan GA. Principles of Bone Biology. 3rd ed., vol. 1. San Diego: Academic Press; 2002. ISBN: 0-12-098652-3.

[40] Fratzl P, Weinkamer R. Nature's hierarchical materials. Prog Mater Sci. 2007; 52: 1263–1334. DOI: 10.1016/j.pmatsci.2007.06.001.

[41] Wegst UGK, Ashby MF. The mechanical efficiency of natural materials. Philos Mag. 2004; 84: 2167–2181. DOI: 10.1080/14786430410001680935.

[42] Gibson EJ. Wood: A natural fibre reinforced composite. Met Mater. 1992; 6: 333–336.

[43] Tampieri A, Sprio S, Ruffini A, Celotti G, Lesci IG, Roveri N. From wood to bone: Multi-step process to convert wood hierarchical structures into biomimetic hydroxyapatite scaffolds for bone tissue engineering. J Mater Chem. 2009; 19(28): 4973–4980. DOI: 10.1039/b900333a.

[44] Minardi S, Pandolfi L, Taraballi F, De Rosa E, Yazdi IK, Liu X, Ferrari M, Tasciotti E. PLGA-mesoporous silicon microspheres for the in vivo controlled temporospatial delivery of proteins. ACS Appl Mater Interfaces. 2015; 7(30): 16364–16373. DOI: 10.1021/acsami.5b03464.

[45] Pankhurst QA, Connolly J, Jones SK, Dobson J. Applications of magnetic nanoparticles in biomedicine. J Phys D Appl Phys. 2003; 36: R167–81. DOI: 10.1088/ 0022–3727/36/13/201.

[46] Ramchand CN, Priyadarshini P, Kopcansky P, Metha RV. Applications of magnetic fluids in medicine and biotechnology. Indian J Pure Appl Phys. 2001; 39: 683–689. DOI: 10.1016/j.jmmm.2006.10.1184.

[47] Meng J, Xiao B, Zhang Y, Liu J, Xue H, Lei J, Kong H, Huang Y, Jin Z, Gu N, Xu H. Super-paramagnetic responsive nanofibrous scaffolds under static magnetic field enhance osteogenesis for bone repair in vivo. Sci Rep. 2013; 3: 2655–2662. DOI: 10.1038/srep02655.

[48] Panseri S, Russo A, Sartori M, Giavaresi G, Sandri M, Fini M, Maltarello MC, Shelyakova T, Ortolani A, Visani A, Dediu V, Tampieri A, Marcacci M. Modifying bone scaffold architecture in vivo with permanent magnets to facilitate fixation of magnetic scaffolds. Bone. 2013; 56: 432–439. DOI: 10.1016/j.bone.2013.07.015.

[49] Shan D, Shi Y, Duan S, Wei Y, Cai Q, Yang X. Electrospun magnetic poly(L-lactide) (PLLA) nanofibers by incorporating PLLA-stabilized Fe_3O_4 nanoparticles. Mater Sci Eng C. 2013; 33: 3498–3505. DOI: 10.1016/j.msec.2013.04.040.

[50] Meng J, Zhang Y, Qi X, Kong H, Wang C, Xu Z, Xie S, Gu N, Xu H. Paramagnetic nanofibrous composite films enhance the osteogenic responses of pre-osteoblast cells. Nanoscale. 2010; 2: 2565–2569. DOI: 10.1039/c0nr00178c.

[51] Hou R, Zhang G, Du G, Zhan D, Cong Y, Cheng Y, Fu J. Magnetic nanohydroxyapatite/PVA composite hydrogels for promoted osteoblast adhesion and proliferation. Colloids Surf B. 2013; 103: 318–325. DOI: 10.1016/j.colsurfb.2012.10.067.

[52] Mertens ME, Hermann A, Bühren A, Olde-Damink L, Möckel D, Gremse F, Ehling J, Kiessling F, Lammers T. Iron oxide-labeled collagen scaffolds for non-invasive MR imaging in tissue engineering. Adv Funct Mater. 2014; 24: 754–762. DOI: 10.1002/adfm.201301275.

[53] Lewinski N, Colvin V, Drezek R. Cytotoxicity of nanoparticles. Small. 2008; 4: 26–49. DOI: 10.1002/smll.200700595.

[54] Singh N, Jenking GJS, Asadi R, Doak SH. Potential toxicity of superparamagnetic iron oxide nanoparticles (SPION). Nano Reviews. 2010; 1: 53–58. DOI: 10.3402/nano.v1i0.5358.

[55] Fresnais J, Yan M, Courtois J, Bostelmann T, Bée A, Berret J-F. Poly(acrylic acid)-coated iron oxide nanoparticles: Quantitative evaluation of the coating properties and applications for the removal of a pollutant dye. J Coll Interf Sci. 2013; 395: 24–30. DOI: 10.1016/j.jcis.2012.12.011.

[56] Castelló J, Gallardo M, Busquets MA, Estelrich J. Chitosan (or alginate)-coated iron oxide nanoparticles: A comparative study. Coll Surf A: Physicochem Eng Asp. 2015; 468: 151–158. DOI: 10.1016/j.colsurfa.2014.12.031.

[57] Yue-Jian C, Juan T, Fei X, Jia-Bi Z, Ning G, Yi-Hua Z, Ye D, Liang G. Synthesis, self-assembly, and characterization of PEG-coated iron oxide nanoparticles as potential MRI contrast agent. Drug Dev Ind Pharm. 2010;36(10): 1235–1244. DOI: 10.3109/03639041003710151.

[58] Tampieri A, D'Alessandro T, Sandri M, Sprio S, Landi E, Bertinetti L, Panseri S, Pepponi G, Goettlicher J, Bañobre-López M, Rivas J. Intrinsic magnetism and hyperthermia in bioactive Fe-doped hydroxyapatite. Acta Biomater. 2012; 8(2): 843–851. DOI: 10.1016/j.actbio.2011.09.032.

[59] Panseri S, Cunha C, D'Alessandro T, Sandri M, Giavaresi G, Marcacci M, Hung CT, Tampieri A. Intrinsically superparamagnetic Fe-hydroxyapatite nanoparticles positively influence osteoblast-like cell behavior. J Nanobiotechnol. 2012; 10: 32–42. DOI: 10.1186/1477-3155-*10*-32.

[60] Clavijo-Jordan V, Kodibagkar VD, Beeman SC, Hann BD, Bennett KM. Principles and emerging applications of nanomagnetic materials in medicine. WIREs Nanomed Nanobiotechnol. 2012; 4: 345–365. DOI: 10.1002/wnan.1169.

[61] Grace KLR, Revell WJ, Brookes M. The effects of pulsed electromagnetism on fresh fracture healing: Osteochondral repair in the rat femoral groove. Orthopedics. 1998; 21: 297–302.

[62] Glazer PA, Heilmann MR, Lotz JC, Bradford DS. Use of electromagnetic fields in a spinal fusion: A rabbit model. Spine. 1997; 22(20): 2351–2356.

[63] Yan QC, Tomita N, Ikada Y. Effects of static magnetic field on bone formation of rat femurs. Med Eng Phys. 1998; 20: 397–402. DOI: 10.1016/S1350-4533(98)00051-4.

[64] Assiotis A, Sachinis NP, Chalidis BE. Pulsed electromagnetic fields for the treatment of tibial delayed unions and nonunions. A prospective clinical study and review of the literature. J Orthop Sur Res. 2012; 7: 24. DOI: 10.1186/1749-799X-7-24.

[65] Chalidis B, Sachinis N, Assiotis A, Maccauro G. Stimulation of bone formation and fracture healing with pulsed electromagnetic fields: Biologic responses and clinical implications. Int J Immunopathol Pharmacol. 2011; 24: 17–20.

[66] Tampieri A, Iafisco M, Sandri M, Panseri S, Cunha C, Sprio S, Savini E, Uhlarz M, Herrmannsdörfer T. Magnetic bio-inspired hybrid nanostructured collagen-hydroxyapatite scaffolds supporting cell proliferation and tuning regenerative process. ACS Appl Mater Interf. 2014; 6(18): 15697–15707. DOI: 10.1021/am5050967.

[67] Torbet J, Ronziere MC. Magnetic alignment of collagen during self-assembly. Biochem J. 1984; 219: 1057–1059.

[68] Higashi T, Yamagishi A, Takeuchi T, Kawaguchi N, Sagawa S, Onishi S, Date M. Orientation of erythrocytes in a strong static magnetic field. Blood. 1993; 82: 1328–1334. DOI: 10.1007/s11626-0030005-0.

[69] Kotani H, Kawaguchi H, Shimoaka T, Iwasaka M, Ueno S, Ozawa H, Nakamura K, Hoshi K. Strong static magnetic field stimulates bone formation to a definite orientation in vitro and in Vivo. J Bone Miner Res. 2002; 17: 1814–1821. DOI: 10.1359/jbmr.2002.17.10.1814.

[70] Xu H-Y, Gu N. Magnetic responsive scaffolds and magnetic fields in bone repair and regeneration. Front Mater Sci. 2014; 8: 20–31. DOI: 10.1007/s11706-014-0232-1.

[71] Ganguly R, Puri IK. Microfluidic transport in magnetic MEMS and bioMEMS. WIREs Nanomed Nanobiotechnol. 2010; 2: 382–399. DOI: 10.1002/wnan.92.

[72] Veiseh O, Gunn JW, Zhang MQ. Design and fabrication of magnetic nanoparticles for targeted drug delivery and imaging. Adv Drug Deliv Rev. 2010; 62: 284–304. DOI: 10.1016/j.addr.2009.11.002.

[73] Sperling RA, Parak WJ. Surface modification, functionalization and bioconjugation of colloidal inorganic nanoparticles. Philos Transact A Math Phys Eng Sci. 2010; 368: 1333–1383. DOI: 10.1098/rsta.2009.0273.

[74] Yiu HH, McBain SC, Lethbridge ZA, Lees MR, Dobson J. Preparation and characterization of polyethylenimine-coated Fe_3O_4-MCM-48 nanocomposite particles as a novel agent for magnet assisted transfection. J Biomed Mater Res A. 2010; 92: 386–392.

[75] Schellenberger E, Schnorr J, Reutelingsperger C, Ungethum L, Meyer W, Taupitz M, Hamm B. Linking proteins with anionic nanoparticles via protamine: Ultrasmall protein-coupled probes for magnetic resonance imaging of apoptosis. Small. 2008; 4: 225–230. DOI: 10.1002/smll.200700847.

[76] Yu MK, Jeong YY, Park J, Park S, Kim JW, Min JJ, Kim K, Jon S. Drug-loaded superparamagnetic iron oxide nanoparticles for combined cancer imaging and therapy in vivo. Angew Chem Int Ed Engl. 2008; 47: 5362–5365. DOI: 10.1002/anie.200800857.

[77] Dilnawaz F, Singh A, Mohanty C, Sahoo SK. Dual drug loaded superparamagnetic iron oxide nanoparticles for targeted cancer therapy. Biomaterials. 2010; 31: 3694–3706. DOI: 10.1016/j.biomaterials.2010.01.057.

[78] Bañobre-Lopez M, Piñeiro-Redondo Y, De Santis R, Gloria A, Ambrosio L, Tampieri A, Dediu V, Rivas J. Poly(caprolactone) based magnetic scaffolds for bone tissue engineering. J Appl Phys. 2011; 109: 07B313. DOI: 10.1063/1.3561149.

[79] Gloria A, Russo T, D'Amora U, Zeppetelli S, D'Alessandro T, Sandri M, Bañobre-Lopez M, Piñeiro-Redondo Y, Uhlarz M, Tampieri A, Rivas J, Herrmannsdörfer T, Dediu VA, Ambrosio L, De Santis R. Magnetic poly(ε-caprolactone)/iron-doped hydroxyapatite nanocomposite substrates for advanced bone tissue engineering. J R Soc Interf. 2013; 10: 20120833. DOI: 10.1098/rsif.2012.0833.

[80] Iafisco M, Sandri M, Panseri S, Delgado-Lopez JM, Gomez-Morales J, Tampieri A. Magnetic bioactive and biodegradable hollow Fe-doped hydroxyapatite coated poly(L-lactic) acid micro–nanospheres. Chem Mater. 2013; 25: 2610–2617. DOI: 10.1021/cm4007298.

[81] Nappini S, Bonini M, Bombelli FB, Pineider F, Sangregorio CL, Baglioi P, Norden B. Controlled drug release under a low frequency magnetic field: Effect of the citrate coating on magnetoliposomes stability. Soft Matter. 2011; 7: 1025–1037. DOI: 10.1039/C0SM00789G.

Chapter 8

The Impact of Graphene Oxide on Bone Regeneration Therapies

Anca Hermenean, Sorina Dinescu,
Mariana Ionita and Marieta Costache

Additional information is available at the end of the chapter

http://dx.doi.org/10.5772/63333

Abstract

Currently, there are several tissue engineering strategies meant to overcome the incomplete or insufficient bone regeneration conditions offered by autologous bone graft or surgery approaches. In the last decade, attention has been focused toward finding the equilibrium between a suitable scaffold with osteoinductive properties, a cell source with evident potential to develop bone tissue and the appropriate pro-osteogenic factors to condition the differentiation process after cell-scaffold implantation. Consequently, this chapter aims to discuss the benefits that graphene and its derivatives, graphene oxide (GO), bring both to the scaffold biomaterial and to the interaction between the material and the cellular component in order to create a favorable micro-environment for efficient osteogenic differentiation process. Several advantages of including GO in the composition of the materials are shown in relation to cell viability, proliferation, attachment, and osteogenic differentiation.

Keywords: graphene oxide, bone regeneration, cell-scaffold interaction, cell adhesion, cytocompatibility

1. Introduction

New materials with outstanding osteoinductive properties and abilities to promote osteogenesis at the implant site are constantly developed for bone tissue engineering applications. One of these new-generation materials with documented pro-osteogenic effects is graphene [1–3]. Graphene and its derivatives are nanomaterials with specific physical and chemical properties compatible with bone regeneration, and therefore, they possess high potential for bone tissue engineering approaches. To date, the information about graphene and its derivatives contribution to bone tissue engineering is relatively limited. In this perspective, superior results were reported after graphene functionalization and immobilization of the derivative on different scaffold biomaterials. This approach was successful probably due to the fact that functional groups can reduce the hydrophobic interactions between graphene and the cellular component [4], thus enhancing improved biocompatibility of the resulted material. In particular, graphene oxide (GO) have been promoted as one of the most valuable graphene derivatives with excellent results in bone regeneration [5, 6]. Nowadays, the beneficial effects of graphene and its derivatives are tested in various biomedical applications—anti-cancer therapy, biosensors, drug delivery, and tissue engineering [7–9].

2. GO impact on material bioactivity and cytocompatibility

A very strong interconnection exists between the structural, physicochemical properties, and cytotoxic potential of the materials. Characteristics such as the flat shape, surface charges, and uncontrolled nanobiodegradability of graphene and its derivatives condition a relative nanocytotoxicity that has been reported [10] and currently represents a challenge for the use of graphene-based nanomaterials in clinical applications. Although a lot of positive observations related to the beneficial effects that graphene and GO have on cell growth, expansion, proliferation, and even differentiation of stem cells, caution and safety issues should still be taken into consideration when materials designed with graphene/GO are included in practical tissue engineering.

Most of the *in vitro* studies, which have aimed to evaluate different material compositions with GO content for biocompatibility, have reported a slight decrease in cell viability after contact with GO [11, 12]. However, cell response in contact with biomaterials can vary depending on the GO concentration and the material form of synthesis. Chng and Pumera study from 2013 [13] revealed that GO degree of cytotoxicity was related to the carbon/oxygen (C/O) ratio and the number and distribution of carbonyl residues on the surface of the material. Additionally, the particular conformation adopted by the GO sheets inside a material structure can have an impact on cell behavior in contact to the material [14]. Particularly, a higher degree of compaction in GO sheets determined a lower viability in dermal fibroblasts. This decrease in viability was also associated with the increase in the levels of reactive oxygen species (ROS) in human dermal fibroblasts [14, 15]. Related to this, the activation of caspase-3 pro-apoptotic marker, as well as the release of lactate dehydrogenase (LDH) by PC12 cells, was also reported when the cells were cultured in highly condensed GO sheets materials. These observations lead to the hypothesis that added in very high concentrations to the scaffold or distributed as a very dense network to support material's structure, GO could actually determine a negative influence upon cell viability and response.

For bone tissue engineering purposes, particularly for orthopedic implants, a composite film based on ultrahigh molecular weight polyethylene (UHMWPE) improved with 0.1–1 wt% graphene nanoplatelets was tested for cytocompatibility with bone cells. The cytotoxicity tests indicated that the increase in graphene nanoplatelets concentration could decrease bone cells viability over 5 days of culture, possibly due to the agglomeration of particles [16].

Other experiments have shown the contrary—that GO added in certain concentrations in the material has no influence upon cell viability or in some cases even has a positive effect on cell proliferation. In this respect, Sahu et al. [17] has published a study dedicated to thermosensitive hydrogel with GO content in regard to cytotoxicity and concluded that the addition of GO in the composition had no pro-inflammatory effects and that the hydrogel was biocompatible. Studies performed on titanium substrates coated with GO [18] also confirmed that graphene derivatives are biocompatible, present low toxicity, and a large dosage loading capacity, thus being able to function as a carrier for delivery of therapeutic proteins.

Conversely, a series of studies highlighted the importance of functionalizing graphene-based materials in order to minimize its potential cytotoxic effects. Graphene is hydrophobic and easily aggregates in solutions with salts, proteins, ions that can produce toxic effects. Covalent or non-covalent modifications can be performed in order to counteract the cytotoxic-susceptible properties of this material [19]. First, it was observed that the addition of polyethylene glycol (PEG) to GO ensures stability in physiological solutions [20]. Another study [21] emphasized that carboxylated graphene displays higher hydrophilicity and reduced cytotoxicity, due to the fact that carboxylation weakens the hydrophobic interactions between graphene and cellular membranes [19].

Based on positive results reported on grapheme derivates, we have recently tested for cytocompatibility nanomaterials based on polysulfone (PS) and different concentrations of carboxylated graphene (PS/G-COOH). Preliminary observations indicated that cells displayed a very good viability and adhesion in contact with these materials and that proliferation rates were improved as compared with control materials (pure polymer materials) (manuscript under revision).

In the same context, our group published a series of studies highlighting the importance of GO present in either bidimensional (2D) or tridimensional (3D) biomaterials for cell viability and proliferation.

When testing the cytocompatibility of chitosan/GO composite films [22], with 0.5, 1, 2.5, and 6 wt% GO content, MC3T3-E1 murine preosteoblasts adapted faster and proliferated more in contact with the chitosan/GO biocomposites with a higher content of GO. The biocomposite chitosan/GO 6 wt% proved to be biocompatible and displayed the most equilibrated ratio between the pro-proliferative and cytotoxic potential. In this case, viability and proliferation potential was assessed at 2, 4, and 7 days both quantitatively by MTT assay and qualitatively by LiveDead assay and by means of fluorescence microscopy. Fluorescence microscopy images revealed that cells progressively proliferated and reached confluent monolayers on all chitosan/GO biocomposite films, but the cellular density was found to be higher on the composite materials with 2.5 and 6 wt% GO content than that on the chitosan/GO composite films with lower GO content or 2D control. Additionally, a particular cell distribution was noticed for 2.5 and 6 wt% GO biomaterials, suggesting that GO could have an influence on cell behavior and distribution. The composites with 2.5 and 6 wt% GO content registered increased cell proliferation than the films with low GO loading and controls, particularly after 7 days of culture, as shown by MTT. Conversely, LDH quantification showed a significantly lower profile for chitosan/GO 6 wt% biocomposite than for control chitosan, thus supporting the hypothesis that increase in GO content in material's composition positively influences cell proliferation.

Further on, similar studies were carried out for graphene oxide/chitosan–polyvinyl alcohol films (CS–PVA/GO) in order to determine the cytocompatibility of these materials and the possible interference of GO with cell viability and proliferation [23]. Scanning electron microscopy (SEM), transmission electron microscopy (TEM), and X-ray diffraction (XRD) were first employed to assess CS–PVA/GO nanocomposites structural and surface properties. Good GO nanosheets dispersion within the polymer matrix and excellent thermal stability and mechanical strength were shown for these composites, while the highest tensile modulus was obtained for CS–PVA/GO 6 wt%. During biocompatibility tests, an interesting cell distribution was highlighted when the GO concentration increased in the composition of the nanomaterials. Cell alignment and behavior were correlated with the observed GO nanosheets small aggregations within the polymer matrix. Simultaneously, no significant cytotoxic potential was reported for the composites even when increasing the GO concentration to 2.5 or 6 wt% and a general increasing profile of cell viability and proliferation was described during 7 days of *in vitro* culture. Particularly, the composite material with 6 wt% GO proved to display the lowest cytotoxic potential by levels of lactate dehydrogenase released in the cell culture media and to favor most efficiently the proliferation of murine preosteoblasts during 1 week of culture in standard conditions. Statistical significant differences were observed in terms of viability and proliferation between nanomaterials with low GO content (0.5 and 1 wt%) and high GO content (2.5 and 6 wt%).

Similar results were obtained for nanofibrous biocomposite scaffolds of PVA/GO [24] using the same MC3T3-E1 preosteoblasts. In this case, cells were able to grow and attach to the surface of the materials and not change in cell viability was indicated when increasing GO concentration up to 5 wt% in the composition.

A composite with particular good results, holding promises for future biomedical application as a filtration membrane, nanocarrier, or support for bone regeneration, is a bidimensional film based on polysulfone (PS) and GO nanosheets [25]. In this case, PS composites with 0.25, 0.5, and 1 wt% GO were compared in terms of cytocompatibility with PS controls. Based on special conditions of synthesis, the GO nanosheets were uniformly distributed within the PS matrix, thus ensuring a more ordered structure, as revealed by XRD analysis. Clear improvement of thermal and mechanical properties of the composites was revealed when GO was added in the matrix. These changes in the structure were correlated with the bioactivity tested for PS/GO nanomaterials. Very low levels of cytotoxicity were detected during 1 week of culture for all compositions, and no relevant increase in LDH levels was found when 0.25–1 wt% GO was added, suggesting that the low cytotoxic potential of the composite was due to the basal cytotoxicity of the PS substrate. Conversely, quantitative data showed a slight increase in cell viability during 7 days of *in vitro* culture, but statistically significant values were obtained only for the composite with 1 wt% GO, when comparing cell viabilities at 7 and

4 days of culture. Additionally, the tendency of cell grouping was emphasized by fluorescence microscopy only for PS/GO 1 wt%, as compared to the other composites and to the PS membrane [25].

Similarly, membranes based on poly(ε-caprolactone) (PCL) reinforced with GO nanoplatelets revealed good results toward use in bone regeneration due to the improvements in bioactivity [26]. PCL/GO nanocomposites showed better mechanical properties than PCL films due to the fiber organization and strengthening offered by GO, reflected also in better bioactivity due to the anionic functional groups on GO surface.

Due to the tridimensional structure of the bone, in certain bone reconstruction applications, a tridimensional porous scaffold is required to mimic bone and to resemble the appropriate conditions for regeneration. Thus, tridimensional materials with mechanical and physical–structural properties close to bone were investigated for biocompatibility and potential for bone tissue engineering. In this respect, the cytocompatibility of chitosan/GO scaffolds improved with 0.5 and 3 wt% GO has been tested both by means of indirect and direct studies [27]. Previous reports have shown that chitosan is particularly attractive for bone reconstruction medical applications due to its good biocompatibility, biodegradability, and ability to support osteoblast attachment and proliferation [28, 29]. Remarkably, the addition of GO to the composition of the scaffolds did not affect cell viability, but even resulted in a lower cytotoxicity of the extract collected from chitosan/GO 3 wt% after 24 h of contact with cells. These observations were correlated with the increasing proliferation profile obtained by MTT assay after 7 days of direct contact between murine preosteoblasts from MC-3T3 line and the materials. The data showed that the addition of 3 wt% GO to the chitosan matrix greatly improved the composite properties and bioactivity, suggesting that GO could have positive effects on cell behavior and metabolic activity [27].

Another combination of chitosan (CS) and GO was used as a template to fabricate hydroxyapatite (HA) nanocomposites resembling bone structure [30]. CS–GO–HA and GO–HA matrices displayed good properties to support murine fibroblast and human osteoblast-*like* cells proliferation, but when compared in terms of viability and bioactivity toward mineralization, chitosan functionalized GO matrix provided better conditions for bone repair.

Preliminary positive results for tridimensional GO-containing scaffolds designed specifically for bone tissue repair were also recently reported for gelatin–poly(vinyl alcohol) biocomposites reinforced with GO [31]. In this case, the combination between a naturally occurring compound (gelatin), a synthetically derived one (polyvinyl alcohol) and GO resulted in a biocomposite with equilibrated physical–chemical properties and low cytotoxic profile that allowed murine preosteoblasts viability.

Further tests are required to select the most appropriate biocomposites to serve as platforms to study osteogenic differentiation and thus to validate the most promising biomaterials with application in bone regeneration therapies.

3. GO effects on cell adhesion

In general, it has been shown that the addition of GO favors the interaction between a cellular component and a material substrate, thus ensuring a positive effect on cell adhesion. Several studies [32, 33, 1] have demonstrated that bone marrow mesenchymal stem cells (BM-MSCs) developed a fusiform phenotype with multiple elongations and focal adhesion points in contact with graphene derivatives. These observations support the idea that GO favors cytoskeleton development and enhances cell adhesion to the material that contains GO. Experimental conditions used for 3D scaffolds based on chitosan ± GO or nylon ± GO [34, 2, 6] also concluded that osteoblasts or preosteoblasts adhered better in the presence of GO to the substrate materials. The mechanism underlying GO enhancement of cell adhesion has not been elucidated yet, but Kim et al. [35] suggested that the initiation of focal adhesions is in direct correlation with the nanotopography conditioned by GO.

From our experience, GO also induced a positive effect on murine preosteoblasts adhesion to polysulfone/GO biofilms [25]. A more developed F-actin cytoskeleton has been identified in the presence of 3 wt% GO by confocal microscopy, as compared to the cell cytoskeleton observed for pure polysulfone or plysulfone with 0.5–1 wt% GO addition.

To support this hypothesis, a substrate based on collagen and GO was developed and tested together with rat BM-MSCs for bioactivity in terms of cell viability, cell adhesion, and cell differentiation to bone cells [36]. An obvious dependency of F-actin fiber distribution with the GO content in the biomaterial was reported in this case, confirming our observations.

Other studies [37] described an increased cell adhesion when using GO in conjunction with fibronectin and titanium substrates. In this case, adhesion was evaluated by looking at focal adhesion molecules expression and localization. Vinculin was found to be highly active in the central and peripheral contact area of the cells cultivated in contact with fibronectin and GO.

Good adhesion of cells to their substrate is crucial for cellular processes such as survival, growth, and activation of molecular pathways involved in proliferation. In particular, it has been shown several times that adhesion to the material is essential to induce the molecular program underlying osteogenic differentiation and maturation to functional osteoblasts and osteocytes capable to produce bone-specific extracellular matrix.

4. GO benefits for cell differentiation processes

Scaffolds with different GO content have been previously reported as good substrates for osteogenic differentiation and consequently, for bone tissue regeneration therapies. The ability of graphene and GO to improve the characteristics of scaffold materials and to promote mesenchymal stem cells adhesion, proliferation, and differentiation toward osteogenic lineages has been intensely studied and demonstrated [3, 38, 1, 2, 39]. Lee et al. [33] have reported a proportional correlation between GO presence in the substrate material and the degree of cell osteogenic differentiation. Particularly, this study has highlighted the possibility that graphene-based substrates behave like concentration platforms for pro-osteogenic induction factors. Nayak et al. [1] have also shown that GO-covered materials accelerated osteogenic differentiation of human mesenchymal stem cells, as compared to the non-GO-treated-substrates. They concluded that the rate of differentiation conditioned by the GO scaffold is comparable to the osteogenic differentiation induced by specific growth factors and inducers in a conditional media.

Great emphasis has been placed on the development of biomaterials that mimic the structure, composition, and properties of endogenous tissue using the biomimetic method [10]. Since the osteogenic process is based on a combination of signals that will promote the nucleation of hydroxyapatite [40–42], it is essential that the bioengineered scaffold has properties that will induce the assembly of bone-*like* apatite, resembling the natural bone [10]. Considering that charged groups can resemble extracellular matrix proteins and induce the mineralization process, functionalization of GO by bioactive molecules such as dopamine and carrageenan [43] or creation of an interface by modification of GO by gelatin [42] resulted in biomimetic mineralization of hydroxyapatite. Correlated to this enhancement in mineralization, higher cell proliferation, adhesion, and osteogenic potential as shown by alkaline phosphatase activity were reported for MC3T3-E1 preosteoblasts cultured in contact with GO–gelatin surface, as compared to the negative controls [42]. Consequently, these observations can further contribute to the development of more efficient cell–scaffold interfaces based on GO properties for successful application in bone surgery.

Although it was confirmed by an increasing number of studies, the molecular mechanism underlying the ability of graphene or GO to induce by itself the osteogenic differentiation process has not yet been elucidated. Xie et al. [44] designed bidimensional and tridimensional graphene-based substrates to comparatively evaluate the crucial molecular events taking place during periodontal ligament stem cells differentiation to bone cells in these substrates. Bone-specific markers such as RUNX2, collagen type I, osteocalcin were found to be upregulated at gene and protein levels of expression in GO substrates, as a proof of differentiation. A combination of physical and chemical properties of graphene act synergistically to control the osteoinductive effect of graphene [44].

Since they did not show significant cytotoxicity during the biocompatibility studies, graphitic nanomaterials based on carbon nanotubes and carboxylated graphenes were evaluated for capacity to stimulate osteogenesis in the perspective of bone regeneration nanomedicine [45]. The study showed that the activation of the osteogenic differentiation program, synthesis of specific bone markers, and mineral deposition was possible for murine preosteoblasts in MC3T3-E1 cells cultivated in contact with these materials.

An interesting approach in order to evaluate the positive effects of GO on cell differentiation to bone was to incorporate GO nanoparticles in the structure of a scaffold designed for bone tissue reconstruction. Hybrid nanoparticles resulted from reduced GO nanosheets and strontium metallic nanoparticles were then incorporated in poly(ε-caprolactone) matrix with the purpose to test the composite for osteoinductive properties [46]. Increased rates of osteoblast proliferation and differentiation were detected for the scaffold containing GO nanoparticles, as compared to the control, and this bioactivity was associated with the release of strontium ions from the system.

Apart from its positive influence on cell viability and proliferation, functionalized graphene or GO proved also to favor efficient osteogenesis. By coating fibrin on the surface of GO, a novel nanocomposite (FGO) resulted as a potential solution for bone tissue engineering applications. Based on the analysis of bone markers' profile, release of calcium ions and alkaline phosphatase activity registered in osteoblast-*like* cells MG-63 cultivated in contact with this material, FGO was confirmed to have osteoinductive properties and to be a good candidate for medical applications [47]. Following the same trend of functionalized GO, another group of researchers [48] developed a gelatin functionalized GO composite with the purpose to use the surface charged proteins to mimic mineralization of hydroxyapatite and to obtain functional bone tissue and matrix. The gelatin–GO surface allowed bioactivity as cell adhesion and proliferation, and additionally, it promoted the formation of osteoid mineral matrix during murine cells osteogenic differentiation when compared to control glass surfaces.

The success and efficiency in bone regenerative medicine applications greatly depend on the structure and properties of the implantable biomaterials, but also on the source and type of cells used to condition regeneration. In the past few years, attention was focused on the use of adult stem cells that display the capacity to differentiate toward bone lineage. In this respect, mesenchymal stem cells became most widely used for bone replacement therapies since it was observed their preferential tendency to differentiate to osteogenic lineage when exposed to mechanically stiff scaffolds resembling bone tissue structure. One study [49] showed that when including GO flakes in the composition of soft collagen scaffolds, the resulted composite acquired the necessary stiffness and properties to support MSCs differentiation to bone-*like* cells. Moreover, enhanced osteogenesis was found in cells exposed to GO composite conditions as a result of good MSCs adhesion to the substrate.

An enhanced cell adhesion to the scaffold appears to be crucial for an efficient osteogenic differentiation process. Preosteoblasts, which were previously shown to strongly adhere to fibronectin/GO surface (Fn-Tigra) developed on titanium materials by electrodropping [37], were also shown to differentiate to mature osteoblasts able to produce osteocalcin, type I collagen, and calcium during 2 weeks of culture in contact with this substrate.

Bioceramics became very important in the context of bone tissue engineering. A group of researchers [50] designed a β-tricalcium phosphate covered in modified GO (β-TCP-GRA) and studied the interaction between this bioceramics, GO and stem cells, for bone reconstruction. This combination was found favorable for bone production, since the bioceramics significantly enhanced human BM-MSCs proliferation and osteogenic differentiation, as shown by alkaline phosphatase gene expression levels. Successful osteogenesis was also reported in the case of graphene nanogrids, which promoted the differentiation of human mesenchymal stem cells isolated from umbilical cord toward bone cells [51].

Mesenchymal stem cells isolated from goat cultivated on graphene-coated plates were also used as a potential platform for testing osteogenic differentiation in the view of bone tissue engineering [52]. This study emphasized the ability of oxidized graphene alone to induce

http://dx.doi.org/10.5772/63333

osteogenesis process in goat MSCs in the absence of osteogenic inducers, thus proving the osteoinducing character of graphenes.

However, a small number of studies have focused until present on the effect of GO on human adipose derived stem cells (hASCs) osteogenic differentiation in 3D biomaterials designed for bone tissue engineering [53, 35]. hASCs have revealed encouraging results for adipose and cartilage tissue engineering and proved to be a valuable and more accessible source of adult stem cells than MSCs isolated from bone marrow. Thus, we have developed a strategy for *in vitro* differentiating hASCs inside chitosan-based biomaterials improved with 0.5–3 wt% GO for 28 days in order to study (i) the correlation between GO concentration and the degree of osteogenic differentiation; (ii) osteogenic markers gene expression evolution by qPCR; (iii) osteogenic markers protein expression by confocal microscopy; and (iv) accumulation of bone-specific extracellular matrix by histological staining in our experimental conditions (manuscript in preparation). Our results suggested that the degree of differentiation is strongly influenced by the content of GO in the material and that these materials are suitable for bone regeneration therapies.

Another hybrid scaffold between chitosan and GO was used as a template material for biomineralization of hydroxyapatite and tested as a possible material for bone tissue engineering. This combination proved to be beneficial for cellular activity including proliferation and attachment to the HAP–CS–GO system. Additionally, the scaffold allowed osteoblast growth and an increasing rate of mineralization during *in vitro* cell differentiation, confirming our results and the potential of chitosan/GO nanomaterials for bone regenerative therapies [54].

In the idea of creating an experimental platform for the evaluation of graphene properties for bone regeneration, Lu et al. [55] developed a self-supporting graphene hydrogel film (SGH), which proved to be cytocompatible and to allow cell adhesion and proliferation.

Nevertheless, the great potential of graphene and its derivatives for biomedical applications and their positive effects on cell viability, proliferation, adhesion, and osteogenic differentiation process have been already well documented. At this point, the challenge remains to elucidate the molecular pathways, which are active in the interaction between graphene and the cellular component and to explore and maximize the potential of graphene/GO-based biomaterials as platforms for bone repair therapies and tissue engineering.

5. *In vivo* GO effects during bone regeneration therapies

Regeneration of large bone defects requires development of bioactive scaffolds with distinct properties of promoting stem cells osteogenic differentiation and inducing the *in vivo* new bone formation. There are just few studies with graphene-based composite materials, which demonstrated potential to stimulate osteogenesis *in vivo* (**Table 1**).

Material	*In vivo* model	Post-implant analysis	Biological effects	References
Nanocomposites of reduced graphene oxide (rGO) and hydroxyapatite (HAp) (rGO/HAp NCs)	Rabbit calvarial defects	4 weeks	• relative mRNA expression levels of interleukin 6 (IL-6) and tumor necrosis factor-α (TNF-α) showed no specific inflammatory responses in the HAp grafts and rGO/HAp grafts • relative micro-CT values for new bone formation were 11.68 ± 8.99, 609.30 ± 308.58 and 1157.83 Å ± 224.52 in the control, Hap grafts, and rGO/HAp grafts • new bone density (%)in the control, HAp grafts, and rGO/HAp grafts were 17.66 (±8.81), 26.80 (±8.32), and 52.85 (±12.04), respectively • conclusion: graphene-based composite materials have potentials to stimulate osteogenesis	[56]
GO-coated titanium implants	Mouse calvarial defects	8 weeks	• BMP-2 delivery using GO-coated Ti found out a higher alkaline phosphatase (ALP) activity in bone-forming cells in vitro compared with bare Ti • substance P (SP), which is known to recruit mesenchymal stem cells (MSCs), was co-delivered using Ti or GO-coated Ti to further promote bone formation • GO-coated Ti induced dual delivery of BMP-2 and SP and increased new bone formation on Ti implanted in the mouse calvaria compared with other groups	[57]
Graphene-oxide-modified β-tricalcium phosphate (β-TCP-GRA) bioceramics	Rabbit calvarial defects	2, 4, and 8 weeks	• micro-CT analysis showed significantly increased new bone formation in the β-TCP-GRA group compared with the β-TCP group; • the volume of the newly formed bone (BV/TV ratio) of the β-TCP-GRA group (26.12 ± 4.44% and 44.83 ± 10.82%) was significantly higher compared with control (16.64 ± 4.57% and 30.41 ± 4.10%) at weeks 4 and 8 post-implant; • trabecular number (Tb.N) in the β-TCP-GRA group (0.39 ± 0.065 and 0.63 ± 0.102) was significantly higher compared with control (0.25 ± 0.049 and 0.41 ± 0.05) at weeks 4 and 8 post-implant; • histomorphometrically analysis of the mineralization area expressed as percentage resulting from the fluorochrome labeling with tetracycline (TE) at 2 weeks, alizarin red (AL) • at 4 weeks, and calcein (CA) at 6 weeks after the implantation surgery, showed increased % of	[50]

Material	*In vivo* model	Post-implant analysis	Biological effects	References
			regeneration and mineralization for β-TCP-GRA group compared with control	
Graphene (GO) flakes suspended in fibrin gels (GO/F) for BMP-2 delivery	Mouse calvarial defects	8 weeks	• micro-CT examination and histological analysis with Goldner's trichrome staining showed that the delivery of various doses of BMP-2 using GO/F resulted in significantly greater bone regeneration than that using F without GO; • a half-dose of BMP-2 delivered by GO/F resulted in bone regeneration similar to that resulting from a full dose of BMP-2 delivered by fibrin gel;	[58]
Graphene hydrogel film	Subcutaneous sites of rats		• stimulate osteogenic differentiation of stem cells, without additional inducer and adequate biodegradability	[55]
Calcium silicate (CS) ceramic reinforced with 1.5 wt% graphene plates (GPs)	Rabbit femur condyle defect	1–3 months	• bone–implant contact ratio reached 84.3 ± 7.4% for GPs/CS coating and 79.6 ± 9.4% for CS coating after 3 months implantation	[59]

Table 1. Platforms to study *in vivo* bone regeneration therapies using graphene-based biomaterials.

Up to date, there is a small number of *in vivo* studies investigating the ability of graphene-based nanomaterial platforms to induce and support production of functional *de novo* bone tissue when practical approaches in bone regenerative medicine require it. Although the implications and benefits for patients experiencing bone defects are of great importance, research toward validation of novel bioimplantable materials designed for bone repair advances in small steps due to safety and ethical requirements. Graphene and its derivatives hold great promise for the synthesis of efficient osteoinductive materials and in-depth research looking at the interplay between graphene effects and molecular pathways active in bone formation will contribute to bringing graphene from bioengineering labs to clinical practice.

Acknowledgements

The authors acknowledge the sources of funding that supported their own studies in the field of graphene-based composites for bone tissue engineering: a grant of the Romanian National Authority for Scientific Research, Executive Agency for Higher Education, Research, Development and Innovation, Project Number PN-II-PCCA-140/2012. Additionally, the studies were financed by the Institute for Research of the University of Bucharest (ICUB), through "Scholarships for Excellence in Research for young researchers, 2015 competition" project.

Author details

Anca Hermenean[1*], Sorina Dinescu[2], Mariana Ionita[3] and Marieta Costache[2]

*Address all correspondence to: anca.hermenean@gmail.com

1 Department of Histology, Faculty of Medicine, Vasile Goldis Western University of Arad, Arad, Romania

2 Department of Biochemistry and Molecular Biology, University of Bucharest, Bucharest, Romania

3 Advanced Polymer Materials Group, University Politehnica of Bucharest, Bucharest, Romania

References

[1] Nayak T.R., Andersen H., Makam V.S., Khaw C., Bae S., Xu X., Ee P.L., Ahn J.H., Hong B.H., Pastorin G., Özyilmaz B. Graphene for controlled and accelerated osteogenic differentiation of human mesenchymal stem cells. ACS Nano. 2011;5:4670–4678.

[2] Depan D., Misra R.D. The interplay between nanostructured carbon-grafted chitosan scaffolds and protein adsorption on the cellular response of osteoblasts: structure function property relationship. Acta Biomater. 2013;9:6084.

[3] Gu M., Liu Y., Chen T., Du F., Zhao X., Xiong C., Zhou Y. Is graphene a promising nanomaterial for promoting surface modification of implants or scaffold materials in bone tissue engineering? Tissue Eng Part B Rev. 2014;20:477–491.

[4] Salavagione H.J., Martinez G., Ellis G. Recent advances in the covalent modification of graphene with polymers. Macromol Rapid Commun. 2011;32:1771.

[5] Depan D., Girase B., Shah J.S., Misra R.D. Structure–process–property relationship of the polar graphene oxide-mediated cellular response and stimulated growth of osteoblasts on hybrid chitosan network structure nanocomposite scaffolds. Acta Biomater. 2011;7:3432.

[6] Misra R.D., Chaudhari P.M. Cellular interactions and stimulated biological functions mediated by nanostructured carbon for tissue reconstruction and tracheal tubes and sutures. J Biomed Mater Res A. 2013;101:528

[7] Fiorillo M., Verre A.F., Iliut M. Graphene oxide selectively targets cancer stem cells, across multiple tumor types: implications for non-toxic cancer treatment, via "differentiation-based nano-therapy". Oncotarget. 2015;6(6):3553–3562.

[8] Pumera M. Graphene in biosensing. Mater Today. 2011;14(7–8):308–315. doi:10.1016/S1369-7021(11)70160-2

[9] Goenka S., Sant V., Sant S. Graphene-based nanomaterials for drug delivery and tissue engineering. J Control Release. 2014;173:75–88.

[10] Shadjou N., Hasanzadeh M. Graphene and its nanostructure derivatives for use in bone tissue engineering: recent advances. 2016. doi:10.1002/jbm.a.35645

[11] Cai X., Tan S., Yu A., Zhang J., Liu J., Mai W. Sodium 1-naphthalenesulfonate-functionalized reduced graphene oxide stabilizes silver nanoparticles with lower cytotoxicity and long-term antibacterial activity. Chem Asian J. 2012;7:1664.

[12] Hong B.J., Compton O.C., An Z., Eryazici I., Nguyen S.T. Successful stabilization of graphene oxide in electrolyte solutions: enhancement of biofunctionalization and cellular uptake. ACS Nano. 2012;6:63.

[13] Chng E.L., Pumera M. The toxicity of graphene oxides: dependence on the oxidative methods used. Chemistry. 2013;19:8227.

[14] Liao K.H., Lin Y.S., Macosko C.W., Haynes C.L. Cytotoxicity of graphene oxide and graphene in human erythrocytes and skin fibroblasts. ACS Appl Mater Interfaces. 2011;3:2607.

[15] Yang K., Li Y., Tan X., Peng R., Liu Z. Behavior and toxicity of graphene and its functionalized derivatives in biological systems. Small. 2013;9:9–10.

[16] Lahiri D., Dua R., Zhang C., de Socarraz-Novoa I., Bhat A., Ramaswamy S., Agarwal A. Graphene nanoplatelet-induced strengthening of ultrahigh molecular weight polyethylene and biocompatibility in vitro. ACS Appl Mater Interfaces. 2012;4(4):2234–2241. doi:10.1021/am300244s

[17] Sahu A., Choi W.I., Tae G. A stimuli-sensitive injectable graphene oxide composite hydrogel. Chem Commun. 2012;48:5280.

[18] La W.G., Park S., Yoon H.H., Jeong G.J., Lee T.J., Bhang S.H., Han J.Y., Char K., Kim B.S. Delivery of a therapeutic protein for bone regeneration from a substrate coated with graphene oxide. Small. 2013;9:4051–4060.

[19] Zhang B., Wang Y., Zhai G. Biomedical applications of the graphene-based materials. Mater Sci Eng C. 2016;61:953–964. doi:10.1016/j.msec.2015.12.073

[20] Liu Z., Robinson J.T., Sun X., Dai H. PEGylated nano-graphene oxide for delivery of water insoluble cancer drugs. J Am Chem Soc. 2008;130(33):10876–10877.

[21] Sasidharan A., Panchakarla L.S., Chandran P., Menon D., Nair S., Rao C.N., Koyakutty M. Differential nano-bio interactions and toxicity effects of pristine versus functionalized graphene. Nanoscale. 2011;3(6):2461–4.

[22] Pandele A.M., Dinescu S., Costache M., Vasile E., Obreja C., Iovu H., Ionita M. Preparation and *in vitro*, bulk, and surface investigation of chitosan/graphene oxide composite films. Polym Compos. 2013;34(12):2116–2124.

[23] Pandele A.M., Ionita M., Crica L., Dinescu S., Costache M., Iovu H. Synthesis, characterization, and *in vitro* studies of graphene oxide/chitosan–polyvinyl alcohol films. Carbohydr Polym. 2014;102:813–820.

[24] Qi Y.Y., Tai Z.X., Sun D.F., Chen J.T., Ma H.B., Yan X.B., Liu B., Xue Q.J. Fabrication and characterization of poly(vinyl alcohol)/graphene oxide nanofibrous biocomposite scaffolds. J Appl Polym Sci. 2013;127:1885–1894.

[25] Ionita M., Vasile E., Crica L.E., Voicu S.I., Pandele A.M., Dinescu S., Predoiu L., Galateanu B., Hermenean A., Costache M. Synthesis, characterization and *in vitro* studies of polysulfone/graphene oxide composite membranes. Compos Part B. 2015;72:108–115.

[26] Wan C.Y., Chen B.Q. Poly(epsilon-caprolactone)/graphene oxide biocomposites: mechanical properties and bioactivity. Biomed Mater. 2011;6(5):055010. doi: 10.1088/1748-6041/6/5/055010

[27] Dinescu S., Ionita M., Pandele A.M., Galateanu B., Iovu H., Ardelean A., Costache M., Hermenean. In vitro cytocompatibility evaluation of chitosan/graphene oxide 3D scaffold composites designed for bone tissue engineering. Biomed Mater Eng. 2014;24(6):2249–2256.

[28] Guo B., Glavas L., Albertsson A.C. Biodegradable and electrically conducting polymers for biomedical applications. Prog Polym Sci. 2013;38:1263–1286.

[29] Lan Levengooda S.K., Zhang M. Chitosan-based scaffolds for bone tissue engineering. J Mater Chem B. 2014;2:3161–3184.

[30] Li M., Wang Y.B., Liu Q., Li Q.H., Cheng Y., Zheng Y.F., Xi T.F., Wei S.C. In situ synthesis and biocompatibility of nano hydroxyapatite on pristine and chitosan functionalized graphene oxide. J Mater Chem B. 2013;1(4):475–484 doi:10.1039/c2tb00053a

[31] Ionita M., Crica L.E., Tiainen H., Haugen H.J., Vasile E., Dinescu S., Costache M., Iovu H. Gelatin–poly(vinyl alcohol) porous biocomposites reinforced with graphene oxide as biomaterials. J Mater Chem B. 2016;4:282–291. doi:10.1039/C5TB02132D

[32] Kalbacova M., Broz A., Kong J., Kalbac M. Graphene substrates promote adherence of human osteoblasts and mesenchymal stromal cells. Carbon. 2010;48:4323–4329.

[33] Lee W.C., Lim C.H., Shi H., Tang L.A., Wang Y., Lim C.T., Loh K.P. Origin of enhanced stem cell growth and differentiation on graphene and graphene oxide. ACS Nano. 2011;5:7334–7341.

[34] Shi X.T., Chang H.X., Chen S., Lai C., Khademhosseini A., Wu H.K. Regulating cellular behavior on few-layer reduced graphene oxide films with well-controlled reduction states. Adv Funct Mater. 2012;22:751.

[35] Kim J., Kim Y.R., Kim Y., Lim K.T., Seonwoo H., Park S. Graphene-incorporated chitosan substrata for adhesion and differentiation of human mesenchymal stem cells. J Mater Chem B. 2013;1:933.

[36] Zhang W.H., Sun H.Y., Mou Y.C., Jiang X.X., Wei L.J., Wang Q.Y., Wang C.Y., Zhou J., Cao J.K. Graphene oxide-collagen matrix accelerated osteogenic differentiation of mesenchymal stem cells. J Biomater Tissue Eng. 2015;5(4):257–266. doi:10.1166/jbt.2015.1314

[37] Subbiah R., Du P., Van S.Y., Suhaeri M., Hwang M.P., Lee K., Park K. Fibronectin-tethered graphene oxide as an artificial matrix for osteogenesis. Biomed Mater. 2014;9(6):065003. doi:10.1088/1748-6041/9/6/065003

[38] Mooney E., Dockery P., Greiser U., Murphy M., Barron V. Carbon nanotubes and mesenchymal stem cells: biocompatibility, proliferation and differentiation. Nano Lett. 2008;8(8):2137–2143.

[39] Bressan E., Ferroni L., Gardin C., Sbricoli L., Gobbato L., Ludovichetti F., Tocco I., Carraro A., Piattelli A., Zavan B. Graphene based scaffolds effects on stem cells commitment. J Transl Med. 2014;c12(1):296.

[40] Hunter G.K., Goldberg H.A. Modulation of crystal formation by bone phosphoproteins: role of glutamic acid-rich sequences in the nucleation of hydroxyapatite by bone sialoprotein. Biochem J. 1994;302:175–179.

[41] Liu H., Xi P., Xie G., Shi Y., Hou F., Huang L., Chen F., Zeng Z., Shao C., Wang J. Simultaneous reduction and surface functionalization of Graphene oxide for hydroxyapatite mineralization. J Phys Chem C. 2012;116:3334–3341.

[42] Liu H., Cheng J., Chen F., Bai D., Shao C., Wang J., Xi P., Zeng Z. Gelatin functionalized graphene oxide for mineralization of hydroxyapatite: biomimetic and in vitro evaluation. Nanoscale. 2014;6:5315–5322.

[43] Cheng J., Liu H., Zhao B., Shen R., Liu D., Hong J., Wei H., Xi P., Chen F., Bai D. MC3T3-E1 preosteoblast cell-mediated mineralization of hydroxyapatite by polydopamine-functionalized graphene oxide. J Bioact Compat Polym. 2015;10:1–13.

[44] Xie H., Cao T., Gomes JV., Neto A.H.C., Rosa V. Two and three-dimensional graphene substrates to magnify osteogenic differentiation of periodontal ligament stem cells. Carbon. 2015;93:266–275. doi:10.1016/j.carbon.2015.05.071

[45] Mahmood M., Villagarcia H., Dervishi E., Mustafa T., Alimohammadi M., Casciano D., Khodakovskaya M., Biris A.S. Role of carbonaceous nanomaterials in stimulating osteogenesis in mammalian bone cells. J Mater Chem B. 2013;1(25):3220–3230. doi:10.1039/c3tb20248h

[46] Kumar S., Chatterjee K. Strontium eluting graphene hybrid nanoparticles augment osteogenesis in a 3D tissue scaffold. Nanoscale. 2015;7(5):2023–2033. doi:10.1039/c4nr05060f

[47] Deepachitra R., Chamundeeswari M., Kumar B.S., Krithiga G., Prabu P., Devi M.P., Sastry T.P. Osteo mineralization of fibrin-decorated graphene oxide. Carbon. 2013;56:64–76. doi:10.1016/j.carbon.2012.12.070

[48] Liu H.Y., Cheng J., Chen F.J., Bai D.C., Shao C.W., Wang J., Xi P.X., Zeng Z.Z. Gelatin functionalized graphene oxide for mineralization of hydroxyapatite: biomimetic and in vitro evaluation. Nanoscale. 2014;6(10):5315–5322. doi:10.1039/c4nr00355a

[49] Kang S., Park J.B., Lee T.J., Ryu S., Bhang S.H., La W.G., Noh M.K., Hong B.H., Kim B.S. Covalent conjugation of mechanically stiff graphene oxide flakes to three-dimensional collagen scaffolds for osteogenic differentiation of human mesenchymal stem cells. Carbon. 2015;83:162–172. doi:10.1016/j.carbon.2014.11.029

[50] Wu C., Xian L., Han P., Xu M., Fang B., Wang J., Chang J., Xiao Y. Graphene oxide modified beta-tricalcium phosphate bioceramics stimulate in vitro and in vivo osteogenesis. Carbon. 2015;93:116–129.

[51] Akhavan O., Ghaderi E., Shahsavar M. Graphene nanogrids for selective and fast osteogenic differentiation of human mesenchymal stem cells. Carbon. 2013;59:200–211.

[52] Elkhenany H., Amelse L., Lafont A., Bourdo S., Caldwell M., Neilsen N., Dervishi E., Derek O., Biris A.S., Anderson D. Graphene supports in vitro proliferation and osteogenic differentiation of goat adult mesenchymal stem cells: potential for bone tissue engineering. J Appl Toxicol. 2015;35(4):367–374. doi:10.1002/jat.3024

[53] Lyu J.Y., Cao C.H., Luo D., Fu Y.X., He Y.S., Zou D.R. Induction of osteogenic differentiation of human adipose-derived stem cells by a novel self-supporting graphene hydrogel film and the possible underlying mechanism. ACS Appl Mater Interfaces. 2015;7(36):20245–20254. doi:10.1021/acsami.5b05802

[54] Depan D., Pesacreta T.C., Misra R.D.K. The synergistic effect of a hybrid graphene oxide-chitosan system and biomimetic mineralization on osteoblast functions. Biomater Sci. 2014;2(2):264–274. doi:10.1039/c3bm60192g

[55] Lu J.Y., He Y.S., Cheng C., Wang Y., Qiu L., Li D., Zou D.R. Self-Supporting graphene hydrogel film as an experimental platform to evaluate the potential of graphene for bone regeneration. Adv Funct Mater. 2013;23(28):3494–3502. doi:10.1002/adfm.201203637.

[56] Lee J.H., Shin Y.C., Lee S.M., Jin O.S., Kang S.H., Hong S.W., Jeong C.M., Huh J.B., Han D.W. Enhanced osteogenesis by reduced graphene oxide/hydroxyapatite nanocomposites. Sci Rep. 5:18833. doi:10.1038/srep18833

[57] La W.G. et al. Delivery of bone morphogenetic protein-2 and substance p using graphene oxide for bone regeneration. Int J Nanomed. 2014;9:107–116.

[58] La W.G., Jung M.J., Yoon J.K., Bhang S.H., Jang H.K., Lee T.J., Yoon H.H., Shin J.Y., Kim B.S. Bone morphogenetic protein-2 for bone regeneration—dose reduction through graphene oxide-based delivery. Carbon. 2014;78:428–438.

[59] Xie Y., Li H., Ding C., Zheng X., Li K. Effects of graphene plates' adoption on the microstructure, mechanical properties, and in vivo biocompatibility of calcium silicate coating. Int J Nanomed. 2015;10:3855–3863.

Chapter 9

The Role of Immune Reactivity in Bone Regeneration

Christian H. Bucher, Hong Lei, Georg N. Duda,
Hans-Dieter Volk and Katharina Schmidt-Bleek

Additional information is available at the end of the chapter

http://dx.doi.org/10.5772/62476

Abstract

Bone is a complex organ with the capacity to regenerate. Even with this healing potential, healing results in fractured bone are unsatisfactory in a considerable patient cohort even with a good treatment regimen. These delayed healing cases encourage further research into possible new treatment approaches. The recently developed field of osteoimmunology addressing the tight interconnectivity of the skeletal system and the immune system could be a promising opportunity in this regard. In this review, the complexity of bone and the bone healing process are highlighted with an emphasis on the early healing phase. Specific immune cell subsets are considered for their potential to enhance bone healing and thus to develop new treatment strategies for patients in need.

Keywords: Regeneration, Fracture, Immune system, Inflammatory reaction, Healing

1. Introduction

1.1. Fracture Incidences

Bone injuries are frequent occurrences in daily life. Considering Germany as an example for a country with a health system guaranteeing treatment for fracture patients at a high standard, fractures of the extremities ranged between 560,000 and 640,000 cases per year over the past 10 years, with around 150,000 fractures of the femur and tibia, respectively (**Figure 1**). The statistical federal ministry recorded 802,662 fractures in Germany in the year 2014 (Statistisches Bundesamt, Wiesbaden, 2016-01-11). These numbers can be split up even further by age, where 38% of the patients with fractures of the extremities were older than 75 years, 33% between the age of 50 and 75 years, 16% between 25 and 50 years, and only 13% were younger than 25 years (**Figure 2A, B**).

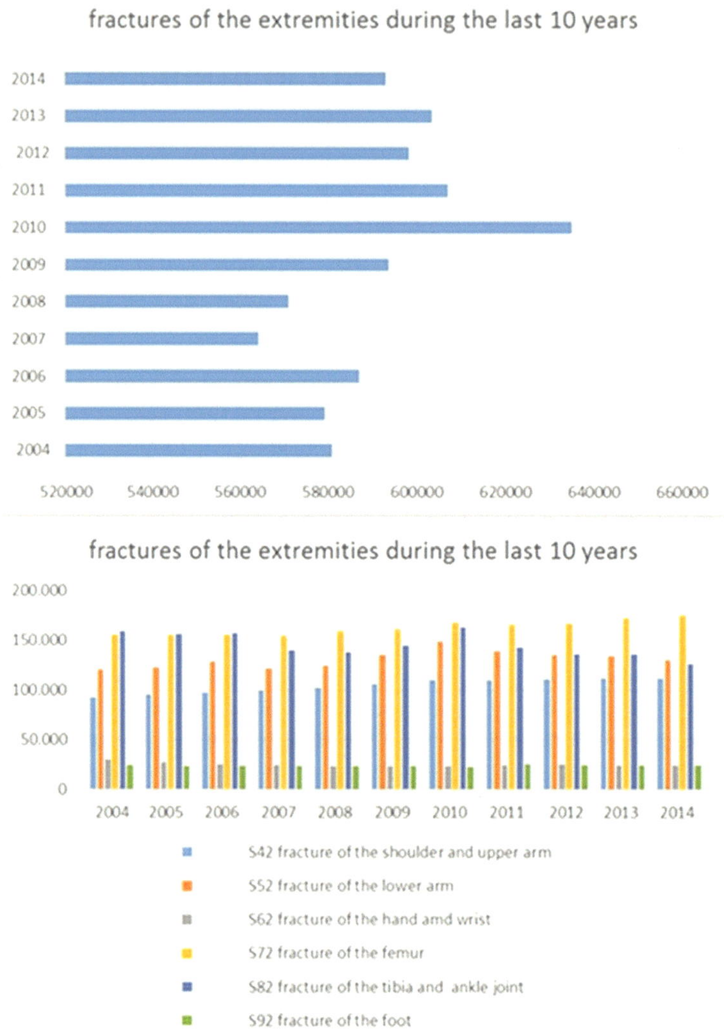

Figure 1. Fracture incidence in Germany (Gesundheitsberichterstattung des Bundes, 2016-01-11)—fractures of hand, arm, shoulder, leg and foot—incidence for 2004–2014.

Even in an environment with a good healthcare system and the normally very good healing potential of bone, 10–20% of all fracture patients still experience a delayed or nonunion after osseous injury [1–3] (**Figure 2C**). To overcome these delays in healing or reduce the nonhealing ratio, further research to gain understanding on the causes of healing delay or lack of healing is essential to enable new treatment strategies that support bone regeneration even under compromised conditions. With respect to the development of our population, the research into fracture treatment strategies becomes even more important as demography predicts an aging of the population. In Europe, it is Germany with the highest percentage of people over 65 years of age, and this percentage is rising (**Figure 2A**). In 1990, about 15% of the Germans were older than 65 years, and in 2011, this percentage had grown to 21% of people being over 65 years

http://dx.doi.org/10.5772/62476

old (Statistisches Bundesamt, Eurostat 2011). This is important because the fracture incidence is higher in elderly people (**Figure 2B**). The demographic projection of the UN World Population Projections for the years up to 2025 foresees an increase of over 50-year-old people of 20%, which equals 219 million people in 2025. Further stratifying this by age groups, the highest growth of 32% is expected for people aged 80 years or older. Consequently, the fracture incidence in elderly will increase by 28% of the 4.5 million fractures estimated for 2025. With this high number of fracture patients with an advanced age, it is eminent to consider age-related alterations that might influence the capacity of osseous tissue to regenerate normally. With increasing age, it is the immune system that undergoes major transformation influencing bone regeneration considerably. To provide adequate treatment options, it is essential to unravel the interactions of the immune and skeletal system.

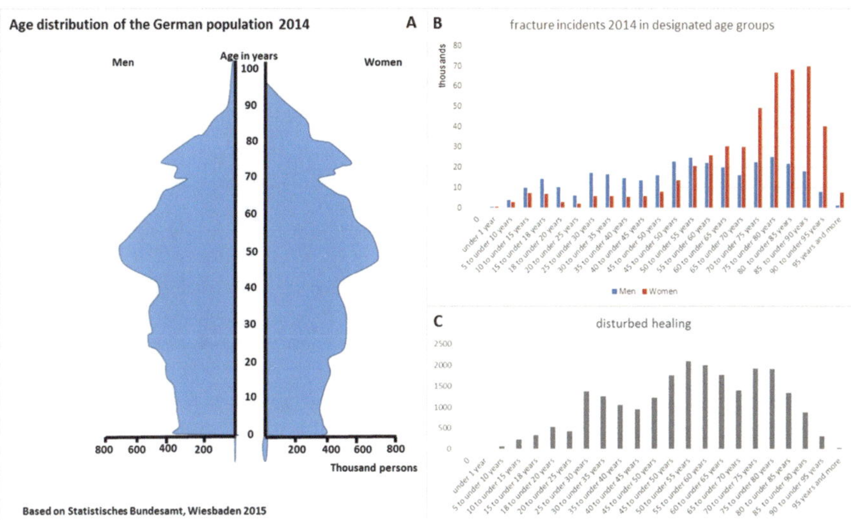

Figure 2. (A) Age distribution in Germany 2014 and (B) fracture incidence according to designated age groups. (C) Unsatisfactory healing results in fracture patients in corresponding age groups are shown, this includes malalignment, delayed healing and pseudarthrosis (nonunion) (M84 classification) (based on Statistisches Bundesamt, Wiesbaden 2016).

1.2. Primary and secondary healing

Bone is a remarkable organ because it is capable of regeneration and complete restoration of the osseous integrity both in form and function. Bone repair and fracture healing are unique because they recapitulate many of the ontological events that occur during the embryological development of the skeleton [4, 5]. To reach the "restitutio ad integrum," bone provides two mechanisms of scarless healing and regeneration: primary and secondary bone healing. Primary bone healing is only possible when the bone fragments are realigned anatomically, and the fracture zone is held under compression by an adequate fixation without a gap between the bony ends (**Figure 3A**). Stable fixation and no relative movement are required when basic multicellular units consisting of cutting cones with osteoclasts and following bone-forming osteoblasts cross the fracture line to directly rebuild bone and thus re-establishing the osseous integrity at the fracture side [6, 7]. During this process, the new bone is directly organized as osteons and oriented along the dominant mechanical loading direction [8, 9]. Primary bone healing was for a long time considered as the best possible healing process and thus was the aim when fractured bone was clinically treated [10].

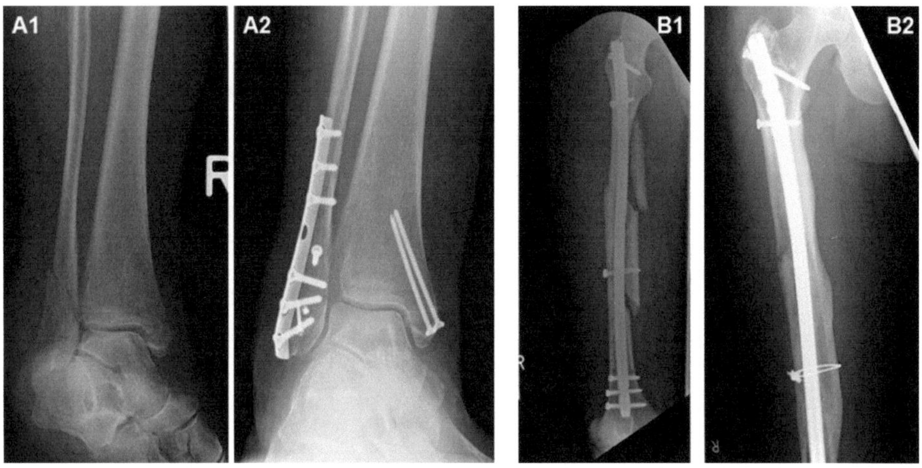

Figure 3. X-ray images from fracture patients: (A) fracture treated with an open reposition and internal fixation (ORIP) procedure with correct anatomical reconstruction of the fracture ends without fracture gap consistency—the bone will heal without callus formation through primary bone healing. (B) Comminuted fracture treated with an internal nail. Several gaps between the fractured bone ends remain and healing takes place by secondary bone healing as the callus visible in the image B2 taken 3 months after treatment clearly shows.

Secondary bone healing occurs whenever a gap persists between the fractured ends or when there is instability and thus interfragmentary movement (**Figure 3B**). This for example is the case if anatomical repositioning is not possible due to comminuted fractures or large bone defects. In secondary bone healing, a substitute tissue is formed to regain stability as fast as possible: an intermediate cartilage callus ensues. While intramembranous bone formation starts to consolidate the injured bone in the periosteal regions of the fracture gap, endochondral ossification processes start with the formation of cartilage islands in the gap between the fracture ends, forming an intermediate soft callus. Cartilage mineralization starts the woven bone formation process, which results in a hard callus. The final remodeling then restores the form of the continuous bone [11]. The intermediate cartilage step that provides a fast regaining of stability and reduces any interfragmentary movements often has a larger diameter than the original bone, especially if, as it would occur in nature, the bone remains untreated. It provides an increased polar moment of inertia against torsion and also withstands bending loads [12, 13]. While the large callus provides an evolutionary advantage to quickly regain mobility, it can be prevented in clinical settings by a stable fixation of the fractured bone [14].

1.3. Fracture treatment

In the wild, a fractured long bone often leads to death of the injured animal. However, it seems that the younger the animal is when the fracture occurs, the higher are the chances of survival [15]. If an animal survives a long bone fracture, the bones most likely heals with a severe misalignment. The potent remodeling capacity of the bones will however strive to restore the mechanically defined form of the bone, which is dictated by the surface strains the bone sense during physiological activities.

In our society, most fractures are treated in such an efficient way that only in rare cases bone fractures lead to death. Fracture treatment in the form of stabilizing the fractured bone goes back at least to 2400 years before Christ as excavated mummies from an Egyptian tomb proved. Prof. G. Elliott Smith discovered the splintered bones during the Hearst Egyptian expedition at Naga-ed-Der in 1903 on two mummies [16]. Both died shortly after the fracture because no healing signs were observed on the bones even though the Egyptians seemed to have reached some proficiency in fracture treatment as other relicts with healed fractures, found later on, could prove. In most cases, healed femoral fractures showed limb shortening or deformation, whereas forearm fractures healed well, demonstrating the challenge of reestablishing weight bearing capacity with the fracture treatment. An Arab surgeon, El Zahrawi (936–1013 AD) described in his treatise "The Surgery" a splinting technique, which was used for a long time, consisting of several layers of bandages combined with splints to provide stability for the fractured limb [17]—a fracture treatment also described by Hippocrates and Celsus [18] and one that is to an extend still valid today.

In the early 1770, first records on internal fracture fixation using ligatures or wire fixation are reported from France [19]. This was followed by the introduction of screws around 1850, again in France [20], and the development of plate fixation reported in 1886 by Hansmann [21] of Hamburg.

Robert Danis (1880–1962) furthered the development of the concept of internal fixation to permit functional rehabilitation. He stated that an osteosynthesis is not entirely successful until it provides immediate mobilization, complete restoration of the form of the bone, and enables primary bone healing without the formation of a callus. This thesis was published in "Danis R.: *Théorie et Pratique de l'Ostéosynthèse*, Paris, Masson, 1949". Between the 15th and 17th of March 1958, a number of orthopedics met in the Kantonsspital of Chur and based on the work of Danis they formulated a number of papers on osteosynthesis and thus the AO—Arbeitsgemeinschaft für Osteosynthesefragen—was founded. The AO has continued to improve the principles of fracture treatment since then and is still a renowned entity in the orthopedic community.

Even with these tremendous progresses in fracture treatment, there are still several open questions concerning the treatment regimen: mal-fixation with too stable or too unstable fixation [22–25], critical gap size [26, 27], a deficit in angiogenesis together with the formation of atrophic pseudarthrosis [28–31], and deficits in the control of the inflammatory cascades [32–34] are challenging clinical situations that still lead to unsatisfactory healing results for patients and surgeons as well.

2. Immune cells and bone regeneration

2.1. Bone – a complex organ

Bone is not simply a hard nonorganic material that functions as an anchor for muscles and tendons providing stability and form for our bodies and enabling movement through the interplay of our musculoskeletal system; it is also protecting vital organs, such as the brain, lungs, and heart, and it is a living organ regulating homeostasis. Additionally, it is an organ that is essential for our immune system, as these cells arise and/or mature from stem cells in the bone marrow, it is also an organ that interacts with our hormonal balance through a multitude of factors, including the hormone osteocalcin [35], and acts as a storage not only for calcium, phosphate, and magnesium but also for growth factors, as for example transforming growth factor-β (TGF-β).

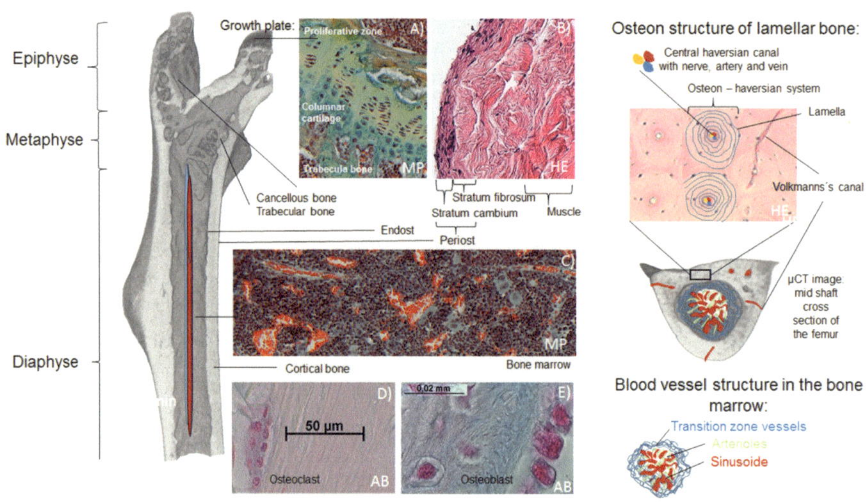

Figure 4. Bone is a complex organ. A long bone can be divided into epi-, meta-, and diaphyseal regions. The epiphyseal region contains the growth plate—the region of length growth of the bone. The epiphyseal zone is broad in young individuals and diminishes with age. Details are shown in a histological image where the transition from cartilage to trabecular bone is shown (A). Bone building cells are the osteoblasts. On the bone surface, they are arranged in palisade formation while synthesizing new bone matrix, the osteoid. They mature while they encase themselves in osteoid and finally mineralized bone matrix and become osteocytes (E). Osteoclasts on the other hand degrade bone; they are large multinucleated cells with a ruffled border directed at the bone surface (D). To emphasize the size difference, scale bars are enclosed in the image of the osteoclast and osteoblast. The bone marrow cavity is filled with bone marrow cells and a network of vessels (C). The vessel structure is explained more in detail with a cross section of long bone on the right-hand side. The cortical bone is covered by the endosteum on the inside and the periosteum on the outside. The periost is a rich source of cells, which are located in the stratum cambium (indicated in the histological out take), here visible by their dark nuclei. The stratum fibrosum covers the stratum cambium and is followed by a fascia and muscle closely adjacent to the bone (B). **Blood vessel structure in the bone marrow**: The bone is highly vascularized, next to a central vein and an artery system of sinusoids, arterials and transient zone vessels pervade the bone marrow cavity as indicated in the cross section of the bone on the right. **Osteon structure of lamellar bone**: The histological out take of the cross section shows the osteon structure of lamellar bone with its Haversian system. The bones are depicted as µCT 3D reconstruction images of mouse femura. Histological stainings are HE, hematoxylin eosin; MP, Movat pentachrome; and Ab, Alcian blue on paraffin- or plastic-embedded sections of long bone samples of mouse and sheep.

Bone healing is a complex process that involves a variety of different cells and signaling molecules, which originate not only from the bone, and here specifically from the periosteum, the cortical or cancellous bone, the endosteum and the bone marrow, but also from surrounding muscle tissue (**Figure 4**). An important supplier for cells and signals is the vasculature and thus the blood as a carrier. Bone is a very well-vascularized organ. Osteons are tube-shaped structures within the bone with an open space for blood vessels, veins, and nerves in the center. Small capillaries are found in the bone marrow near the endosteum, which continue into arterioles and sinusoids (with fenestrated basal membranes) towards the center where a large artery and central sinusoid transverse longitudinally through the bone marrow space [36]. Through the vessel connectivity, any osseous injury is prone to be influenced by systemic effects and vice versa to influence the systemic homeostasis. For example, the callus formation of injured bone is heightened in patients with traumatic brain injury. In this case, systemic changes caused by the brain injury influence the bone healing, most likely due to a competition for nutrients between the two injury sites and an altered hormone homeostasis [37, 38]. Another systemic effect that is most likely communicated to the bone is a change in the inflammatory state of an injured person—a higher systemic inflammatory reactivity will disturb the bone healing process and prolong the healing time necessary to achieve bridging [39]. Upon fracture, the vascular system of the bone is disrupted at the injury site, and it is imperative that revascularization swiftly occurs in order for a successful healing process. Tissue formation relies on the supply through the vasculature with oxygen, nutrients, signaling molecules and cells [29, 31, 40–42]. Restoration of the vasculature also enables cell recruitment of circulating regenerative cells towards the fracture site [41–44].

The cells partaking in the bone healing process do not only originate from the bone itself, but they also migrate out of different cell sources, which contribute finally to the healing process. A rich cell source for cells contributing to bone healing after injury is the periosteum as well as the bone marrow from where cells are attracted to migrate towards the injury site [45–47]. The muscle surrounding the fractured bone is also a valuable source for growth factors and stem cells, promoting revascularization and thus the bone healing process [48].

On analyzing bone healing, it is important to keep in mind that there are several different compartments involved, including the bone itself, the medullary cavity, the surrounding muscle and connective tissue, the blood supply, the metabolism, and the immune system.

2.2. Fracture healing

The fracture healing process itself is a strictly controlled complex process composed of consecutive and partly overlapping phases, which progress towards rebuilding bone integrity in form and function. Different cell types (immune cells, progenitor cells, and mesenchymal cells) [11] and their signaling molecules (cytokines, growth factors, and chemokines) [49] are partaking during a successful regenerative process.

Several growth factors involved in the healing cascade are currently under investigation to develop new therapeutic approaches to enhance bone healing: fibroblast growth factor [50], insulin-like growth factor [51], platelet-derived growth factor [52], transforming growth factor-β [53], vascular endothelial growth factor [50], and growth and differentiation factor 5 [54,

55]. However, the only growth factors so far clinically applied to further bone healing are bone morphogenetic protein 2 and 7 [56, 57].

The bone healing process can be roughly divided according to the healing steps into an inflammatory phase, a soft callus phase, and a hard callus phase (**Figure 5**). Upon closer observation, however, it becomes apparent that the healing process is more complicated than that. A more in-depth sequence of the healing cascade would be hematoma phase, proinflammatory phase, hypoxic phase, anti-inflammatory phase, revascularization phase, organized connective tissue phase, cartilage phase, hypertrophic cartilage phase, revascularization phase, cartilage mineralization phase, woven bone formation phase and remodeling phase [58].

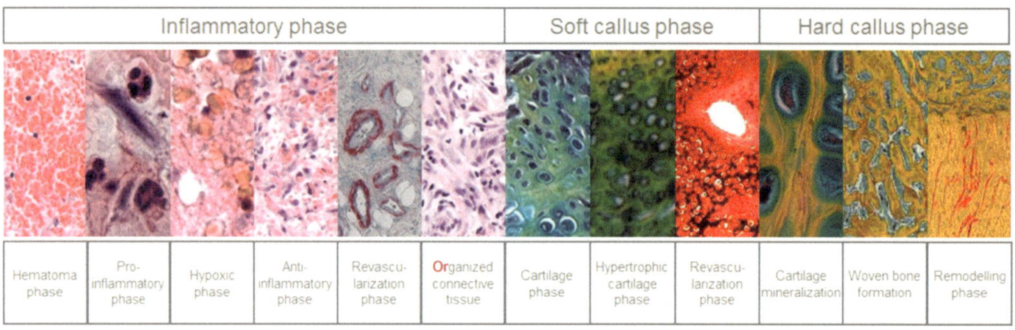

Figure 5. Fracture healing cascade: On closer examination, the inflammatory phase can be divided into at least six consecutive and partly overlapping phases showing the transition from the hematoma (red blood cells with some lymphocytes with dark stained nuclei) towards fibrocytes in the organized connective tissue (hematoxylin–eosin staining, different magnifications and an immunohistological staining for alpha smooth muscle for the revascularization phase). Soft callus phase can be divided into three phases (Movat pentachrome staining and Safranin van Kossa staining for the revascularization). The hard callus phase is divided into cartilage mineralization, woven bone formation and remodeling (Movat pentachrome staining).

Due to the complexity of the bone healing cascade with the multitude of different cell types involved and the plethora of tightly interacting and simultaneously highly controlled signaling molecules aiming to rebuild an organ consisting of periosteum, cortical bone, endosteum, and bone marrow in a way that optimally withstands the ruling mechanical strains, the process of bone regeneration is so far not understood. Therefore, research is compelled to use heuristic approaches to gain a more in-depth understanding and in conclusion develop new treatment approaches for patients in need.

2.3. Osteoimmunology

For a long time, bone homeostasis was explained with the balanced interaction of bone-forming osteoblasts and bone resorbing osteoclasts (**Figure 4**), however, this simple concept has changed. The interconnectivity of the skeletal system and the immune system has come into the focus of current research, consecutively leading to the founding of the new research field of "osteoimmunology." This new research field aims to elucidate the complex interactions between these two systems in health and disease and already more and more knowledge has accumulated [59–63], enabling us to consider new treatment possibilities for regeneration in general and also specifically for bone [64]. The opportunity to control the inflammatory cascade to stimulate successful bone healing has now been confirmed [32–34, 65].

Both cell systems, the skeletal system and the immune system, originate in the bone marrow. They share progenitor cells (e.g. osteoclasts/macrophages) and signaling pathways, and due to their colocalization, which often cross react with each other. This is apparent for example when considering the RANK/RANKL/OPG system, the system controlling osteoclast differentiation/activity and thus bone resorption. Activated T cells and osteoblasts are able to express the membrane-bound and the soluble form of RANKL (receptor activator of nuclear factor kappa-B ligand) promoting osteoclastogenesis. B cells and osteoblasts produce and secrete OPG (osteoprotegerin), a decoy receptor blocking the RANK-RANKL ligation, thus inhibiting osteoclastogenesis [59, 62, 66]. This example illustrates that immune cells are involved in bone homeostatic processes directing either bone resorption or bone apposition.

Due to the interdependency of the two systems, any considered treatment option of immune modulation must take into account that by affecting the immune system the skeletal systems could also be targeted unintentionally.

2.4. The initial inflammatory phase

Vessels are disrupted and bleeding occurs upon injury and the fracturing of bone. The infiltrating blood coagulates and forms the initial hematoma in the fracture gap. The formation of a fracture hematoma in the early healing phase is an indispensable step for successful healing because it develops an angiogenic and osteogenic potential [29, 67]. The removal of the early fracture hematoma can delay bone healing as it has been demonstrated in animal studies, where the transplantation of a fracture hematoma can lead to ectopic bone formation [68, 69], demonstrating its osteogenic potential. The coagulation process and a simultaneous proinflammatory reaction are phylogenetically connected [70]. During evolution, the closure of a breached outer shell and the defense against possible pathogenic intruders were performed by one cell, the amebocytes, capable of clotting and a defensive immune response. This connection has survived evolutionary diversification of the clotting system and the immune system—both reactions still occur simultaneously upon bleeding. The amebocytes can still be found today in living fossils, such as the horse shoe crab [70]. Their immune response is so potent that it is used to monitor endotoxin levels within solutions by pharmaceutical companies. The limulus amebocyte lysate (LAL) test is capable of detecting contaminations as low as one part per trillion [71]. In evolutionary younger organisms, this highly effective immune cell is being replaced by a whole array of immune cells, which can be divided into an innate immunity and an adapted immunity, the latter is only found in vertebrates (**Figure 6**). Each of these is composed of various different cells: macrophages, neutrophils/granulocytes, mast cells, natural killer cells, dendritic cells and the complement system belong to the innate immune system, whereas T and B cells and the humoral immunity belong to the adaptive immune system. The cells of the adaptive immune system provide their host with a long lasting and protective immunity by maturing from naïve T and B cells to effector cells, when they come in contact with their cognate antigen, and in some cases to memory cells, which allow a rapid immune response upon recurrent infection with an antigen previously encountered by the host. It has to be pointed out that the immune system is not only a barrier for extracellular microbes but also a regulatory system for body homeostasis. The immune system senses alteration in the environment, for instance damaged or aged cells [72, 73], expressing Toll-like receptors and other pattern-recognition receptors (PRRs).

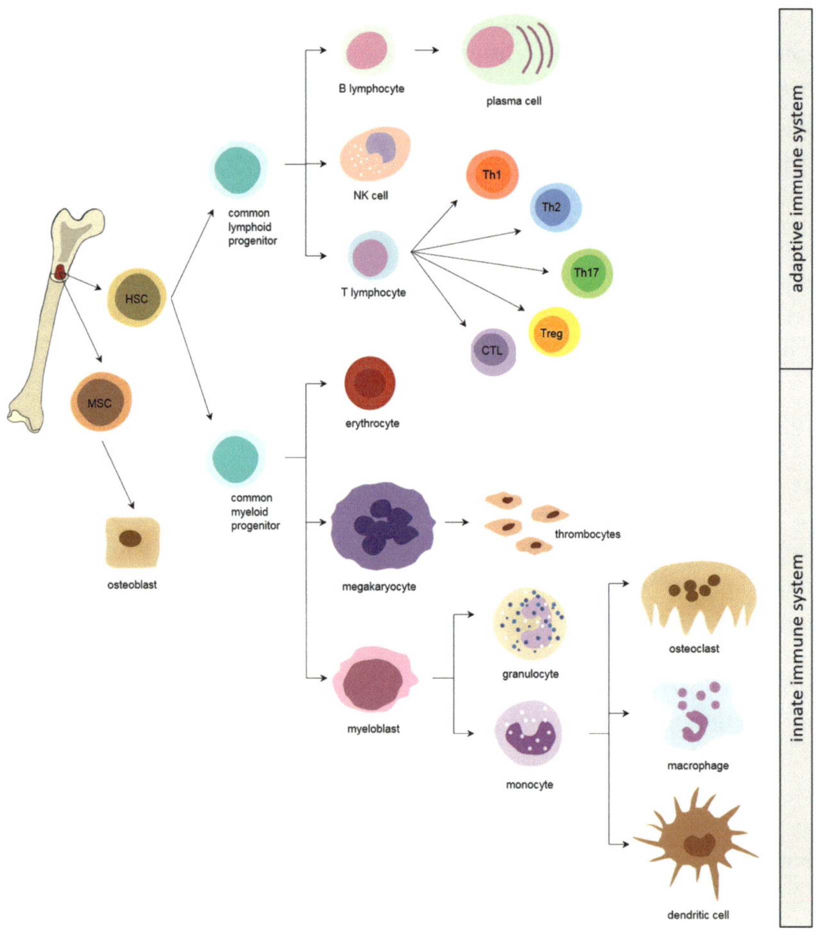

Figure 6. Diversity of cells of the immune system. Cells from the bone marrow give rise to the immune cells of the innate and adaptive immune system and also to the osteoblasts and osteoclasts of the skeletal system.

During fracture healing, both the cells of the innate and the adaptive immunity are involved, and immune cells play essential roles during all the fracture healing phases [74–77]. The initial inflammatory reaction ensuing upon hematoma formation initiates the healing cascade and thus can significantly affect the healing outcome [33, 34]. This initial inflammatory reaction is characteristic for bone, tightly controlled and different from other tissue healing with scar formation [32]. In fracture repair, the anti-inflammatory signaling is up-regulated between 24 and 36 hours after injury to terminate the proinflammatory reaction needed to attract necessary cells to the injury side [32, 33]. In parallel, the angiogenic signaling is up-regulated to initiate the essential revascularization process. The timely down-regulation of the initial proinflammatory reaction has been shown to be important as a prolonged proinflammatory reaction delays the bone healing process [29, 33].

The complexity of the initial immune reaction becomes even more apparent when considering cytokines expressed by immune cells during the different stages of the bone healing cascade. Tumor necrosis factor-α (TNF-α) has been reported to peak 24 hours after injury and return to baseline levels afterwards. During the remodeling phase, TNF-α shows a second expression peak during normal bone healing [64]. It is suggested that the first wave is due to activated tissue-resident cells, like macrophages, triggered through PRRs, and the second wave directly and indirectly by activated T cells. Looking closer into the role of this factor during bone healing is has been shown that too little, but also too much TNF-α leads to a delay in bone healing [78–80]. This demonstrates that the cytokine pattern has to be tightly controlled during the regenerative healing cascade to lead to a satisfactory healing outcome. Interleukin (IL)-17 is another cytokine that has been acknowledged to influence bone formation. On one hand, this cytokine has been reported to enable osteoblast formation [81], thus supporting bone formation; on the other hand, in the context of osteoporosis treatment, evidence occurred that IL-17 furthered osteoclastogenesis [82], thus supporting bone degradation. Contradictory reports can also be found for IL-6, which enhances fracture healing [83, 84] but reduces the mechanical strength of noninjured bone [85]. The microenvironment seems to be highly important for determination of the effect the cytokines have on the bone healing process, a fact that indicates the difficulties in using inflammatory cytokines to improve bone healing. The balanced immune response is highly important for a successful bone regenerative cascade [32, 33, 67].

Upon injury and disruption of the blood vessels, the nutrient and oxygen supply as well as the transport of metabolic waste is interrupted. The early tissue in the fracture gap consisting of the hematoma becomes hypoxic because oxygen is no longer provided by the vasculature. Therefore, cells trapped in the hematoma have to switch towards an anaerobic energy supply. The use of the remaining glucose in glycolysis to produce adenosine triphosphate (ATP), the energy molecule of the cellular metabolism, without the consecutive citrate cycle, results in lactate, an acid that consecutively lowers the pH value during the initial healing phase. Simultaneously, the sodium and potassium concentrations rise. These conditions present a milieu that is difficult for some cells, such as progenitor cells [86]. However, innate immune cells are well equipped to deal with these conditions and thus can be seen as the first responders to an injury. They express a range of cytokines that attract scavenger cells to clear the detritus that ensued upon tissue disruption and also direct the cells needed for the regenerative process towards the injury side. They readily switch from an aerobic energy supply towards an anaerobic and are often activated upon injury. Not only macrophages but also some T cell subsets are the most important actors during this first response [87, 88]. Hypoxia is a strong inducer of hypoxia inducible factor 1α (HIF1α), a transcription factor that is important for revascularization, cell migration, energy metabolism and growth factor expression, and therefore involved in the regenerative bone healing cascade [89]. HIF1α is expressed by most innate and adaptive immune cells, including macrophages and lymphocytes; they stabilize HIF1α and are being influenced by HIF1α in their immune cell function [90].

The swift up-regulation of a proinflammatory reaction upon injury activates immune cells, which are capable to withstand the unfavorable environment and initiate the healing cascade through a very specific and highly controlled release of cytokines. Hypoxia is an important trigger for the transcription factor HIF1α that in turn initiates gene expression to instigate revascularization. For this process to succeed, effective anti-inflammatory signaling has to begin to terminate the initial proinflammatory reaction. During this initial phase, the track for a successful healing is thus determined, and it becomes apparent that a skewed first reaction leads to a delayed healing by consecutively retarding the following healing steps.

2.5. Challenging immune constraints

The interdependency of the immune and skeletal system indicates that there is a change in the interaction as the immune system changes with the advancement of age. Due to the memory function of the adaptive immunity in vertebrates, the naïve T and B cell population diminishes upon aging, whereas the compartment of memory T and B cells grows. More and more lymphocytes encounter their antigens and the library of known pathogens enlarges. Recent studies could show that CD8 positive terminally differentiated memory and effector cells (CD8+ T_{EMRA} cells) have a negative impact on bone healing and osteogenic differentiation of stem cells [91, 92]. Elderly people with a longer exposure time to antigens thus are prone to experience delayed healing.

Mice, a common laboratory animal to investigate bone healing, are mostly kept under sterile conditions. If these animals are housed under less sterile conditions, their immune cell composition changes so that after 4 weeks of semi-sterile housing the percentage of memory and effector (CD8+) T cells was markedly enhanced. If bone healing is compared between sterile raised mice and those exposed mice, our group could show that the regenerative capacity was reduced [91, 93]. This is an important aspect that should be kept in mind during future research questions, which are analyzed in mice.

Nonsteroidal anti-inflammatory drugs (NSAIDs) offer pain relief and are commonly used also on fracture patients. As the name already indicates, these selective cyclooxygenase-2 (COX-2) inhibitors have anti-inflammatory functions. After reviewing the importance of the initial inflammatory reaction, the question arises whether this pain medication could delay fracture healing or not. Indeed there are numerous reports that state that NSAIDs delay healing [94–98]. The effect, however, depends on the dose and time frame of application and seems to be more pronounced in older nonselective anti–COX-2 agents [99]. Clinically, NSAIDs are a valuable alternative to opioids (painkillers directly addressing the nervous system) and still remain in use also in fracture patients for short-term pain relief.

Several diseases have also been reported to delay bone healing through a changed immune response. Diabetic-related delay of fracture healing has been linked to higher TNF-α levels [100]. A weakened immune response in diabetic patients results in a dampened chemotactic function and defective macrophage activity—two factors that are needed in a successful bone healing cascade [101]. A systemic disease with a high impact on the immune system is human immunodeficiency virus (HIV), and these patients have a bone phenotype with a high prevalence of osteoporosis and fragility fractures [102]. The impact on fracture healing, however, is unclear and difficult to determine due to the highly active antiretroviral therapy that these patients receive [102, 103]. Transplant patients receiving severe immune suppressive medication also show a higher risk for fractures and delayed healing outcomes. In contrast to these examples – where the immune system is weakened – conditions where a patient has a heightened immune answer or is already in a chronic proinflammatory systemic state, such as rheumatoid and arthritis patients, the prolonged proinflammatory reaction can result in delays in fracture healing [104–106].

Currently, the patient's immune status is not being evaluated when a fracture treatment is considered. However, this could help in the future to stratify patients who would benefit from an immune modulatory intervention to prevent a delay in fracture healing. This would especially be true in elderly patients because being bed-ridden for longer periods of time enhances frailty considerably.

2.6. Specific immune cell subsets that have been identified as important players in the bone regenerative process

In fracture healing, immune cells from the innate immune system and from the adaptive immune system are involved with specific and essential roles. Main cell types of the adaptive immunity are B and T cells with highly specific antigen receptors. Another important aspect of the adaptive immune system is its memory that enables its fast reaction towards recurring pathogen invasion. Adaptive immune cells can be activated not only through their antigen receptors, but also probably more important for the bone healing process through signals released by the innate immune system. From the innate immune system, especially macrophages have been in the current focus of osteoimmunology.

2.6.1. Macrophages

Macrophages are an important part of the innate immune system; they are among the first responders in case of an injury. Not only do they prevent pathogen invasion, but they also help in clearing ensuing cell debris [107]. However, their role in bone healing is even more complex and even today we have not yet unraveled their participation completely. Tissue-resident macrophages have been determined as key players in the orchestration of the recovery process towards a re-establishment of tissue integrity [108]. It was only in 1992 that it was recovered that macrophages are capable of a phenotype change from a proinflammatory type towards a prohealing phenotype [109]. The proinflammatory phenotype is named M1 or classically activated macrophage, and the second phenotype is termed M2 or alternatively activated macrophage. Since then, these "M2" macrophages have been associated with the resolution of wound healing *in vivo* in chronic leg ulcers [110], atherosclerotic lesions [111], traumatic spinal cord injury [112] and inflammatory renal disease [113]. It turned out that the M2 population is more divers and therefore subclassifications have been introduced: M2a (anti-inflammatory), M2b (immune-regulatory) and M2c (remodeling) [114]. In bone healing, the prominent macrophage phenotype during the initial phase is M1. Upon attenuating of the proinflammatory phase, the macrophage phenotype changes towards the M2 phenotype [77]. In a proof of concept study in mice, we were able to show that an induction of the M2 phenotype early in the fracture healing cascade can enhance bone healing [77].

2.6.2. *Regulatory T cells*

The T cell population is highly divers and probably pleiotropic as well as interchangeable. Among the T cells, there seem to be subpopulations supporting the fracture healing process and also other subpopulations, which have negative effects on the healing process. CD4+ and CD8+ T cell subsets have been addressed in this context. CD4+ T cells have been shown to increase osteogenic differentiation in human mesenchymal stem cell cultures in *in vitro* assays using their conditioned medium, whereas this effect was missing when observing CD8+ T cells [115]. The osteogenic effect of CD4+ T cells was further supported through their positive effects during wound healing [116], however without a more specific determination of the responsible CD4+ T cell subset. In later studies, regulatory T cells came more and more into the focus as a CD4+ T cell subset with positive effects on bone healing. Mice with an increased percentage of regulatory T cells showed higher bone mass and decreased bone resorption when compared to wild type mice [117, 118]. Regulatory T cells support osteoblast differentiation and have a negative impact on osteoclast differentiation and function [119]. In a skull defect model in mice, it was possible to enhance bone healing through the addition of regulatory T cells in combination with applied autologous bone graft [120]. Currently under investigation is the possibility of a direct interaction of regulatory T cells and bone-forming cells or their progenitor cells, the mesenchymal stromal/stem cells. This interaction is supported by the fact that mesenchymal stromal/stem cells, as osteoblast precursors, and regulatory T cells use similar suppression mechanisms for an immune response [121]. The direct interaction between regulatory T cells and bone-forming cells as well as mesenchymal stromal/stem cells could proceed through coordination of the CD39-CD73-(adenosine)-ADOR pathway. This purinergic signaling would potentiate the differentiation of mesenchymal stromal/stem cells and thus facilitate bone regeneration [122]. Another direct interaction between osteoblasts and regulatory T cells could be the induction of IDO (indoleamine 2,3-dioxygenase) and HO-1 (heme oxygenase-1) by regulatory T cells [123] or the fact that regulatory T cells can inhibit CD40L and thus regulating the RANKL-OPG balance in favor of osteoblast differentiation [124].

2.6.3. *T helper 17 cells*

The lead cytokine expressed by Th17 (T helper 17) is IL-17. The dual effect of IL-17 on osteoclasts and osteoblasts has been mentioned before. However, these cells are of interest as novel therapeutics targeting IL-12, IL-23, IL-17, and IL-17 receptor and which are now used to successfully treat psoriasis by either repressing Th17 differentiation (IL-12/IL-23) or by directly targeting IL-17. Psoriasis has two manifestations, one in skin (psoriasis vulgaris) and one in bone (psoriasis arthritis), and the immune modulatory treatment shows positive results in both [125]. Th-17 cell differentiation is induced by IL-1β, IL-6 and TGF-β [126, 127], with TGF-β being responsible for an increase in responsiveness of Th17 cells to IL-23. IL-23 is necessary for stabilization, survival and proliferation of Th17 cells [128]. This IL-23/Th17 axis is the target of the immune modulatory therapies currently introduced. For example, a cytokine neutralizing antibody against the p40 subunit of IL-23 inhibiting Th17 differentiation and survival, which in consequence lowers IL-17 concentrations, underwent clinical trials [129, 130].

2.6.4. CD8 + T_{EMRA} cells

A direct crosstalk between activated T cells and bone-forming cells can be assumed during the healing process. Among these T cells, CD8+ T_{EMRA} cells were confirmed to have a negative effect on the bone regenerative process. High expression levels of TNF-α and interferon-γ (IFN-γ) of CD8+ T cells decreased the osteogenic differentiation capacity *in vitro* [91]. CD8+ T_{EMRA} cells can be triggered to express these cytokines without antigen-presenting cells and do not necessarily need costimulatory molecules like CD80/86-CD28 but are activated by bystander responsiveness [131–133]. These cells accumulate in the fracture hematoma due to their tissue homing qualities and they occur in higher numbers in patients experiencing a delayed healing [91]. In the clinical setting, the recognition of a delayed or missing bone healing is so far only possible when these healing disturbances become visible in X-ray or computed tomography evaluations of the fractured bone. An early identification of patients at risk of a delayed or disturbed fracture healing is still missing. CD8+ T_{EMRA} cells could proof to be a marker for delayed healing risk in patients, since these cells also show elevated values in peripheral blood. Predicting patients with an extended need for special fracture treatment could thus just be done by analyzing the CD8+ T_{EMRA} percentage in peripheral blood early on in the healing process.

2.6.5. Outlook

Not only the interaction of the skeletal and immune system in fracture healing is not well understood so far, the immune reaction in itself is also still not unraveled. Aside from the complexity of the cytokine pattern guiding the regenerative process, the plasticity of the immune cells is still a vast challenge: M1 macrophage phenotype changing towards M2, Th1 changing towards Th2 response, regulatory T cells changing into Th17 cells and vice versa, to mention only a few aspects that still have to be understood. First approaches have been successful in influencing the fracture treatment through immune modulation (NSAIDs or IL-23 neutralization antibodies) but the possibilities are far from being exploited. A stratification of patients can help to decide, which treatment is optimal for which patient, especially with respect to the current immune status of these patients. With the numbers of delayed healing fracture patients still vastly unknown and possibly massively underestimated, and the demographic prognostic of a substantial increase in the elderly population during the next years, the need for further treatment options is rising together with the necessity of enhanced basic research in the field of osteoimmunology.

Acknowledgements

This work has been supported through the German Research Foundation (FG 2195—DFG SCHM2977 and DFG DU298) and the Berlin-Brandenburg Center for Regenerative Therapies. We like to acknowledge Dr. Serafeim Tsitsilonis for providing X-ray images of fracture treatment examples from the orthopedic and trauma department of the Charité – Universitätsmedizin Berlin and Dr. Hanna Schell for providing histological images to visualize bone anatomy.

Author details

Christian H. Bucher[1], Hong Lei[2], Georg N. Duda[1], Hans-Dieter Volk[2] and Katharina Schmidt-Bleek[1*]

*Address all correspondence to: katharina.schmidt-bleek@charite.de

1 Julius Wolff Institut, Charité – Universitätsmedizin Berlin, Berlin, Germany

2 Institute of Medical Immunology, Charité –Universitätsmedizin Berlin, Berlin, Germany

References

[1] Haas NP. [Callus modulation--fiction or reality?]. Chirurg 2000;71: 987–8.

[2] Dimitriou R, Tsiridis E, Giannoudis PV. Current concepts of molecular aspects of bone healing. Injury 2005;36: 1392–404.

[3] Bostrom MP, Camacho NP. Potential role of bone morphogenetic proteins in fracture healing. Clin Orthop Relat Res 1998;355 Suppl: S274–82.

[4] Einhorn TA. The cell and molecular biology of fracture healing. Clin Orthop Relat Res 1998;355 Suppl: S7–21.

[5] Ferguson C, Alpern E, Miclau T, Helms JA. Does adult fracture repair recapitulate embryonic skeletal formation? Mech Dev 1999;87: 57–66.

[6] Burger EH, Klein-Nulend J, Smit TH. Strain-derived canalicular fluid flow regulates osteoclast activity in a remodelling osteon--a proposal. J Biomech 2003;36: 1453–9.

[7] Smit TH, Burger EH, Huyghe JM. A case for strain-induced fluid flow as a regulator of BMU-coupling and osteonal alignment. J Bone Miner Res 2002;17: 2021–9.

[8] Smit TH, Burger EH. Is BMU-coupling a strain-regulated phenomenon? A finite element analysis. J Bone Miner Res 2000;15: 301–7.

[9] Parfitt AM. Osteonal and hemi-osteonal remodeling: the spatial and temporal framework for signal traffic in adult human bone. J Cell Biochem 1994;55: 273–86.

[10] Perren SM. Fracture healing. The evolution of our understanding. Acta Chir Orthop Traumatol Cech 2008;75: 241–6.

[11] Schmidt-Bleek K, Petersen A, Dienelt A, Schwarz C, Duda GN. Initiation and early control of tissue regeneration - bone healing as a model system for tissue regeneration. Expert Opin Biol Ther 2014;14: 247–59.

[12] Gerstenfeld LC, Alkhiary YM, Krall EA, Nicholls FH, Stapleton SN, Fitch JL, Bauer M, Kayal R, Graves DT, Jepsen KJ, Einhorn TA. Three-dimensional reconstruction of fracture callus morphogenesis. J Histochem Cytochem 2006;54: 1215–28.

[13] Epari DR, Schell H, Bail HJ, Duda GN. Instability prolongs the chondral phase during bone healing in sheep. Bone 2006;38: 864–70.

[14] Epari DR, Kassi JP, Schell H, Duda GN. Timely fracture-healing requires optimization of axial fixation stability. J Bone Joint Surg Am 2007;89: 1575–85.

[15] Bulstrode C, King J, Roper B. What happens to wild animals with broken bones? Lancet 1986;1: 29–31.

[16] Smith GE. The most ancient splints. Br Med J 1903.

[17] Spink MS, Lewis GL. Albucasis on Surgery and Insturments. London; University of California Press, 1973; 1-850. Print.

[18] Milne JS. The apparatus used by the Greeks and the Romans in the setting of fractures and the reduction of dislocations. Interstate Med J 1909;16: 48-60.

[19] Evans PE. Cerclage fixation of a fractured humerus in 1775. Fact or fiction? Clin Orthop Relat Res 1983;174: 138–42.

[20] Cucuel R. Des vis métalliques enfoncées dans le tissue des os pour le traitement de certaines fractures. Rev Medicochir Paris 1850;8: 113.

[21] Hansmann C. Eine neue Methode der Fixirung der Fragmente bei complicirten Fracturen. Verh Dtsch Ges Chir 1886;15: 134.

[22] Mehta M, Strube P, Peters A, Perka C, Hutmacher D, Fratzl P, Duda GN. Influences of age and mechanical stability on volume, microstructure, and mineralization of the fracture callus during bone healing: is osteoclast activity the key to age-related impaired healing? Bone 2010;47: 219–28.

[23] Lienau J, Schmidt-Bleek K, Peters A, Weber H, Bail HJ, Duda GN, Perka C, Schell H. Insight into the molecular pathophysiology of delayed bone healing in a sheep model. Tissue Eng Part A 2010;16: 191–9.

[24] Schell H, Thompson MS, Bail HJ, Hoffmann JE, Schill A, Duda GN, Lienau J. Mechanical induction of critically delayed bone healing in sheep: radiological and biomechanical results. J Biomech 2008;41: 3066–72.

[25] Schell H, Epari DR, Kassi JP, Bragulla H, Bail HJ, Duda GN. The course of bone healing is influenced by the initial shear fixation stability. J Orthop Res 2005;23: 1022–8.

[26] Reichert JC, Saifzadeh S, Wullschleger ME, Epari DR, Schutz MA, Duda GN, Schell H, van Griensven M, Redl H, Hutmacher DW. The challenge of establishing preclinical models for segmental bone defect research. Biomaterials 2009;30: 2149–63.

[27] Clements JR, Carpenter BB, Pourciau JK. Treating segmental bone defects: a new technique. J Foot Ankle Surg 2008;47: 350–6.

[28] Fassbender M, Strobel C, Rauhe JS, Bergmann C, Schmidmaier G, Wildemann B. Local inhibition of angiogenesis results in an atrophic non-union in a rat osteotomy model. Eur Cell Mater 2011;22: 1–11.

[29] Lienau J, Schmidt-Bleek K, Peters A, Haschke F, Duda GN, Perka C, Bail HJ, Schutze N, Jakob F, Schell H. Differential regulation of blood vessel formation between standard and delayed bone healing. J Orthop Res 2009;27: 1133–40.

[30] Carano RA, Filvaroff EH. Angiogenesis and bone repair. Drug Discov Today 2003;8: 980–9.

[31] Keramaris NC, Calori GM, Nikolaou VS, Schemitsch EH, Giannoudis PV. Fracture vascularity and bone healing: a systematic review of the role of VEGF. Injury 2008;39 Suppl 2: S45-57.

[32] Schmidt-Bleek K, Schell H, Lienau J, Schulz N, Hoff P, Pfaff M, Schmidt G, Martin C, Perka C, Buttgereit F, Volk HD, Duda G. Initial immune reaction and angiogenesis in bone healing. J Tissue Eng Regen Med 2014;8: 120-30.

[33] Schmidt-Bleek K, Schell H, Schulz N, Hoff P, Perka C, Buttgereit F, Volk HD, Lienau J, Duda GN. Inflammatory phase of bone healing initiates the regenerative healing cascade. Cell Tissue Res 2012;347: 567–73.

[34] Kolar P, Gaber T, Perka C, Duda GN, Buttgereit F. Human early fracture hematoma is characterized by inflammation and hypoxia. Clin Orthop Relat Res 2011;469: 3118–26.

[35] Schuh-Huerta SM, Pera RA. Reproductive biology: bone returns the favour. Nature 2011;472: 46–7.

[36] Acar M, Kocherlakota KS, Murphy MM, Peyer JG, Oguro H, Inra CN, Jaiyeola C, Zhao Z, Luby-Phelps K, Morrison SJ. Deep imaging of bone marrow shows non-dividing stem cells are mainly perisinusoidal. Nature 2015;526: 126–30.

[37] Locher RJ, Lunnemann T, Garbe A, Schaser K, Schmidt-Bleek K, Duda G, Tsitsilonis S. Traumatic brain injury and bone healing: radiographic and biomechanical analyses of

bone formation and stability in a combined murine trauma model. J Musculoskelet Neuronal Interact 2015;15: 309–15.

[38] Tsitsilonis S, Seemann R, Misch M, Wichlas F, Haas NP, Schmidt-Bleek K, Kleber C, Schaser KD. The effect of traumatic brain injury on bone healing: an experimental study in a novel in vivo animal model. Injury 2015;46: 661–5.

[39] Kleber C, Becker CA, Malysch T, Reinhold JM, Tsitsilonis S, Duda GN, Schmidt-Bleek K, Schaser KD. Temporal profile of inflammatory response to fracture and hemorrhagic shock: proposal of a novel long-term survival murine multiple trauma model. J Orthop Res 2015;33: 965–70.

[40] Hankenson KD, Dishowitz M, Gray C, Schenker M. Angiogenesis in bone regeneration. Injury 2011;42: 556–61.

[41] Otsuru S, Tamai K, Yamazaki T, Yoshikawa H, Kaneda Y. Circulating bone marrow-derived osteoblast progenitor cells are recruited to the bone-forming site by the CXCR4/stromal cell-derived factor-1 pathway. Stem Cells 2008;26: 223–34.

[42] Farrington-Rock C, Crofts NJ, Doherty MJ, Ashton BA, Griffin-Jones C, Canfield AE. Chondrogenic and adipogenic potential of microvascular pericytes. Circulation 2004;110: 2226–32.

[43] Matsumoto T, Kuroda R, Mifune Y, Kawamoto A, Shoji T, Miwa M, Asahara T, Kurosaka M. Circulating endothelial/skeletal progenitor cells for bone regeneration and healing. Bone 2008;43: 434–9.

[44] Pignolo RJ, Shore EM. Circulating osteogenic precursor cells. Crit Rev Eukaryot Gene Expr 2010;20: 171–80.

[45] Gruber R, Mayer C, Bobacz K, Krauth MT, Graninger W, Luyten FP, Erlacher L. Effects of cartilage-derived morphogenetic proteins and osteogenic protein-1 on osteochondrogenic differentiation of periosteum-derived cells. Endocrinology 2001;142: 2087–94.

[46] Colnot C. Skeletal cell fate decisions within periosteum and bone marrow during bone regeneration. J Bone Miner Res 2009;24: 274–82.

[47] Park D, Spencer JA, Koh BI, Kobayashi T, Fujisaki J, Clemens TL, Lin CP, Kronenberg HM, Scadden DT. Endogenous bone marrow MSCs are dynamic, fate-restricted participants in bone maintenance and regeneration. Cell Stem Cell 2012;10: 259–72.

[48] Shah K, Majeed Z, Jonason J, O'Keefe RJ. The role of muscle in bone repair: the cells, signals, and tissue responses to injury. Curr Osteoporos Rep 2013;11: 130–5.

[49] Ai-Aql ZS, Alagl AS, Graves DT, Gerstenfeld LC, Einhorn TA. Molecular mechanisms controlling bone formation during fracture healing and distraction osteogenesis. J Dent Res 2008;87: 107–18.

[50] Willems WF, Larsen M, Giusti G, Friedrich PF, Bishop AT. Revascularization and bone remodeling of frozen allografts stimulated by intramedullary sustained delivery of FGF-2 and VEGF. J Orthop Res 2011;29: 1431–6.

[51] Granero-Molto F, Myers TJ, Weis JA, Longobardi L, Li T, Yan Y, Case N, Rubin J, Spagnoli A. Mesenchymal stem cells expressing insulin-like growth factor-I (MSCIGF) promote fracture healing and restore new bone formation in Irs1 knockout mice: analyses of MSCIGF autocrine and paracrine regenerative effects. Stem Cells 2011;29: 1537–48.

[52] Al-Zube L, Breitbart EA, O'Connor JP, Parsons JR, Bradica G, Hart CE, Lin SS. Recombinant human platelet-derived growth factor BB (rhPDGF-BB) and beta-tricalcium phosphate/collagen matrix enhance fracture healing in a diabetic rat model. J Orthop Res 2009;27: 1074–81.

[53] Lee JY, Kim KH, Shin SY, Rhyu IC, Lee YM, Park YJ, Chung CP, Lee SJ. Enhanced bone formation by transforming growth factor-beta1-releasing collagen/chitosan microgranules. J Biomed Mater Res A 2006;76: 530–9.

[54] Moore YR, Dickinson DP, Wikesjo UM. Growth/differentiation factor-5: a candidate therapeutic agent for periodontal regeneration? A review of pre-clinical data. J Clin Periodontol 2010;37: 288–98.

[55] Wulsten D, Glatt V, Ellinghaus A, Schmidt-Bleek K, Petersen A, Schell H, Lienau J, Sebald W, Ploger F, Seemann P, Duda GN. Time kinetics of bone defect healing in response to BMP-2 and GDF-5 characterised by in vivo biomechanics. Eur Cell Mater 2011;21: 177–92.

[56] Zwingenberger S, Nich C, Valladares RD, Yao Z, Stiehler M, Goodman SB. Recommendations and considerations for the use of biologics in orthopedic surgery. BioDrugs 2012;26: 245–56.

[57] Schmidt-Bleek K, Willie BM, Schwabe P, Seemann P, Duda GN. BMPs in bone regeneration: Less is more effective, a paradigm-shift. Cytokine Growth Factor Rev 2016;27: 141-8.

[58] Schmidt-Bleek K, Kwee BJ, Mooney DJ, Duda GN. Boon and bane of inflammation in bone tissue regeneration and its link with angiogenesis. Tissue Eng Part B Rev 2015;4: 354-64.

[59] Takayanagi H. Osteoimmunology: shared mechanisms and crosstalk between the immune and bone systems. Nat Rev Immunol 2007;7: 292–304.

[60] Lorenzo J, Choi Y, Horowitz M, Takayanagi H. Osteoimmunology. First Edition. London: Elsevier; 2011.

[61] Lorenzo J, Horowitz M, Choi Y. Osteoimmunology: interactions of the bone and immune system. Endocr Rev 2008;29: 403–40.

[62] Walsh MC, Kim N, Kadono Y, Rho J, Lee SY, Lorenzo J, Choi Y. Osteoimmunology: interplay between the immune system and bone metabolism. Annu Rev Immunol 2006;24: 33–63.

[63] Nakashima T, Takayanagi H. Osteoimmunology: crosstalk between the immune and bone systems. J Clin Immunol 2009;29: 555–67.

[64] Mountziaris PM, Spicer PP, Kasper FK, Mikos AG. Harnessing and modulating inflammation in strategies for bone regeneration. Tissue Eng Part B Rev 2011;17: 393-402.

[65] Hoff P, Gaber T, Schmidt-Bleek K, Senturk U, Tran CL, Blankenstein K, Lutkecosmann S, Bredahl J, Schuler HJ, Simon P, Wassilew G, Unterhauser F, Burmester GR, Schmidmaier G, Perka C, Duda GN, Buttgereit F. Immunologically restricted patients exhibit a pronounced inflammation and inadequate response to hypoxia in fracture hematomas. Immunol Res 2011;51: 116-22.

[66] Li Y, Toraldo G, Li A, Yang X, Zhang H, Qian WP, Weitzmann MN. B cells and T cells are critical for the preservation of bone homeostasis and attainment of peak bone mass in vivo. Blood 2007;109: 3839–48.

[67] Kolar P, Schmidt-Bleek K, Schell H, Gaber T, Toben D, Schmidmaier G, Perka C, Buttgereit F, Duda GN. The early fracture hematoma and its potential role in fracture healing. Tissue Eng Part B Rev 2010;16: 427–34.

[68] Mizuno K, Mineo K, Tachibana T, Sumi M, Matsubara T, Hirohata K. The osteogenetic potential of fracture haematoma. Subperiosteal and intramuscular transplantation of the haematoma. J Bone Joint Surg Br 1990;72: 822–9.

[69] Park SH, SilvaM, Bahk WJ, McKellop H, Lieberman JR. Effect of repeated irrigation and debridement on fracture healing in an animal model. J Orthop Res 2002;20: 1197–204.

[70] Opal SM. Phylogenetic and functional relationships between coagulation and the innate immune response. Crit Care Med 2000;28: S77-80.

[71] Madrigal AC. The Blood Harvest. Washington: The Atlantic, 2014. Web.

[72] Pugin J. How tissue injury alarms the immune system and causes a systemic inflammatory response syndrome. Ann Intensive Care 2012;2: 27.

[73] Kono H, Rock KL. How dying cells alert the immune system to danger. Nat Rev Immunol 2008;8: 279–89.

[74] Singh A, Mehdi AA, Srivastava RN, Verma NS. Immunoregulation of bone remodelling. Int J Crit Illn Inj Sci 2012;2: 75–81.

[75] Neil Granger D, Senchenkova E. Inflammation and microcirculation. In: Neil Granger D, Granger JP, editor. Integrated Systems Physiology: From Molecule to Function #8. San Rafael (CA): Morgan & Claypole Life Sciences, 2010. Print.

[76] Konnecke I, Serra A, El Khassawna T, Schlundt C, Schell H, Hauser A, Ellinghaus A, Volk HD, Radbruch A, Duda GN, Schmidt-Bleek K. T and B cells participate in bone repair by infiltrating the fracture callus in a two-wave fashion. Bone 2014;64: 155–65.

[77] Schlundt C, El Khassawna T, Serra A, Dienelt A, Wendler S, Schell H, van Rooijen N,Radbruch A, Lucius R, Hartmann S, Duda GN, Schmidt-Bleek K. Macrophages in bone fracture healing: their essential role in endochondral ossification. Bone 2015; doi: 10.1016/j.bone.2015.10.019.

[78] Guo R, Yamashita M, Zhang Q, Zhou Q, Chen D, Reynolds DG, Awad HA, Yanoso L, Zhao L, Schwarz EM, Zhang YE, Boyce BF, Xing L. Ubiquitin ligase Smurf1 mediates tumor necrosis factor-induced systemic bone loss by promoting proteasomal degradation of bone morphogenetic signaling proteins. J Biol Chem 2008;283: 23084–92.

[79] Gerstenfeld LC, Cho TJ, Kon T, Aizawa T, Tsay A, Fitch J, Barnes GL, Graves DT, Einhorn TA. Impaired fracture healing in the absence of TNF-alpha signaling: the role of TNF-alpha in endochondral cartilage resorption. J Bone Miner Res 2003;18: 1584–92.

[80] Lehmann W, Edgar CM, Wang K, Cho TJ, Barnes GL, Kakar S, Graves DT, Rueger JM, Gerstenfeld LC, Einhorn TA. Tumor necrosis factor alpha (TNF-alpha) coordinately regulates the expression of specific matrix metalloproteinases (MMPS) and angiogenic factors during fracture healing. Bone 2005;36: 300–10.

[81] Nam D, Mau E, Wang Y, Wright D, Silkstone D, Whetstone H, Whyne C, Alman B. T-lymphocytes enable osteoblast maturation via IL-17F during the early phase of fracture repair. PLoS One 2012;7: e40044.

[82] Yuan FL, Li X, Lu WG, Zhao YQ, Li CW, Li JP, Sun JM, Xu RS. Type 17 T-helper cells might be a promising therapeutic target for osteoporosis. Mol Biol Rep 2012;39: 771–4.

[83] Yang X, Ricciardi BF, Hernandez-Soria A, Shi Y, Pleshko Camacho N, Bostrom MP. Callus mineralization and maturation are delayed during fracture healing in interleukin-6 knockout mice. Bone 2007;41: 928–36.

[84] Li Y, Backesjo CM, Haldosen LA, Lindgren U. IL-6 receptor expression and IL-6 effects change during osteoblast differentiation. Cytokine 2008;43: 165–73.

[85] Rozen N, Lewinson D, Bick T, Jacob ZC, Stein H, Soudry M. Fracture repair: modulation of fracture-callus and mechanical properties by sequential application of IL-6 following PTH 1–34 or PTH 28–48. Bone 2007;41: 437–45.

[86] Street J, Winter D, Wang JH, Wakai A, McGuinness A, Redmond HP. Is human fracture hematoma inherently angiogenic? Clin Orthop Relat Res 2000: 224–37.

[87] Gaber T, Haupl T, Sandig G, Tykwinska K, Fangradt M, Tschirschmann M, Hahne M, Dziurla R, Erekul K, Lautenbach M, Kolar P, Burmester GR, Buttgereit F. Adaptation of human CD4+ T cells to pathophysiological hypoxia: a transcriptome analysis. J Rheumatol 2009;36: 2655–69.

[88] Fangradt M, Hahne M, Gaber T, Strehl C, Rauch R, Hoff P, Lohning M, Burmester GR, Buttgereit F. Human monocytes and macrophages differ in their mechanisms of adaptation to hypoxia. Arthritis Res Ther 2012;14: R181.

[89] Gaber T, Dziurla R, Tripmacher R, Burmester GR, Buttgereit F. Hypoxia inducible factor (HIF) in rheumatology: low O2! See what HIF can do! Ann Rheum Dis 2005;64: 971–80.

[90] Palazon A, Goldrath AW, Nizet V, Johnson RS. HIF transcription factors, inflammation, and immunity. Immunity 2014;41: 518–28.

[91] Reinke S, Geissler S, Taylor WR, Schmidt-Bleek K, Juelke K, Schwachmeyer V, Dahne M, Hartwig T, Akyuz L, Meisel C, Unterwalder N, Singh NB, Reinke P, Haas NP, Volk HD, Duda GN. Terminally differentiated CD8+ T cells negatively affect bone regeneration in humans. Sci Transl Med 2013;5: 177ra36.

[92] Horwitz EM. Advancing regenerative medicine the translational way. Sci Transl Med 2013;5: 177fs9.

[93] Schlundt C., Schell H., Goodman S.B., Vunjak-Novakovic G., Duda G.N., Schmidt-Bleek K. Immune modulation as a therapeutic strategy in bone regeneration. J Exp Orthop 2015;2: 1.

[94] Zhang X, Schwarz EM, Young DA, Puzas JE, Rosier RN, O'Keefe RJ. Cyclooxygenase-2 regulates mesenchymal cell differentiation into the osteoblast lineage and is critically involved in bone repair. J Clin Invest 2002;109: 1405–15.

[95] Zhang X, Morham SG, Langenbach R, Young DA, Xing L, Boyce BF, Puzas EJ, Rosier RN, O'Keefe RJ, Schwarz EM. Evidence for a direct role of cyclo-oxygenase 2 in implant wear debris-induced osteolysis. J Bone Miner Res 2001;16: 660–70.

[96] Seidenberg AB, An YH. Is there an inhibitory effect of COX-2 inhibitors on bone healing? Pharmacol Res 2004;50: 151–6.

[97] Giordano V, Giordano M, Knackfuss IG, Apfel MI, Gomes RD. Effect of tenoxicam on fracture healing in rat tibiae. Injury 2003;34: 85–94.

[98] Simon AM, Manigrasso MB, O'Connor JP. Cyclo-oxygenase 2 function is essential for bone fracture healing. J Bone Miner Res 2002;17: 963–76.

[99] Boursinos LA, Karachalios T, Poultsides L, Malizos KN. Do steroids, conventional non-steroidal anti-inflammatory drugs and selective Cox-2 inhibitors adversely affect fracture healing? J Musculoskelet Neuronal Interact 2009;9: 44–52.

[100] Ko KI, Coimbra LS, Tian C, Alblowi J, Kayal RA, Einhorn TA, Gerstenfeld LC, Pignolo RJ, Graves DT. Diabetes reduces mesenchymal stem cells in fracture healing through a TNFalpha-mediated mechanism. Diabetologia 2015;58: 633–42.

[101] Forslund JM, Archdeacon MT. The pathobiology of diabetes mellitus in bone metabolism, fracture healing, and complications. Am J Orthop (Belle Mead NJ) 2015;44: 453–7.

[102] Richardson J, Hill AM, Johnston CJ, McGregor A, Norrish AR, Eastwood D, Lavy CB. Fracture healing in HIV-positive populations. J Bone Joint Surg Br 2008;90: 988–94.

[103] Gardner RO, Bates JH, Ng'oma E, Harrison WJ. Fracture union following internal fixation in the HIV population. Injury 2013;44: 830–3.

[104] Timmen M, Hidding H, Wieskotter B, Baum W, Pap T, Raschke MJ, Schett G, Zwerina J, Stange R. Influence of antiTNF-alpha antibody treatment on fracture healing under chronic inflammation. BMC Musculoskelet Disord 2014;15: 184.

[105] Bogoch ER, Moran EL. Bone abnormalities in the surgical treatment of patients with rheumatoid arthritis. Clin Orthop Relat Res 1999: 8–21.

[106] Nagira K, Hagino H, Yamashita Y, Kishimoto Y, Teshima R. Insufficiency fracture at the distal diaphysis of the radius after synovectomy combined with the Sauve-Kapandji procedure in a patient with rheumatoid arthritis. Mod Rheumatol 2010;20: 511–3.

[107] Janeway CA, Jr., Medzhitov R. Innate immune recognition. Annu Rev Immunol 2002;20: 197–216.

[108] Chazaud B. Macrophages: supportive cells for tissue repair and regeneration. Immunobiology 2014;219: 172–8.

[109] Stein M, Keshav S, Harris N, Gordon S. Interleukin 4 potently enhances murine macrophage mannose receptor activity: a marker of alternative immunologic macrophage activation. J Exp Med 1992;176: 287–92.

[110] Krishnamoorthy L. The role of macrophages in human wound healing and their response to a tissue engineered dermal replacement in human chronic wounds. University of Glasgow: MD thesis, 2006. Web.

[111] Khallou-Laschet J, Varthaman A, Fornasa G, Compain C, Gaston AT, Clement M, Dussiot M, Levillain O, Graff-Dubois S, Nicoletti A, Caligiuri G. Macrophage plasticity in experimental atherosclerosis. PLoS One 2010;5: e8852.

[112] Kigerl KA, Gensel JC, Ankeny DP, Alexander JK, Donnelly DJ, Popovich PG. Identification of two distinct macrophage subsets with divergent effects causing either neurotoxicity or regeneration in the injured mouse spinal cord. J Neurosci 2009;29: 13435–44.

[113] Spiller K, Nassiri S., Witherel CE., Anfang RR., Ng J., Nakazawa KR., Vunjak-Novakovic G. Sequential delivery of immunomodulatory cytokines to facilitate the M1-to-M2 transition of macrophages and enhance vascularization of bone scaffolds. Biomaterials 2014; 37: 194-207.

[114] Mantovani A, Sica A, Sozzani S, Allavena P, Vecchi A, Locati M. The chemokine system in diverse forms of macrophage activation and polarization. Trends Immunol 2004;25: 677–86.

[115] Grassi F, Cattini L, Gambari L, Manferdini C, Piacentini A, Gabusi E, Facchini A, Lisignoli G. T cell subsets differently regulate osteogenic differentiation of human

mesenchymal stromal cells in vitro. J Tissue Eng Regen Med 2013; doi: 10.1002/term. 1727.

[116] Park JE, Barbul A. Understanding the role of immune regulation in wound healing. Am J Surg 2004;187: 11S-16S.

[117] Pacifici R. Osteoimmunology and its implications for transplantation. Am J Transplant 2013;13: 2245–54.

[118] Zaiss MM, Frey B, Hess A, Zwerina J, Luther J, Nimmerjahn F, Engelke K, Kollias G, Hunig T, Schett G, David JP. Regulatory T cells protect from local and systemic bone destruction in arthritis. J Immunol 2010;184: 7238–46.

[119] Zaiss MM, Axmann R, Zwerina J, Polzer K, Guckel E, Skapenko A, Schulze-Koops H, Horwood N, Cope A, Schett G. Treg cells suppress osteoclast formation: a new link between the immune system and bone. Arthritis Rheum 2007;56: 4104–12.

[120] Liu Y, Wang L, Kikuiri T, Akiyama K, Chen C, Xu X, Yang R, Chen W, Wang S, Shi S. Mesenchymal stem cell-based tissue regeneration is governed by recipient T lymphocytes via IFN-gamma and TNF-alpha. Nat Med 2011;17: 1594–601.

[121] Glenn JD, Whartenby KA. Mesenchymal stem cells: emerging mechanisms of immunomodulation and therapy. World J Stem Cells 2014;6: 526–39.

[122] Lei H, Schmidt-Bleek K, Dienelt A, Reinke P, Volk HD. Regulatory T cell-mediated anti-inflammatory effects promote successful tissue repair in both indirect and direct manners. Front Pharmacol 2015;6: 184.

[123] Oliveira V, Agua-Doce A, Duarte J, Soares MP, Graca L. Regulatory T cell maintenance of dominant tolerance: induction of tissue self-defense? Transpl Immunol 2006;17: 7–10.

[124] Canavan JB, Afzali B, Scotta C, Fazekasova H, Edozie FC, Macdonald TT, Hernandez-Fuentes MP, Lombardi G, Lord GM. A rapid diagnostic test for human regulatory T-cell function to enable regulatory T-cell therapy. Blood 2012;119: e57-66.

[125] Sukhov A, Adamopoulos IE, Maverakis E. Interactions of the immune system with skin and bone tissue in psoriatic arthritis: a comprehensive review. Clin Rev Allergy Immunol 2016; doi: 10.1007/s12016-016-8529-8.

[126] Bettelli E, Carrier Y, Gao W, Korn T, Strom TB, Oukka M, Weiner HL, Kuchroo VK. Reciprocal developmental pathways for the generation of pathogenic effector TH17 and regulatory T cells. Nature 2006;441: 235–8.

[127] Weaver CT, Harrington LE, Mangan PR, Gavrieli M, Murphy KM. Th17: an effector CD4 T cell lineage with regulatory T cell ties. Immunity 2006;24: 677–88.

[128] Mangan PR, Harrington LE, O'Quinn DB, Helms WS, Bullard DC, Elson CO, Hatton RD, Wahl SM, Schoeb TR, Weaver CT. Transforming growth factor-beta induces development of the T(H)17 lineage. Nature 2006;441: 231–4.

[129] Leonardi CL, Kimball AB, Papp KA, Yeilding N, Guzzo C, Wang Y, Li S, Dooley LT, Gordon KB, investigators Ps. Efficacy and safety of ustekinumab, a human interleukin-12/23 monoclonal antibody, in patients with psoriasis: 76-week results from a randomised, double-blind, placebo-controlled trial (PHOENIX 1). Lancet 2008;371: 1665–74.

[130] Papp KA, Langley RG, Lebwohl M, Krueger GG, Szapary P, Yeilding N, Guzzo C, Hsu MC, Wang Y, Li S, Dooley LT, Reich K, investigators Ps. Efficacy and safety of ustekinumab, a human interleukin-12/23 monoclonal antibody, in patients with psoriasis: 52-week results from a randomised, double-blind, placebo-controlled trial (PHOENIX 2). Lancet 2008;371: 1675–84.

[131] Pearl JI, Ma T, Irani AR, Huang Z, Robinson WH, Smith RL, Goodman SB. Role of the Toll-like receptor pathway in the recognition of orthopedic implant wear-debris particles. Biomaterials 2011;32: 5535–42.

[132] Zhang Q, Raoof M, Chen Y, Sumi Y, Sursal T, Junger W, Brohi K, Itagaki K, Hauser CJ. Circulating mitochondrial DAMPs cause inflammatory responses to injury. Nature 2010;464: 104–7.

[133] Li H, Hong S, Qian J, Zheng Y, Yang J, Yi Q. Cross talk between the bone and immune systems: osteoclasts function as antigen-presenting cells and activate CD4+ and CD8+ T cells. Blood 2010;116: 210–7.

Chapter 10

Progress in Bioactive Metal and, Ceramic Implants for Load-Bearing Application

Mohammed Elbadawi, James Meredith,
Lynne Hopkins and Ian Reaney

Additional information is available at the end of the chapter

http://dx.doi.org/10.5772/62598

Abstract

The field of biomaterials is an exuberant and enticing field, attracting interest across a number of scientific disciplines. Synthetic materials such as metals and ceramics have helped civilisation accomplish many feats, and this can also be said for the achievements in orthopaedic applications. Metals and ceramics have achieved success in non-load-bearing applications and attempts are made to translate the accomplishments into weight-bearing applications. For this, a material needs to be porous but with sufficient strength to withstand daily loading; however, both properties are mutually exclusive. The implant must also avoid causing adverse reactions and toxicity and, preferably, bond to the surrounding tissues. Metals such as stainless steels and chromium-cobalt alloys have been used due to their excellent mechanical properties that can withstand daily activities, but retrospective studies have alluded to the possibilities of significant adverse reaction when implanted within the human body, caused by the elution of metal ions. Lessons from metals have also demonstrated that materials with significantly higher mechanical properties will not necessarily enhance the longevity of the implant—such is the complexity of the human body. Ceramics, on the other hand, exhibit excellent biocompatibility, but their mechanical properties are a significant hindrance for load-bearing use. Thus, the chapter herein provides a select overview of contemporary research undertaken to address the aforementioned drawbacks for both metals and ceramics. Furthermore, the chapter includes a section of how metals and ceramics can be combined in a multi-material approach to bring together their respective properties to achieve a desirable characteristics.

Keywords: Bioactive Metals, Osseointegration, High Strength, Fabrication, Ceramics

1. Introduction

The orthopaedic implant market is expected to grow from its current $30 billion value due to the rising demands for orthopaedic implant procedures in a universally aging civilisation. A plethora of synthetic materials capable of encouraging bone growth are available in the market, referred to as bioactive materials. The clinical success rates of bioactive orthopaedic implant validate the concerted research undertaken to enhance their abilities, underpinned by their propensity to alleviate pain, expedite recovery, and ameliorate quality of life for the patient. Applicable artificial implants can be in the form of plates, rods, screws, or scaffolds (a porous structure used to substitute missing osseous tissue). Indeed, artificial implants can be fabricated from metals, ceramics, polymers, and composites; however, due to the complexity of the human skeleton, no one class of materials is suited for all applications. Moreover, bioactive materials are not without their drawbacks. The aim of this chapter is to provide an overview of how material science and engineering techniques are employed to maximise their potential and thus ensuring long-term efficiency.

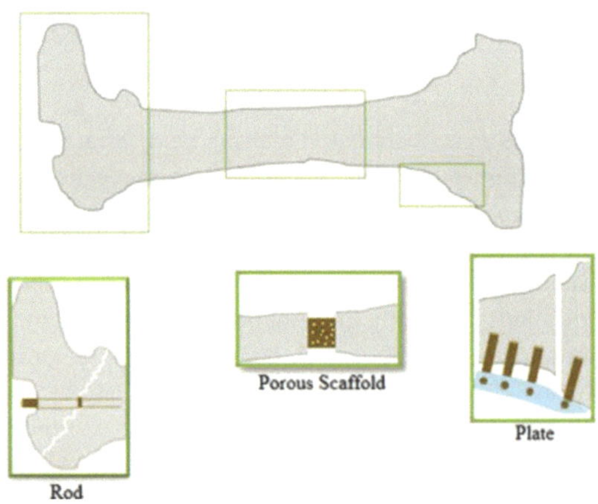

Figure 1. Schematic to show how implants are used for load-bearing applications.

1.1. Background

Bone resides in a perpetual resorption-regeneration state dictated by osseous cells and, like the skin, has a natural tendency to heal when fractured over time. There are instances when the healing cannot be accomplished, such as non-union fractures, which leads to medical intervention. Bone grafting is considered a strong candidate in such cases. A graft can either be natural or synthetic in its form but serves the purpose of encouraging the bone to grow. Bone grafts can be retrieved from the patients' own skeleton (autograft) or from a donor (allograft); however, concerns including but not limited to histocompatibility, disease transfer, and lack of availability necessitate the use of synthetic materials—of which metals and ceramics have been extensively researched.

Synthetic materials can exert several responses within physiological environment. If no adverse reaction occurs, then the material is said to be biologically compatible, or "biocompatible." This can further be subdivided into two groups: bioinert and bioactive, where the former is used to refer to a material that does not interact with the surrounding tissues. A bioactive implant can elicit an efficacious reaction that induces a phenomenon where a bone-like layer is formed around the implant providing an initial rapid and robust bond between the bone and implant that can culminate in complete integration. This type of response is technically referred to as *osseointegration*. Materials can recruit pre-existing bone cells to lay the groundwork for the integration, which is referred to as *osteoconduction*. Others stimulate undifferentiated cells into bone cells are referred to as *osteoinduction*. Implants eliciting such a response are associated with high success rates in clinical settings. Such exceptional attributes are inherent in some materials, and others need additional processing to implement the trait. An assortment of bioactive materials is capable of dissolving gradually within the human body, under physiological environment. The concept of a synthetic material inducing bone growth and vanishing, so to speak, when a new bone is remodelled is very attractive as it can avoid added patient inconvenience and healthcare costs. Materials that can dissolve or degrade under the physiological conditions are referred to as "biodegradable" or "bioresorbable." The aim for bioresorbable materials in load-bearing applications is for the implant to bear the majority of the load when implanted, and as the bone heals and more bone tissue is formed, the load is shared between the implant and healing tissues. As the scaffold is resorbed and consequently weakened, the healing bone sustains the majority of the load until the scaffold is completely resorbed and bone is fully restored. Preferably, if the graft resorption occurs in tandem with bone regeneration, structural weakness can be mitigated and minimising premature graft failure. A porous structure is also favoured because opportunities for bone to grow within the implant (as opposed to solely on the surface) can be achieved that leads to enhanced osseointegration and early implant stabilisation. Therefore, designing an artificial implant should incorporate as many of the aforementioned attributes.

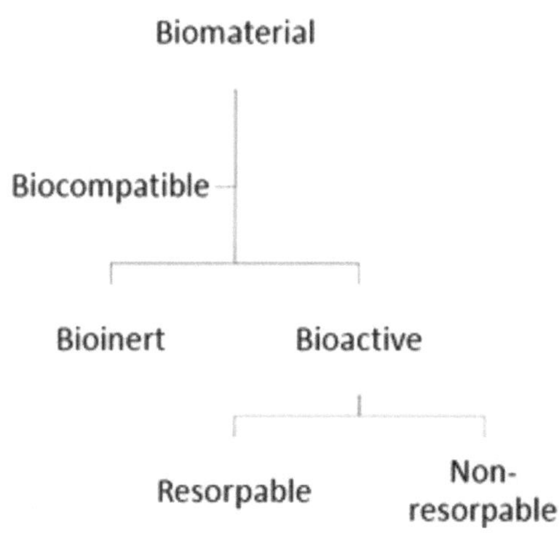

Figure 2. Figure depicting the hierarchy of biocompatible materials.

A material's characteristics (e.g. its resorbability in the body, and at what rate) is ultimately determined by their composition and the fabrication process employed. The overall process involves multiple steps that determine the structure and properties of the final product, ranging from structural modifications at the atomic level through to the gross level visible to the eye, such as colour and surface roughness. All materials have their atoms arranged in some manner, which can be altered through, for example, heat treatment. If the arrangement is homogenous throughout the material's microstructure, then it is referred to as homogenous, or single phase. However, if two or more discrete zones are evident within the microstructure, then the additional zones will be referred to as secondary, tertiary, etc., phases. Alternatively, a complete change in atomic orientation can occur, resulting in a transition of phases. Greek letters are used to denote between different phases of a material, e.g. α-titanium, β-tricalcium phosphate, etc.

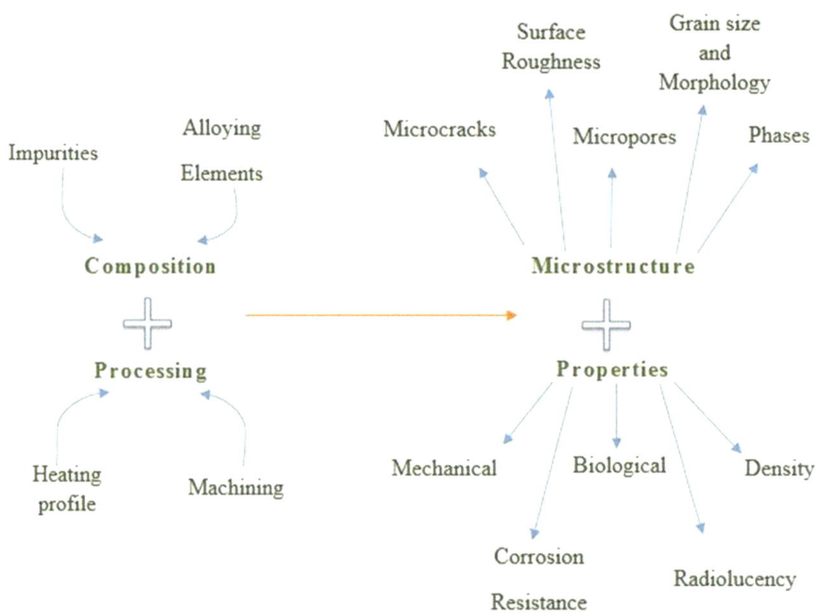

Figure 3. Figure illustrating examples for composition, processing, microstructure, and properties.

Metals are a popular choice for synthetic implants and their strength lies in the various processing routes available—owing to their mechanical properties. Their mechanical properties are either comparable or exceed that of bone. Contrarily, their chemical makeup is a limiting factor for both load and non-load-bearing orthopaedic implants. Ceramics, on the other hand, offer far more options with respect to their excellent bioactivity, but the manufacturing processes are a limiting factor that prevents them from producing the mandatory physical and mechanical properties for load-bearing applications. Therefore, the scientific interest varies for metals and ceramics. The chapter herein draws from contemporary research to provide examples of how material engineering is capitalised to tackle the challenges faced.

http://dx.doi.org/10.5772/62598

2. Metals

In general, metals possess a versatility that extends their application beyond that of other material classes, ranging from mechanical strength to bioactivity. A favourable characteristic of metals is the diversity of both the manufacturing processes available for shaping complex, porous structures, and the range of properties attainable. Metals show appreciable plasticity that allows them to be shaped either cold (ambient temperatures) or hot (high temperatures). Equally, altering their chemical composition can be achieved through a number of engineering routes. Alloying, from Old French to "combine," is a useful method of altering a metal's characteristics, including mechanical and chemical characteristics. Essentially, conventional methods entail two metals melted and combined together. A *solvent* metal (the parent metal) is combined with a *solute* metal where mixing occurs at the atomic level. The chemical outcome results in either a homogenous distribution of the combined atoms, or heterogeneous mixture with dissimilar atomic orientation.

Not all metals can be alloyed together due to factors such as atomic size, electrochemical behaviour, and valency, as well as temperature discrepancies.[1] As stated, the new changes at the atomic level can lead to profound changes to the metal's properties, such as mechanical, thermal, and wear-resistance behaviours. Moreover, subsequent fabrication processes are able to influence the final performance of the metals such as shaping, work hardening, and coating. Modifications can be made only on the surface, without a global change to the metal's structure. Treatments to the surface are effective in improving biological properties and can be both straightforward as well as cost-effective.

Metals used for implants are frequently formed from iron-, titanium-, and cobalt-based alloys. However, common iron- and cobalt-based implants (steel and cobalt-chromium alloys, respectively) are bioinert and possess mechanical properties that are deleterious to implant fixation. Titanium-based implants can be made bioactive through alloying and surface treatments, and their mechanical properties are less detrimental than steel and cobalt-chromium. Furthermore, a few metals yield degradable behaviour under physiological environment. The section herein illustrates examples of biodegradable and non-biodegradable metals, starting with the metal considered as the gold standard of metallic implants.

2.1. Non-degradable metals

2.1.1. Titanium

Titanium (Ti) and its alloys, such as the widely used Ti-6Al-4V (shortened to TAlV; contains aluminium and vanadium contents), have long been the favoured alloy for load-bearing applications [1]. While priced higher than other metals, titanium contains standout properties that make it a suitable choice for implants such as high specific strength, good corrosion resistance and biocompatibility. The latter two are attributed to the titanium oxide (TiO_2) layer

[1] As an example, the boiling temperature of magnesium is lower than the melting temperature of titanium and attempts to use the melt-driven alloy process results in partial evaporation of magnesium.

produced in the presence of oxygen that reforms within milliseconds when damaged [2]. Ti and its alloys exhibit high strength and good biocompatibility in contrast to 316L stainless steel, cobalt-chromium implants (Co-Cr). Pure titanium is stronger but also lighter with respect to steel; however, it possesses a stiffness (referred to as elastic or Young's modulus) that is several times higher than cortical bone.[2] The problem therein produces a phenomenon known as "stress shielding"—where the implant absorbs the applied stress instead of the bone which leads to the tissue resorption (i.e. dissolved). The dynamic state of bone regeneration-resorption is dictated by stress, among other factors. Tissue resorption around the implant leads to loosening and consequently a surgical revision is needed. Therefore, to ensure the longevity of titanium-based implants, the stiffness should be reduced as much as possible.

Alloying of Ti allows the compressive strength and weight benefit to be maintained above the threshold value but reduces the elastic modulus of the implant to lessen the effects of stress shielding. Furthermore, although non-modified pure Ti is unable to, TAlV can in fact bond with tissues, further securing the implant to the host's bone. Additionally, the alloy exhibits mechanical properties that are more suited for implantation than ceramics and, considering that pure titanium exhibited no cytoxicity, was conjectured to do the same. Clinical application of the alloy include fixation plates, fasteners (screws, nails, etc.), and bone replacement; however, it has been documented that aluminium and vanadium ion release from the surface can induce a plethora of side effects, such as neuropathy, Alzheimer's disease, and immunological responses, to name a few [1, 3].

In search of new alloying elements, potential metals have been evaluated in vitro, in their pure form. Niobium (Nb) and zirconium (Zr) were found to have low toxicity and higher cell proliferation detected with respect to other alloying elements, such as aluminium and molybdenum [1]. Thus, a surge of interest was generated in Ti alloys that incorporated both Zr and Nb (termed TNZ alloys). The improved biocompatibility of the TNZ alloys stems from the fact that the added elements produce a metal with ions that are less likely to elute from the implant surface as the elements are less soluble than aluminium and vanadium in biological fluids. In addition, the spontaneous coating formed (technically referred to as self-passivation) that provides greater protection to the substrate [4].

For load-bearing applications, TNZ alloys display excellent fatigue results that make them compelling for long-term load-bearing application. They could also be fabricated with a lower Young's modulus with adequate compressive strength and exhibit superior cold-forming ability with respect to other TAlV. Moreover, the alloys are cheaper to manufacture. Most of these qualities can be attributed to the rich β-phase found in TNZ. As mentioned, metals can be composed of more than one phase. Titanium can exist in a number of forms, of which the β-phase (not ordinarily seen at ambient temperatures), has been demonstrated to possess a lower elastic moduli than its counterparts, including the ($\alpha + \beta$) phase produced in Ti-6Al-4V [4–6]. Furthermore, studies have demonstrated how porous TNZ alloys can be fabricated with a physical structure and mechanical strength suitable for load-bearing applications. Indeed,

[2] The human bone is truly a complex structure. It comprises of two sections referred to as cancellous and cortical bone. The latter has the greater mechanical properties and thereof is used as a reference for load-bearing.

TNZ has inherited the versatility seen in other Ti-based alloys and is a likely candidate to replace TAlV [7–9].

Surface treatments are an alternative to ensuring a firm bone-implant bond, and can be applied to both dense and porous titanium. Considering that host tissues first point of contact is with the surface, such treatments are designed to avoid altering the bulk properties of the material and, as is the case in titanium, can be an alternative to avoiding toxicological concerns. They can be designed, however, in combination with desirable bulk attributes to further enhance biological properties. There are more than one surface treatments available that can be used to coat both dense and porous titanium, such as plasma surface modification [10] and hydrothermal treatments [11, 12] that result in an improvement to the coverage of the bone around the implant. One interesting method is ultraviolet (UV) light treatment to bioinert pure titanium. The treatment is technically simple as it does not require any additional chemical, high temperatures, or mechanical processing [13, 14], and can be applied to a range of Ti and its alloys [15]. The process involves a chemical reaction where hydrocarbons that form on the surface of titanium under ambient conditions are reduced and results in an osteoinductive metal with good osteoconductive properties. Furthermore, the coverage of bone tissue on the implant was found to be almost 100%, which is unprecedented for a titanium implant, and thus the term "superosteoconductive" has been coined for such an accomplishment [14, 16, 17]. UV-light treatment was also found to prompt a similar biological effect on chromium-cobalt alloys [17].

2.1.2. Other non-biodegradable metals

Titanium belongs to a group of metals known as refractory metals that are acknowledged for their excellent corrosion resistance and, incredibly, biocompatibility—such as tantalum and niobium [18, 19]. Both metals have displayed improved bone-implant binding with respect to titanium, with tantalum (Ta) exhibiting rapid bond-binding abilities. Surface adhesion can be further enhanced using hydrothermal treatments that form a Ta-OH layer, which is effective for bonding to bone [20–22] without adverse effects. Porous Ta can be engineered using methods such as solid-free form (see next section) and conventional powder methods, with porosity of up to 85%, and pore sizes ranging from 400 to 600 μm. The compressive strength and elastic modulus can also be tailored to that of cortical bone values [23, 24]. Short-term clinical trials have shown immediate weight-bearing capabilities, as well as a high volume of patient satisfaction in multiple orthopaedic implants [25]. Current limitations of the tantalum are its high cost and high density (preventing development of larger implants). Tantalum also displays a high melting temperature (>3000°C) that makes it difficult for processing using traditional alloying methods, and thus relies on powder metallurgic[3] routes for shaping.

Niobium (Nb) has been largely used as an alloying element and a coating due to its excellent biocompatibility but has been researched recently as a possible implant candidate in its pure form due to its attractive properties [26]. Unsurprisingly, Nb can be surface treated to become

[3] Techniques were extremely high temperatures needed for traditional alloying can be circumvented. Briefly, the metal is mixed in its powder form, followed by compaction into a desired shape and sintered.

bioactive and thus form a bone-implant bonding. With regards to load-bearing applications, Nb can be combined with zirconia to form a metal-ceramic composite which is capable of bearing high loads; however, more work is needed to determine the potential of pure niobium [27].

2.2. Biodegradable metals

2.2.1. Magnesium

Unequivocally, refractory metals offer a flexibility as orthopaedic implants that are difficult to match; however, for temporary implantations, bioresorbable materials are preferred as they can prevent a second surgery. Magnesium (Mg), on the other hand, does exhibit biodegradable capabilities in physiological conditions due to the presence of chlorides that react with the surface's chemical structure. Degradation of magnesium occurs through corrosion where Mg^{2+} ions are released and hydrogen gas is produced. Incidentally, Mg^{2+} is one of the essential minerals found in our body [28], of which over half the average is located in our bone cells—and deficiencies of the element results in several bone deformities. In addition, the release of Mg^{2+} results in mineralised bone formed on the surface, with in vivo tests demonstrating strong bone-implant bonding [29]. Moreover, in its dense form, the mechanical properties are more akin with cortical bone, and, at 44 GPa, the elastic modulus of magnesium is much lower than Ti and its alloys [30]. Current interest in magnesium is directed towards fasteners and fixation plates; however, based on contemporary research, it may be conceivable to advance its usage towards bone substitution.

Although biodegradability is a sought-after property, this is found to be rapid and uncontrollable in Mg, which causes the implant to lose much of its mechanical strength rapidly due to the rate of corrosion [31]. In vitro studies of Mg have demonstrated that cracks are generated through pits created by corrosion. Furthermore, the hydrogen gas released during corrosion further exacerbates implant failure by causing brittleness to the metal [32], in what can be referred to as "self-corroding," along with damaging the surrounding cells. Fortunately, the surface of magnesium is covered by a partial oxide film when exposed to air and aqueous environments and is said that corrosion attacks are more likely to occur in interruptions in the film [33]. Therefore, taking advantage of this phenomenon can be used to combat corrosion.

Alloying is again a favourable method in addressing the corrosion-assisted failure of Mg. There are about 25 metals with an appropriate atomic size, but realistically, only a few are considered to be appropriate alloying elements, due to the restriction in solubility. This number is further reduced when considering the use of adverse-free elements. Mg can be alloyed with calcium, strontium, and zinc, which are a plausible choice from a biological perspective considering that all three alloying elements are naturally present within the human body, with both Ca and Sr involved in bone metabolism [34]. Remarkably, all three have been implicated in the retardation of corrosion in both short-term in vitro and in vivo studies, with a synergistic effect observed when Ca and Sr are incorporated simultaneously, with respect to their individual binary Mg alloys [35]. Such mechanisms included improvement to the surface coverage of the oxide film, and higher resistance to corrosion via microstructural changes (via a reduction to

http://dx.doi.org/10.5772/62598

the grain size). There are reports, however, that suggest that excess amount of calcium can lead to a decrease corrosion resistance due to the formation of an intermetallic phase, Mg_2Ca [36], hence, tailoring the degradation rate can be made to suit the lifespan of an implant. Further work is needed to elucidate the optimum composition for a suitable strike between good strength and corrosion.

Surface treatment options with emphasis on altering the chemical structure of the surface have not been studied to the same extend as titanium. Nevertheless, improving the thickness of the oxide layer can be achieved through alkaline and heat treatment on the surface, with results indicating a slower degradation rate without observable cytotoxic effects.

Corrosion pits are able to intensify crack propagation under loading. Defects formed during manufacturing can also worsen corrosion resistance [37], which is further attenuated in porous Mg due to the increased surface area (i.e. more area for the chlorine to react with the surface). Therefore, in order to be seen as a candidate for bone replacement, the aforementioned setbacks will need further investigations. Porous magnesium continues to be a matter of intensive research.

2.2.2. Other biodegradable metals

Intriguingly, magnesium is joined by both iron and zinc as part of the resurrection of biodegradable metallic implants seen over the past three decades. The metals also degrade via corrosion. Iron (Fe) from an engineering perspective offers many advantages—such as low cost, availability, and durability, to name a few. Fe is also one of the essential elements that the human body requires, which further boosts its appeal. With respect to Mg, Fe and its alloys exhibit a significantly lower degradation rate in physiological fluid [38] and higher mechanical properties [39], with an elastic modulus of ~210 GPa, which once more, can be reduced drastically by incorporating pores [40]. The degradation rate of iron can be controlled using manganese or silicon alloying elements, to either increase or reduce the rate, respectively [38, 41]. Alternatively, Fe can be prepared as a porous structure to manipulate the degradation rate.

Zinc has a biodegradability that is in between pure Mg and pure Fe and hence could offer an alternative option for biodegradable implants. Zn is generally used as an alloying element to improve magnesium's properties, including corrosion and biological, and is also important for numerous protein functions in the body [42, 43]. This has led to the notion of zinc as a possible orthopaedic implant. Pure zinc has a low strength, plasticity, and hardness that limit its usage as a biomedical implant, and thus it relies on alloying techniques to improve its strength. Unsurprisingly, investigations were conducted on incorporating magnesium, calcium, and strontium, and all were found to augment the mechanical strength of zinc [44, 45]. From an engineering perspective, zinc-based alloys possess a low melting point and low reactivity in molten state, thus can be prepared by simple melting techniques. As of yet, most research is concentrated on the use of zinc as a fixation implant, but with Zn-Mg alloys boasting a compressive yield strength double that of femoral cortical bone, its potential as a load-bearing scaffold is very promising.

2.3. Summary of metals with bioactivity

In summary, metals possess a versatility that extends their application surpassing other material classes. New techniques are being developed and added to the existing large repertoire, and clever processing tricks are used to address reservations that exist with traditional methods, such cost and complexity. The emergence of metals that can be relied on to degrade by way of corrosion as metallic grafts is encouraging, and further research could surprisingly open more avenues. There are over 90 metals found on the periodic table; however, only a select few find recurring usage as alloying elements, particularly those found naturally in the human body. However, there are concerns regarding the metallic ions released into the human body that can have debilitating consequences in the long term.

3. Ceramics and glasses

Bioactive ceramics and glasses are brittle in nature with poor tensile and fracture toughness properties, which limits their application as orthopaedic implants. However, their excellent biological properties and no cytoxicity cannot be discounted, and accordingly, there is ardent interest in producing bone graft substitutes using bioactive ceramics and glasses. In contrast to metals, there are a number of bioresorbable ceramics and bioactive glasses (BG) with excellent osseointegration where degradation occurs as a consequence of dissolution (solution-mediated) and cell-mediate degradation. Hydroxyapatite (HA) is the mineral component of human bone[4] and, alongside a number of other calcium phosphates (CaP), can induce bone regeneration. CaP are a non-toxic group of ceramics with excellent bioactivity, which can be modified based on the calcium-to-phosphate ratio present resulting in a different structure. For example, a Ca/P ratio of 1.66 is associated with hydroxyapatite, whereas a Ca/P ratio of 1.5 results in a CaP with a significantly faster rate of degradation, known as tricalcium phosphate. Synthetic HA, ($Ca_{10}(PO_4)_6(OH)_2$), can be synthesised in a number of ways, where the quantity of raw materials, as well as heat treatment applied, can modify the Ca/P ratio. Other ceramics are also biocompatible with the human body and have been extensively used as orthopaedic implants, such as alumina (Al_2O_3) and zirconia (ZrO_2), but despite having high strength and excellent corrosion resistance, they are not bioactive. BGs have excellent bioactivity, where implantation of the material is able to bind to bone by producing a layer of carbonated HA between the glass and the host's bone [46]. In general, they have better biological properties as they are both osteoinductive and osteoconductive (see chapter introduction). Clinical indications for ceramics and bioactive glasses include vertebral arthrodesis, tibial osteotomy, and for filling femur, tibia, and humerus voids caused by fractures, resection, or tumour resection. Ceramisys' ReproBone™ and Keramat's Keramedic® are commercially available ceramic bone substitutes.

[4] In its carbonated form.

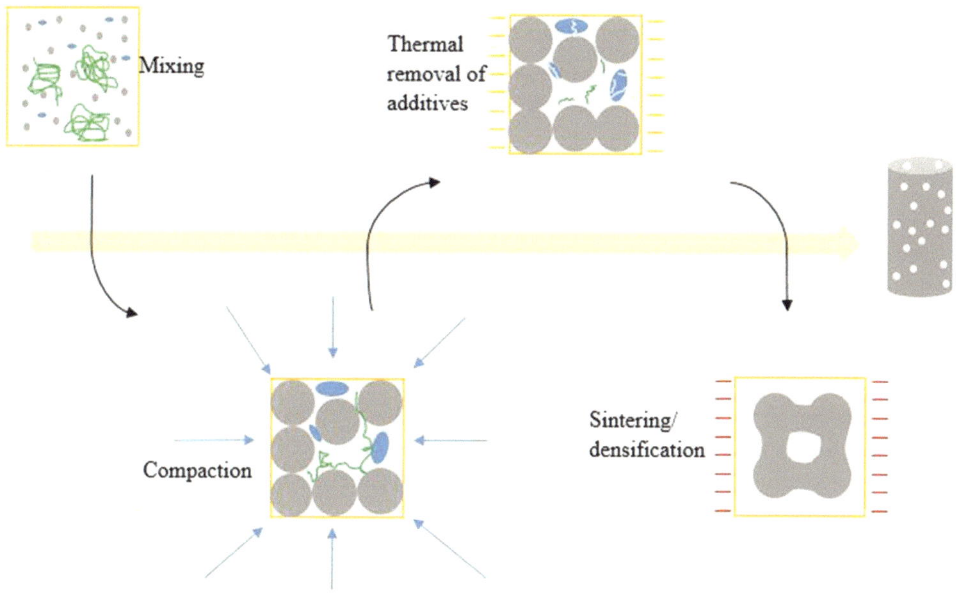

Figure 4. Schematic to illustrate the steps involved in forming ceramics using additives.

3.1. Fabrication of porous grafts

Dense hydroxyapatite displays a compressive strength that is markedly higher than cortical bone, and although it degrades at a rate well below the threshold for clinical use, it can be expedited with the implementation of pores. The quid pro quo for increased resorption due to porosity results in a substantial loss in mechanical strength. Moreover, as brittle materials with no appreciable plastic deformation (as anyone who has dropped a ceramic plate or glass beaker can attest to!), shaping of ceramics and glasses is difficult. Consequently, the outcome is a catastrophic failure in material due to microstructural flaws introduced throughout the processing stages. One possible solution is to use near-net shaping methods. Ceramic and glass in their powder form are combined with additives that introduces plasticity leading to complex, porous shapes produced. The powders are then evolved into a single solid mass through heating to remove the additives, and then subsequently heated at elevated temperatures to densify the solid mass—a process known as sintering. Plasticised ceramics with additives and a solvent are referred to as slurry or pastes. It has to be noted that removal of the non-ceramic contents presents its own problems.

Of relevance is not only complex shaping of the ceramics but the degree of porosity. Porosity and mechanical strength are mutually exclusive. The inclusion of pores contributes towards structural failure, as they are sites for crack initiators and propagation. Traditional fabrication routes have resulted in a porous scaffold with compressive strength well below the prescribed value. Such techniques are also difficult for producing a porous structure in a controllable manner because the pores are formed randomly. Moreover, the pores generated tend to have a spherical or ellipsoidal shape, where both pore morphologies experience tensile forces under compression loading—and it is the tensile forces established that give rise to crack nucleation. Preferably, engineering a scaffold where the majority of pores are in the shape of a columnar profile (i.e. parallel and aligned) is desired as the tensile forces are limited [47], and thus improve mechanical integrity. Moreover, a scaffold with interconnected pore channels leads to enhanced bone-binding abilities, hence is also sought after in pore designs. Therefore, there is pressing concern in seeking new fabrication routes with well-defined pore architecture. The knowledge can then perhaps be used to better the commercially available scaffolds. The section hereafter details innovative methods used to improve the compressive strength.

3.1.1. Freeze casting

Freeze casting is a novel method that provides a highly porous ceramic with a well-controlled structure. Initially developed for highly dense ceramics. A porous scaffold with an aligned interconnectivity can be attained, with the added option for a hybrid porous structure if needed [48]. Freezecasting is a cost-effective method that provides a wide range of porosity in ceramics [48] and does not require the use of complicated equipment with minimal additives needed. The method entails preparing a colloidal slurry of ceramic powder with a liquid (aqueous or not), then pouring it into a mould where one end is attached to a cooling mechanism able to initiate freezing. The frozen solvent acts as a temporary binder holding the suspension together before demoulding [49]. During the freezing step, the liquid portion pushes and packs the ceramic particles as the ice crystals grow until further packing cannot occur. The frozen slurry is subjected to sublimation (i.e. converted from solid to gas state) in a freeze-dryer where the ice crystal remnants form the porous phase of the structure. The final step is sintering of the powder. Freezing liquids have a tendency to expel impurities and ceramic solutes rather than incorporating them into the crystal lattice during crystal growth which results in a preferential arrangement where spaces between ice grains are enriched with solutes [50].

One distinguishable benefit of the technique is that benign liquids can be used [51], including water and camphene without the use of solid polymeric additives, which can limit pre-sintering defects (although they can be incorporated for additional modification or improving the green strength of the scaffold). Each liquid vehicle allows for further modification of the final product as different liquids can produce a different crystal structure when frozen, thus different pore morphologies can be achieved. Opting for camphene can further reduce the complexity and the overall cost of the technique as it can form its frozen crystals at room temperature and therefore does not require complex operations below 0°C. Other processing parameters, including freezing rate, time, and holding temperature, can be adjusted to control the scaffold, along with solid loading and particle size. Particles have an extra role in that the particle surface is able to influence the nucleation of the ice crystals, thus particle morphology can be assigned to generate different pores.

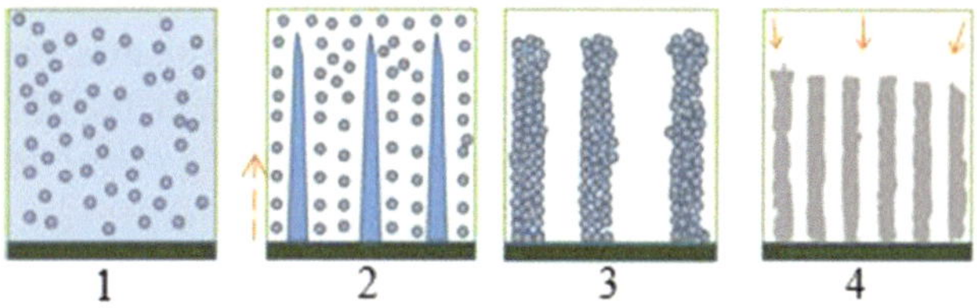

1. Ceramic particles in a suspension
2. Freezing stage
3. Sublimation
4. Densification

Figure 5. A schematic of the steps involved in freeze casting. The dashed arrow represents the direction of crystal growth, and the solid arrows represent the direction of densification.

With freeze casting, the removal of non-ceramic segments diminishes the drying stresses and shrinkage that are detected in other fabrication methods, therefore subsequently mitigating cracks and other defects observed before sintering [52]. Moreover, the technique allows for complex shapes to be generated, including a graded porosity where the scaffold comprises of regions with varying porous morphology [53], which is more representative of human bone. The process does not depend on chemical but on physical interaction and accordingly can be used to engineer other materials, such as bioactive glasses—or composites of bioactive glass/ceramic [54–56].

A remarkable compromise between porosity and compressive strength can be obtained using freeze casting, with recent research illustrating pore sizes ranging from 200 to 500 μm with a relatively high compressive strength comparable to that of cortical bone [49, 51, 57]. The controllable manner of porosity, as well as a high solid loading[5] of ceramic powder, is a contributory factor [58]. Equally impressive, high levels of porosity and powder loading were achieved in glass-only casts, in conjunction with compressive strength comparable to that of cortical bone [56]—hence, freeze casting is an encouraging technique for load-bearing applications.

3.1.2. *Solid free form*

Solid free form (SFF) is a relatively new technique developed towards the end of the last century and has gained tremendous attraction because of their ability to address key barriers faced by conventional fabrication methods. Although significant measures have been taken in mould-based fabrication routes with respect to mechanical properties, the lack of realising complex geometries, high spatial resolution of scaffold architecture, and labour-intensive procedures are considered a hindrance. Fortunately, SFF methods, also referred to as rapid prototyping or additive manufacturing, are able to address such shortcomings. SFF is an assortment of computer-controlled processes that build a scaffold from powders based on an iterative method, using a 3-dimensional (3D) computer-aided design (CAD). The computer-

[5] A high solid loading, or ceramic content, equates to improved powder packing and subsequently a densified structure with minimum unwanted gaps.

ised assistance delivers excellent reproducibility of outstanding spatial resolution. The CAD design can be based on an accurate reconstruction of the fractured site, using popular non-invasive imaging modalities such as computed tomography and magnetic resonance imaging scans, obtaining the geometry of the defect site. Thus, the techniques eliminate the need for post-processing machining of the scaffold to the desired, or incorporating "pockets" for the addition of protein carriers for a synergetic effect on healing rate if needed. The final outcome is a reduction in surgical time and cost before surgery, despite SFF techniques themselves are, by and large, more expensive than the conventional techniques used to manufacture bioceramics.

As mentioned in the previous section, SFFs can be used to engineer metallic structure, which is a testimony to their versatility. There are distinct methods for SFFs to assemble an implant, which are divided into two classes: extrusion based or powder based. In general, the latter offers improved flexibility for complex 3D shapes and their internal architecture but it is the former, extrusion based, that has been known to realise high compressive strengths sufficient for load-bearing use. Notably, a technique known as robocasting, colloidal HA pastes with compressive strengths reaching approximately 300 MPa were achieved, whereas direct ink writing and freeze-form extrusion fabrication attained 136 MPa and 140 MPa, respectively, for bioactive glass (13–93). All three SFF techniques are capable of attaining porosity of over 40%, but the range of pore size is restricted with respect to other techniques [59–61]. Direct ink writing fabrication of the primordial 45S5 Bioglass® has also been attempted, but the compressive strength was insufficient for bearing loads [62]. SFFs are rapid and can incorporate other processing conditions such as porogens for additional customisation [63, 64]. The high spatial finesse of SFF leads to superior mechanical properties because of their structured architecture [65]. Although bespoke grafts for clinical use can be developed, whether such complex geometries are able to maintain their structural strength will need to be investigated. SFF are still in their early stages and their potential is yet to be realised.

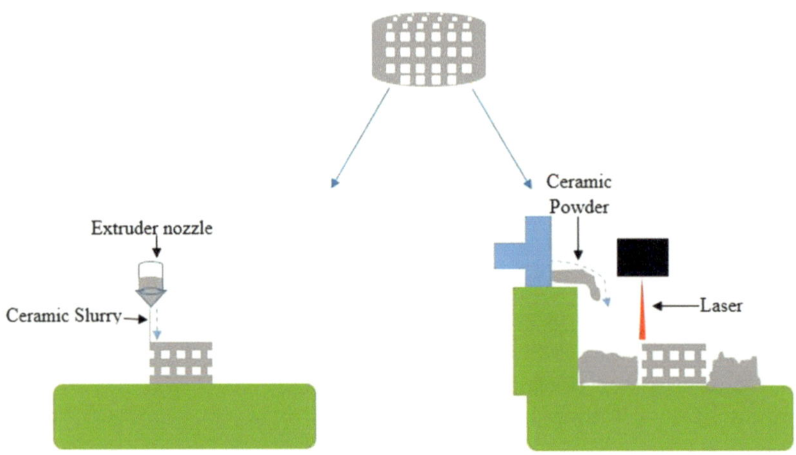

Figure 6. Schematic representing the two forms of solid free form.

3.2. Ionic substitution

Ionic substation, also known as doping, is analogous to alloying in metal in that essentially, elements are incorporated to produce a material where the base is still a ceramic but with a modified (and desirable) atomic structure that consequently results in altered properties. Doping of CaP is a simple technique, and more than one ionic substitution can be readily incorporated to occur simultaneously (i.e. double- or multi-substitution). Doping with fluorine is particularly favoured due to the improvement to both mechanical and biological properties in contrast to un-doped hydroxyapatite.

3.3. Summary

The strength can be enhanced if microstructural defects can be avoided, and hence the pressing concern is to seek a fabrication route that can eliminate such flaws. The section introduced examples of engineering routes capable of attaining sought-after compressive strengths, and despite their difference, the resultant research has elucidated structured porosity results in improved mechanical attributes.

Strengthening bioresorbable ceramic and glass can be achieved through minimising the processing steps in obtaining the final design, and/or minimal inclusion of non-ceramic components. The techniques described reveal that arranged pores are less susceptible to early fracturing. Such techniques carry a positive outlook and whence the fabrication methods have been perfected, they can be applied to other bioactive materials not mentioned in this section, such as calcium silicates. Incorporation of pores in a tightly controlled manner is of scientific interest because of the results on mechanical and biological properties are affected by pore morphology, and an aligned porous structure that allows for a high compressive strength to be achieved.

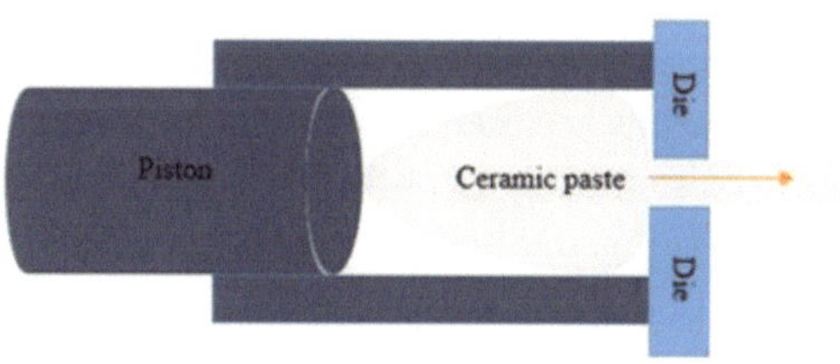

Figure 7. Extrusion schematic.

The fabrication of such pore architecture using traditional ceramic extrusion is of significant interest to the author. Extrusion is the technique of choice for imparting high strengths to ceramic in the catalyst support industry, and the aim is to transfer the accomplishment to bioactive ceramics. Essentially, a ceramic paste is forced through a honeycomb die followed by removal of additives and sintering. The desirable columnar and interconnected pores can be generated spanning the length of the scaffold as the cross-sectional features are maintained throughout the paste; and the die opted for can be designed to alter pore size, shape, and orientation. Large pressures can be generated to extrude a high solid-loading (67+ wt%)

ceramic paste that also compacts and reorients the ceramic particles for improved particle packing—thus minimising defects associated with shrinkage during drying and sintering.

4. Combined metal-ceramic approach

The human bone is fundamentally a biological composite composed of two phases where one instils strength and the other flexibility. Hence, it infers the use of synthetic composites. In principle, synthetic composites can be used to prevent elution of alloying elements in metals by applying a coating. If an enhanced bioactivity is desired throughout the implant then powder blending can be employed to embed CaP throughout the implant. The aim, once again, is to engineer an implant with both excellent mechanical properties and excellent osseointegration. Composites differ from alloying or ionic substitution in that the two amalgamated materials maintain their individualistic properties. Therefore, synthetic composites can provide an alternate route to developing new bioactive materials for load-bearing applications. The section herein provides examples of how osseointegration is improved in metallic implants through coating and powder blending.

4.1. Ceramic-metal composites

Combining ceramics and metals can be achieved through many routes, including coatings and powder blending. To reiterate, the first contact made between implant and the host occurs on the surface of the material, and thus, coating an implant can alter the host's response. This is an alternative method to addressing the ions released from metallic implants as coating with, for example, a CaP layer prevents the release of the harmful ions, effectively acting as a shield. Such coatings can be achieved either through physical or wet-chemical deposition methods. As the name suggests, physical deposition coats the designated substrate using a physical process that vaporises a solid form of CaP under vacuum (to eliminate contamination and ensure directional control). The atoms are then transferred to the surface where condensation of the vaporised atoms occurs culminating in a film coating of the substrate. Suffice it to say, this method of coating is costly as some methods require high power, and not to mention extra care is needed to ensure the method of vaporisation does not conduce decomposition of the specific CaP desired. Moreover, the physical deposition techniques are associated with "line-of-sight" coating, where the vaporised atoms coat the surface that is in-plane, and complex shapes with corners and holes are not well coated, if at all. Wet-chemical deposition on the other hand is less complex and better suited for coating intricate shapes. These techniques involve immersing or spraying a solution of highly saturated CaP to form the coating. The process does not require the same level of high temperatures allowing for organic components, such as antibiotics, to be incorporated into the process.

The two coating categories offer a range of techniques that allows for a range of possibilities —such as coating multi-doped HA, nano-range thickness, controlled porosity, and incorporating polymers, to name a few. Similarly, the substrates can be dense or porous, biodegradable, or non-biodegradable. In any case, the key considerations for a coating is to ensure excellent long-term adhesion with the surface of the implant and to resist delamination due to stresses caused during the processing stage, or stresses caused by degradation under physiological milieu that will expose the substrate surface. Additionally, the purity of the CaP will need to upheld and not decompose during the process, and in the case of load-bearing application, the mechanical properties are met. Hydroxyapatite and its doped derivatives have been comprehensively used to coat metals in order to alter their biological responses—such as imparting bioactivity to a pure Ti scaffold to elicit tissue bonding [66], and on Mg and its alloys to reduce their rapid corrosion and safeguard against localised toxicity of hydrogen gas [67, 68]. Coatings are able to act as a protective layer and stop the dissolution of harmful alloying elements, in the case of Ti-6Al-4V alloys, and can also be added to ceramic-metal composites (see Section 4.3). Relatively straightforward techniques with low temperature and low energy consumption requirement, as well as environmentally conscious are available—such as electrolytic deposition—and have been experimented with positive outcomes. Nevertheless, the added processing steps of applying the coating result in the overall fabrication process incurring costs.

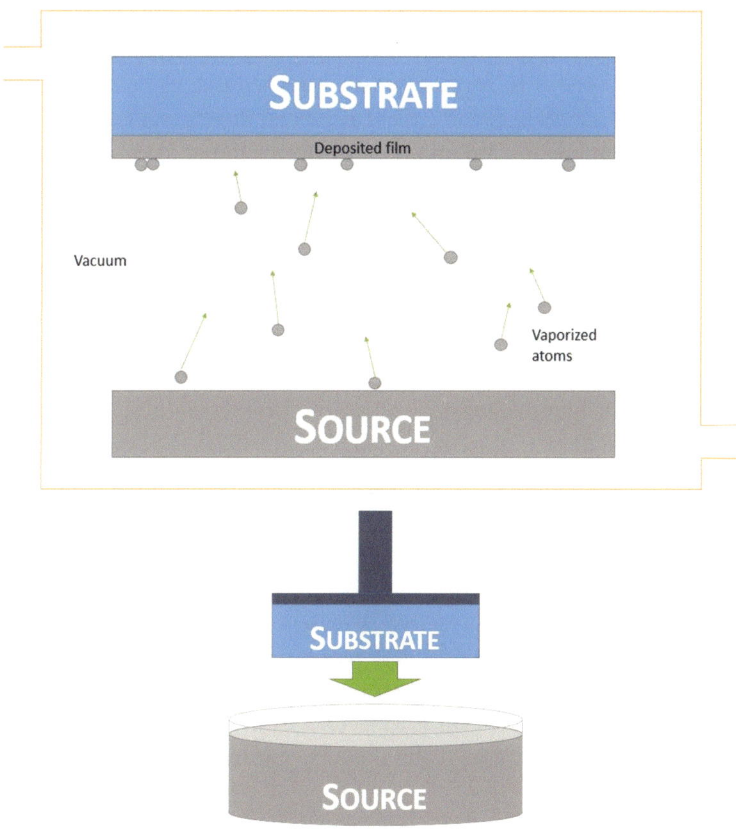

Figure 8. A representative of (a) physical and (b) wet deposition.

Other forms of ceramic-metal composites can be attained through the powder blending route. Metallic powders of iron and magnesium can be homogenously mixed with CaP powders, followed by consolidation and densification. This can be an ideal method if the strategy is to impart the desired qualities (e.g. ductility) throughout a porous structure rather than purely on the surface. Considerations such as mixing time and sintering temperatures need to be determined without resulting in contaminations by milling apparatus[6] or decomposition of CaP, respectively. In order to avoid the latter issue, Choy et al. [69] used microwave synthesis of a Ti-CaP composite to avoid using high temperatures, where materials absorb electromagnetic energy that are produced by the microwave and subsequently convert it into heat energy. Additional benefits of the technique include fast reaction rate and efficient energy transformation. A Ti-CaP composite with excellent mechanical properties comparable to cortical bone was fabricated by mixing and reacting Ti with two precursors of HA (calcium carbonate and dicalcium phosphate dihydrate in this case). Interestingly, it was discovered that the in situ synthesis method chosen resulted in the presence of Ti, HA, TTCP, and $CaTiO_3$, indicating that the calcium precursors were able to react indiscriminately with the Ti. Incidentally, $CaTiO_3$ was claimed to facilitate apatite formation in vitro.[7]

4.2. Same material composites

A titanium-magnesium porous composite is one example of two metals combined, and can be achieved in a number of ways to form a semi-biodegradable metallic implant—including powder blending, melt infiltration casting, or as a layered structure. Porosity and compressive strength suitable for bearing loads are attainable, but this depends on the amount of magnesium, which is significantly altered in situ as corrosion of Mg takes place.

5. Conclusion

Contemporary research in bioactive metals and ceramics for load-bearing application is focused on bridging the gap between mechanical properties and biocompatibility. The fabrication techniques detailed in this chapter have demonstrated that great strides have been made and in doing so, can potentially be applied to improve on existing orthopaedic implants. The chapter also presented materials that are yet to be used in load-bearing application, such as zinc and niobium, but have great potential in doing so. With regards to metals, mitigating the toxicity of their respective ions is the major focus. This can be achieved through alloying with elements that are less toxic, or improving the coating on the implant to ensure ion release is minimised. Emerging biodegradable metals, such as magnesium and iron, are highly promising as they can reduce the overall healthcare cost. These metals degrade in the body through corrosion, and, as they are naturally found in the body, they can be excreted. The message from bioactive metals is that if the metal is naturally found in the body, then it is

---

[6] Wear from the container for example in which the powders are mixed can form into the mixture.

[7] Intriguingly, this is a clear example of how an attempt to address an issue results in more questions and possibilities in biomaterial engineering.

corroded and thus resorbed. If not, then if binding should occur, improved binding is achieved if a ceramic coating is formed, for example, TiO_2 on titanium-based implant. This is interesting considering that metals such as titanium and tantalum are extracted in their oxide form and are followed by arduous processing to achieve high levels of purity, for only osseous tissues to show preference to their oxide form. Perhaps if certain steps necessary for achieving high purity can be avoided, then this could lessen the costs associated with the manufacturing steps, and thus implant fabrication.

Many ceramics and glasses display excellent bioactivity and are toxic-free. This is to be expected considering that they have been synthesised based on the composition of natural bone. Forming ceramics and glass into complex shapes is difficult irrespective of the application due to their inherent properties; however, progress is being made to eliminate such factors. The chapter on ceramics and glasses focused predominantly on fabrication routes with "ideal" porous structure. Such techniques have elucidated to how compressive strength for load-bearing application is attainable in porous CaP if excellent control over the physical properties can be achieved. However, the bone exhibits multiple stress states which will all need to be addressed before clinical application is considered. To achieve desirable flexural (bending) strength and fracture toughness, the fabrication method could use a CaP reinforced with ceramics that possess high toughness and flexural strength. Reinforcing dense β-TCP composite with varying amounts of the bioactive TiO_2 is known to increase the fracture toughness and flexural strength similar to that of cortical bone. Recent progress showed that an eight-fold increase in compressive strength in HA reinforced with TiO_2 above the required amount, with respect to TiO_2-free HA. Alternatively, hydroxyapatite rod-like particulates, also known as whiskers, can be incorporated into the CaP matrix. Although a form of CaP, the whiskers are able to preserve their morphology during sintering, forming a distinct phase from the surrounding CaP. When dispersed throughout the microstructure, whiskers improve the fracture resistance by deflecting microcrack propagation, as well as absorbing the energy generated by the microcrack. Factors such as the aspect ratio, whisker orientation, and content volume influence their effectiveness. Incidentally, natural bone exhibits crack deflection behaviour. Therefore, in theory, fabricating CaP using freeze casting or extrusion with reinforced whiskers or TiO_2 can enhance flexural strength and/or fracture toughness, and thus CaP implants can be made suitable for multiple stress states.

The final section of the chapter presented examples of how ceramics and materials can be combined to produce synthetic implants with excellent bioactivity and mechanical properties. A CaP coating can be applied to titanium or magnesium to impart bioactivity or improve corrosion resistance, respectively. However, the extra process required additional costs.

Titanium-based materials still remain as the exemplary implant for load-bearing application. The fatigue resistance and analysis of multiple stress responses of biodegradable materials have not been concluded, and indeed, there are concerns with their ability to reach the benchmark set by titanium-based materials. However, if they can be engineered to withstand the initial load and allow for natural bone to remodel, then what synthetic material currently available (and possibly for the very long foreseeable future) is able to outperform the natural bone? Furthermore, the great diversity in bone morphology means that there is no ideal scaffold and thus each application requires a bespoke graft with matching mechanical properties, which will need to be addressed.

It is evident from this chapter that material engineers are exhausting their resources and developing ingenious methods in the process to improving bioactive implants. There are issues regarding the rate of degradation of bioresorbable implants; however, different materials (e.g. magnesium and zinc) degrade at varying rates. It will be interesting to see if technology can allow for a multi-layered bioresorbable implant can be engineered (the different layers corresponding to different bioresorbable materials). Investigations into finding ways of degrading titanium could be interesting. The conjecturing of future directions in the field is limitless and thus it can be said with confidence that the future of the field is very encouraging.

Author details

Mohammed Elbadawi[1*], James Meredith[1], Lynne Hopkins[2] and Ian Reaney[2]

*Address all correspondence to: melbadawi1@sheffield.ac.uk

1 Department of Mechanical Engineering, University of Sheffield, Sheffield, United Kingdom

2 Department of Material Science and Engineering, University of Sheffield, United Kingdom

References

[1] Stenlund P., et al., *Bone response to a novel Ti–Ta–Nb–Zr alloy.* Acta Biomaterialia, 2015. 20: p. 165–175.

[2] Velten D., et al., *Preparation of TiO2 layers on cp-Ti and Ti6Al4V by thermal and anodic oxidation and by sol–gel coating techniques and their characterization.* Journal of Biomedical Materials Research, 2002. 59(1): p. 18–28.

[3] Aguilar C., et al., *Synthesis and characterization of Ti–Ta–Nb–Mn foams.* Materials Science and Engineering: C, 2016. 58: p. 420–431.

[4] Henriques V., et al., *Production of Ti–13Nb–13Zr alloy for surgical implants by powder metallurgy.* Journal of Materials Science Letters, 2010. 45(21): p. 5844–5850.

[5] Bai Y., et al., *Characterization, corrosion behavior, cellular response and in vivo bone tissue compatibility of titanium-niobium alloy with low Young's modulus.* Materials Science & Engineering. C, Materials for Biological Applications, 2016. 59: p. 565.

[6] Ozan S., et al., *Development of Ti–Nb–Zr alloys with high elastic admissible strain for temporary orthopedic devices.* Acta Biomaterialia, 2015. 20: p. 176–187.

[7] Rao X., Chu C.L., and Zheng Y.Y., *Phase composition, microstructure, and mechanical properties of porous Ti–Nb–Zr alloys prepared by a two-step foaming powder metallurgy method.* Journal of the Mechanical Behavior of Biomedical Materials, 2014. 34: p. 27–36.

[8] Wang X., et al., *Porous TiNbZr alloy scaffolds for biomedical applications.* Acta Biomaterialia, 2009. 5(9): p. 3616–3624.

[9] Sheremetyev V., et al., *Functional fatigue behavior of superelastic beta Ti-22Nb-6Zr(at%) alloy for load-bearing biomedical applications.* Materials Science and Engineering C, 2016. 58: p. 935–944.

[10] Chu P.K., et al., *Plasma-surface modification of biomaterials.* Materials Science and Engineering: R: Reports, 2002. 36(5–6): p. 143–206.

[11] Hamada K., et al., *Hydrothermal modification of titanium surface in calcium solutions.* Biomaterials, 2002. 23(10): p. 2265–2272.

[12] Takemoto S., et al., *Corrosion behavior and surface characterization of titanium in solution containing fluoride and albumin.* Biomaterials, 2005. 26(8): p. 829–837.

[13] Tsukimura N., et al., *Synergistic effects of UV photofunctionalization and micro-nano hybrid topography on the biological properties of titanium.* Biomaterials, 2011. 32(19): p. 4358–4368.

[14] Hori N., et al., *Effects of UV photofunctionalization on the nanotopography enhanced initial bioactivity of titanium.* Acta Biomaterialia, 2011. 7(10): p. 3679–3691.

[15] Ishijima M., et al., *Enhancing osteoblast-affinity of titanium scaffolds for bone engineering by use of ultraviolet light treatment.* Biomedical Research (Japan), 2015. 36(1): p. 55–62.

[16] Hori N., et al., *Electrostatic control of protein adsorption on UV-photofunctionalized titanium.* Acta Biomaterialia, 2010. 6(10): p. 4175–4180.

[17] Att W., et al., *The effect of UV-photofunctionalization on the time-related bioactivity of titanium and chromium–cobalt alloys.* Biomaterials, 2009. 30(26): p. 4268–4276.

[18] Matsuno H., et al., *Biocompatibility and osteogenesis of refractory metal implants, titanium, hafnium, niobium, tantalum and rhenium.* Biomaterials, 2001. 22(11): p. 1253–1262.

[19] Levine B.R., et al., *Experimental and clinical performance of porous tantalum in orthopedic surgery.* Biomaterials, 2006. 27(27): p. 4671–4681.

[20] Godley R., StarosvetskyD., and GotmanI., *Bonelike apatite formation on niobium metal treated in aqueous NaOH.* Official Journal of the European Society for Biomaterials, 2004. 15(10): p. 1073–1077.

[21] Gao H., et al., *Bioactive tantalum metal prepared by micro-arc oxidation and NaOH treatment.* Journal of Materials Chemistry B, 2014. 2(9): p. 1216–1224.

[22] Kokubo T., et al., *REVIEW Bioactive metals: preparation and properties.* Official Journal of the European Society for Biomaterials, 2004. 15(2): p. 99–107.

[23] Balla V., et al., *Tantalum—a bioactive metal for implants.* The Journal of The Minerals, Metals & Materials Society (TMS), 2010. 62(7): p. 61–64.

[24] Arabnejad S., et al., *High-strength porous biomaterials for bone replacement: a strategy to assess the interplay between cell morphology, mechanical properties, bone ingrowth and manufacturing constraints.* Acta Biomaterialia, 2016. 30: p. 345–356.

[25] Long W.J. and Scuderi G.R., *Porous tantalum cones for large metaphyseal tibial defects in revision total knee arthroplasty: a minimum 2-year follow-up.* The Journal of Arthroplasty, 2009. 24(7): p. 1086–1092.

[26] Johansson C.B. and Albrektsson T., *A removal torque and histomorphometric study of commercially pure niobium and titanium implants in rabbit bone.* Clinical Oral Implants Research, 1991. 2(1): p. 24–29.

[27] Bartolomé J.F., et al., *In vitro and in vivo evaluation of a new zirconia/niobium biocermet for hard tissue replacement.* Biomaterials, 2016. 76: p. 313–320.

[28] Mochizuki A. and Kaneda H., *Study on the blood compatibility and biodegradation properties of magnesium alloys.* Materials Science & Engineering C, 2015. 47: p. 204–210.

[29] Berglund I.S., et al., *Peri-implant tissue response and biodegradation performance of a Mg–1.0Ca–0.5Sr alloy in rat tibia.* Materials Science and Engineering: C, 2016. 62: p. 79–85.

[30] Pompa L., et al., *Surface characterization and cytotoxicity response of biodegradable magnesium alloys.* Materials Science and Engineering: C, 2015. 49: p. 761–768.

[31] Jafari S., Singh Raman R.K., and Davies C.H.J., *Corrosion fatigue of a magnesium alloy in modified simulated body fluid.* Engineering Fracture Mechanics, 2015. 137: p. 2–11.

[32] Atrens A., Liu M., and Zainal Abidin N.I., *Corrosion mechanism applicable to biodegradable magnesium implants.* Materials Science & Engineering B, 2011. 176(20): p. 1609–1636.

[33] Atrens A., et al., *Advances in Mg corrosion and research suggestions.* Journal of Magnesium and Alloys, 2013. 1(3): p. 177–200.

[34] Guan, R.-g., et al., *Development and evaluation of a magnesium–zinc–strontium alloy for biomedical applications—alloy processing, microstructure, mechanical properties, and biodegradation.* Materials Science & Engineering C, 2013. 33(7): p. 3661–3669.

[35] Bornapour M., et al., *Magnesium implant alloy with low levels of strontium and calcium: the third element effect and phase selection improve bio-corrosion resistance and mechanical performance.* Materials Science & Engineering C, 2014. 35: p. 267–282.

[36] Harandi S.E., et al., *Effect of calcium content on the microstructure, hardness and in-vitro corrosion behavior of biodegradable Mg-Ca binary alloy.* Materials Research, 2013. 16: p. 11–18.

[37] Singh Raman R.K., S. Jafari, and S.E. Harandi, *Corrosion fatigue fracture of magnesium alloys in bioimplant applications: a review.* Engineering Fracture Mechanics, 2015. 137: p. 97–108.

[38] Xu Z., Hodgson M.A., and Cao P., *A comparative study of powder metallurgical (PM) and wrought Fe–Mn–Si alloys.* Materials Science and Engineering: A, 2015. 630: p. 116–124.

[39] Schinhammer M., et al., *Design strategy for biodegradable Fe-based alloys for medical applications.* Acta Biomaterialia, 2010. 6(5): p. 1705–1713.

[40] Čapek J., et al., *Microstructural, mechanical, corrosion and cytotoxicity characterization of the hot forged FeMn30(wt.%) alloy.* Materials Science and Engineering C, 2016. 58: p. 900–908.

[41] Fântânariu M., et al., *A new Fe–Mn–Si alloplastic biomaterial as bone grafting material: In vivo study.* Applied Surface Science, 2015. 352: p. 129–139

[42] Zakiyuddin A. and LeeK., *Effect of a small addition of zinc and manganese to Mg–Ca based alloys on degradation behavior in physiological media.* Journal of Alloys and Compounds, 2015. 629: p. 274–283.

[43] Zhou Y.-L., et al., *Microstructures, mechanical and corrosion properties and biocompatibility of as extruded Mg–Mn–Zn–Nd alloys for biomedical applications.* Materials Science and Engineering: C, 2015. 49: p. 93–100.

[44] Kubásek J., et al., *Structure, mechanical characteristics and in vitro degradation, cytotoxicity, genotoxicity and mutagenicity of novel biodegradable Zn-Mg alloys.* Materials Science & Engineering. C, Materials for Biological Applications, 2016. 58: p. 24.

[45] Liu X., et al., *Effects of alloying elements (Ca and Sr) on microstructure, mechanical property and in vitro corrosion behavior of biodegradable Zn–1.5Mg alloy.* Journal of Alloys and Compounds, 2016. 664: p. 444–452.

[46] Hoppe A., Güldal N.S., and Boccaccini A.R., *A review of the biological response to ionic dissolution products from bioactive glasses and glass-ceramics.* Biomaterials, 2011. 32(11): p. 2757–2774.

[47] Huang T.S., et al., *Porous and strong bioactive glass (13–93) scaffolds fabricated by freeze extrusion technique.* Materials Science & Engineering C, 2011. 31(7): p. 1482–1489.

[48] Liu R., XuT., and Wang C.-A., *A review of fabrication strategies and applications of porous ceramics prepared by freeze-casting method.* Ceramics International, 2016. 42(2, Part B): p. 2907–2925.

[49] Deville S., Saiz E., and Tomsia A.P., *Freeze casting of hydroxyapatite scaffolds for bone tissue engineering.* Biomaterials, 2006. 27(32): p. 5480–5489.

[50] Pawelec K., et al., *Ice-templated structures for biomedical tissue repair: from physics to final scaffolds.* Applied Physics Reviews, 2014. 1(2): p. 021301-1 – 021301-13

[51] Wegst U.G.K., et al., *Biomaterials by freeze casting*. Philosophical Transactions of the Royal Society A, 2010. 368(1917): p. 2099–2121.

[52] Macchetta A., Turner I.G., and Bowen C.R., *Fabrication of HA/TCP scaffolds with a graded and porous structure using a camphene-based freeze-casting method*. Acta Biomaterialia, 2009. 5(4): p. 1319–1327.

[53] Tang Y., et al., *Two-step freeze casting fabrication of hydroxyapatite porous scaffolds with bionic bone graded structure*. Ceramics International, 2013. 39(8): p. 9703–9707.

[54] Mozafari M. and Moztarzadeh F., *Synthesis, characterisation and biocompatibility evaluation of sol–gel derived bioactive glass scaffolds prepared by freeze casting method*. Ceramics International, 2014. 40(4): p. 5349–5355.

[55] Mallick K.K., *Freeze casting of porous bioactive glass and bioceramics*. Journal of the American Ceramic Society, 2009. 92: p. S85–S94.

[56] Liu X., Rahaman M., and Fu Q., *Oriented bioactive glass (13–93) scaffolds with controllable pore size by unidirectional freezing of camphene-based suspensions: microstructure and mechanical response*. Acta Biomaterials, 2011. 7(1): p. 406–416.

[57] Deville S., *Freeze-casting of porous ceramics: a review of current achievements and issues*. Advanced Engineering Materials, 2008. 10(3): p. 155–169.

[58] Soon Y.-M., et al., *Compressive strength and processing of camphene-based freeze cast calcium phosphate scaffolds with aligned pores*. Materials Letters, 2009. 63(17): p. 1548–1550.

[59] Dellinger J.G., Wojtowicz A.M., and Jamison R.D., *Effects of degradation and porosity on the load bearing properties of model hydroxyapatite bone scaffolds*. Journal of Biomedical Materials Research Part A, 2006. 77(3): p. 563–571.

[60] Fu Q., Saiz E., and Tomsia A.P., *Direct ink writing of highly porous and strong glass scaffolds for load-bearing bone defects repair and regeneration*. Acta Biomaterialia, 2011. 7(10): p. 3547–3554.

[61] Huang T.S., et al., *Porous and strong bioactive glass (13–93) scaffolds fabricated by freeze extrusion technique*. Materials Science and Engineering: C, 2011. 31(7): p. 1482–1489.

[62] Eqtesadi S., et al., *A simple recipe for direct writing complex 45S5 Bioglass® 3D scaffolds*. Materials Letters, 2013. 93: p. 68–71.

[63] Leong K.F., Cheah C.M., and Chua C.K., *Solid freeform fabrication of three-dimensional scaffolds for engineering replacement tissues and organs*. Biomaterials, 2003. 24(13): p. 2363–2378.

[64] Cesarano J., et al., *Customisation of load-bearing hydroxyapatite lattice scaffolds*. International Journal of Applied Ceramic Technology, 2005. 2(3): p. 212–220.

[65] Doiphode N., et al., *Freeze extrusion fabrication of 13–93 bioactive glass scaffolds for bone repair*. Official Journal of the European Society for Biomaterials, 2011. 22(3): p. 515–523.

[66] Gopi D., Shinyjoy E., and Kavitha L., *Influence of ionic substitution in improving the biological property of carbon nanotubes reinforced hydroxyapatite composite coating on titanium for orthopedic applications.* Ceramics International, 2015. 41(4): p. 5454–5463.

[67] Zhang J., et al., *Effect of the addition CNTs on performance of CaP/chitosan/coating deposited on magnesium alloy by electrophoretic deposition.* Materials Science and Engineering C, 2016. 58: p. 992–1000.

[68] Zomorodian A., et al., *Biofunctional composite coating architectures based on polycaprolactone and nanohydroxyapatite for controlled corrosion activity and enhanced biocompatibility of magnesium AZ31 alloy.* Materials Science & Engineering C, 2015. 48: p. 434–443.

[69] Choy M., et al., *Microwave assisted-in situ synthesis of porous titanium/calcium phosphate composites and their in vitro apatite-forming capability.* Composites Part B: Engineering, 2015. 83: p. 50–57.

Section 3

Tissue Engineering

Chapter 11

Bioreactor-Based Bone Tissue Engineering

Inga Marijanovic, Maja Antunovic, Igor Matic,
Marina Panek and Alan Ivkovic

Additional information is available at the end of the chapter

http://dx.doi.org/10.5772/62546

Abstract

The aim of this chapter is to describe the main issues of bone tissue engineering. Bone transplants are widely used in orthopedic, plastic and reconstructive surgery. Current technologies like autologous and allogenic transplantation have several disadvantages making them relatively unsatisfactory, like donor site morbidity, chronic pain, and immunogenicity and risk hazard from infectious disease. Therefore, regenerative orthopedics seeks to establish a successful protocol for the healing of severe bone damage using engineered bone grafts. The optimization of protocols for bone graft production using autologous mesenchymal stem cells loaded on appropriate scaffolds, exposed to osteogenic inducers and mechanical force in bioreactor, should be able to solve the current limitations in managing bone injuries. We discuss mesenchymal stem cells as the most suitable cell type for bone tissue engineering. They can be isolated from a variety of mesenchymal tissues and can differentiate into osteoblasts when given appropriate mechanical support and osteoinductive signal. Mechanical support can be provided by different cell scaffolds based on natural or synthetic biomaterials, as well as combined composite materials. Three-dimensional support is enabled by bioreactor systems providing several advantages as mechanical loading, homogeneous distribution of cells and adequate nutrients/waste exchange. We also discuss the variety of osteoinductive signals that can be applied in bone tissue engineering. The near future of bone healing and regeneration is closely related to advances in tissue engineering. The optimization of protocols of bone graft production using autologous mesenchymal stem cells loaded on appropriate scaffolds, exposed to osteogenic inducers and mechanical force in bioreactor, should be able to solve the current limitations in managing bone injuries.

Keywords: bioreactor, bone, stem cells, differentiation, scaffold

1. Introduction

Tissue engineering is a multidisciplinary field that applies basic concepts and techniques of life science and engineering. It is generally understood as a process of taking human or animal tissues, isolating cells from the tissues, culturing the isolated cells in a supporting material, i.e., scaffold to fabricate cell-scaffold complex, and transplanting the fabricated cell-scaffold complex into human or animal subject. It is applied to fabricate almost every human organ including artificial skin, artificial bone, artificial cartilage, artificial cornea, artificial blood vessels and artificial muscles.

Bone is one of the few organs/tissues capable of spontaneous regeneration rather than simple repair. In other words, after disruption of its structure (fracture), its unique microanatomy and biological properties enable complete structural restoration without the creation of fibrotic scar tissue. However, in certain clinical situations where extensive injury, disease or malformation cause such large defects, it is necessary to resort to bone reconstruction, restoration and/or regeneration by a surgical procedure that replaces missing bone, i.e., by bone grafting. A bone graft is an implanted material that promotes bone healing alone or in combination with other material(s), through osteogenesis, osteoinduction and osteoconduction, in combination or alone [1].

The selection of an ideal bone graft relies on several factors such as tissue viability, defect size, graft size, shape and volume, biomechanical characteristics, graft handling, cost, ethical issues, biological characteristics and associated complications. The materials used in bone grafting can be divided into several major categories, including autografts, allografts, and xenografts. Synthetic and biologically based, tissue-engineered biomaterials and combinations of these substitutes are other options. Altogether, tissue-engineered bone graft requires the optimal selection of cells that are seeded on biomaterial-based scaffolds and exposed to specific biochemical and physical signals known to induce osteogenesis. The development of the successful bone tissue-engineering protocols depends very much on our understanding of bone structure, physiology and development.

Bone is a dynamic biological tissue consisting of metabolically active cells. The cell component of bone consists of the precursor cells (progenitors), osteoblasts, osteoclasts, osteocytes and bone marrow hematopoietic elements. Osteoblasts are metabolically active mature bone-forming cells. They secrete osteoid, non-mineralized organic corpuscle that in turn undergoes mineralization process. Osteocytes are mature osteoblasts trapped within the bone matrix. Every osteocyte extends network of cytoplasmic tubules to the blood vessels and other cells. These cells are involved in the control of extracellular calcium. Osteoclasts are large multi-nucleated cells that degrade bone. Beside cells, bone is also composed of organic and inorganic elements. Approximately 20% of the weight of bone is water until the weight of dry inorganic bone makes calcium phosphate (65–70%) and the organic matrix of fibrous proteins and collagen (30–35%). Bone formation models in vitro are based on the fact that cell differentiation and function can be modelled according to factors that are important for embryonic development. Stem cells represent the building blocks of our bodies, functioning as the natural units of embryonic generation during development and adult regeneration following tissue damage. Stem cells are undifferentiated cells that can, under certain influence, differentiate into specialized cells and tissues. During development, the potency of stem cells decreases from totipotent stem cells (morula stage), capable of differentiating into all embryonic and extra embryonic tissues, to pluripotent stem cells (PSCs) (blastocyst stage), forming all embryonic tissues, and to multi- or unipotent adult stem cells (ASCs), forming tissues within their germ layer or tissue compartment [2]. Here, we discuss clinically relevant multipotent ASCs found in various adult tissues. Adult stem cells, also called somatic stem cells, in adult organism act as repair system for the body, replenishing adult tissues, prompt tissue homeostasis throughout life and ensure tissue regeneration following damage and they have great potential in regenerative medicine. Mesenchymal stem cells replenish connective tissues including bone. Therefore, they are the first choice among ASCs for regeneration of bone tissue.

Osteogenic differentiation *in vitro* is induced by ascorbic acid, b-glycerophosphate and dexamethasone. Ascorbic acid is essential for the development of osteoblasts, serves as a cofactor in the synthesis of collagen and stimulates the production of extracellular matrix, proliferation and differentiation of cells. b-Glycerophosphate serves as a source of phosphate for the formation of calcium phosphate *in vitro*. It is also responsible for the formation of three-dimensional bone nodules between cells as proof of realized osteoblast phenotype. Dexamethasone (DEX) is composed by a synthetic glucocorticoid, which regulates the expression of osteoblast genes, enhances differentiation *in vitro*, alkaline phosphatase activity and mineralization of bone. Understanding of osteoblast differentiation provided us the information on key pathways' components and enabled us the induction of differentiation using different recombinant proteins like BMP-2, -6 to -9. Also, mechanical stimulation promotes osteoblast differentiation and induces mineralization of extracellular matrix. Mechanical stimulation can be achieved using steady and dynamic fluid flow in bioreactors. For this purpose, different dynamic culture systems have been developed. These systems improve nutrient delivery to the cells and generate shear stress that promotes cell differentiation into osteoblastic phenotype. Bioreactors for bone engineering applications are broadly classified in few main categories, including rotating wall vessels, spinner flasks, perfusion bioreactors and compression systems. In addition to these, combinations of different bioreactors types have been explored in order to better mimic the bone physiological environment *in vitro*, such as for example compression bioreactors with added perfusion [3]. The process of bone tissue engineering in three-dimensional dynamic bioreactor system is a recapitulation of bone healing process *in vivo* in which progenitor cells, due to signals in the microenvironment, are stimulated to differentiate into osteoblasts [4].

2. Cells in bone engineering

2.1. MSCs as the best choice

The important step in bone engineering is the choice of human cell sources that can efficiently produce bone grafts when attached to proper mechanical support with the addition of osteogenic supplements. Cell types that can be potentially used in bone engineering are primary osteogenic cells isolated from adult bone tissue and periosteum, embryonic stem cells (ESCs), induced PSCs (iPSCs) and ASCs.

The selection of appropriate cell source for bone tissue engineering depends on several factors such as:

- Possibility of application of patient's own (autologous) cells or another person's (allogeneic) cells;
- Availability and ease of tissue harvesting with minimal donor site morbidity;
- Efficiency of cell isolation and cell yield;
- Potential of cell proliferation;
- Use of cells that have both osteogenic and vasculogenic potential to support the formation of vascularized bone;
- Homogeneity of the obtained cell population;
- Control of induction of osteogenic phenotype;
- Phenotype stability and cell safety;
- Automation and good manufacturing practices production.

Among the mentioned candidates, mesenchymal stem cells (MSCs), as a member of the ASC group, currently possess characteristics that make them the most appropriate cell source for bone tissue engineering. Unlike ESCs which are pluripotent and have unlimited potential for proliferation *in vitro* [5], MSCs possess multilineage differentiation potential and have limited proliferation capacity [6, 7]. In bone tissue engineering, ESCs gained enormous value as a cell source for the derivation of multiple lineages present in adult bone, such as osteogenic cells, vascular cells, osteoclasts, nerve cells and others. Despite increasing interest in the application of ESCs in bone regeneration strategies, use of this cell source is limited due to political issues and ethical concerns as well as safety reasons. The primary concern is the source from which ESCs are derived. The most commonly referenced pluripotent cells are ESCs derived from the inner cell mass of blastocyst which results in destruction of the embryo [8]. It has also become clear that pluripotency is a double-edged sword; the same plasticity that permits hESCs to generate hundreds of different cell types also makes them difficult to control. Transplantation of hESCs into immune-deficient mice leads to the formation of differentiated tumors comprising all three germ layers, resembling spontaneous human teratomas [9, 10]. Karyotype abnormalities have been observed in ESCs as well as in human iPSCs [11]. Therefore, further studies are needed to ensure the stability and safety of ESC-derived progenitor populations before their potential use in clinical applications. Because these particular cells have created an ethical debate, the researchers have investigated fetal stem cells derived from voluntary interruption of pregnancy as a potential cell source for bone tissue engineering [12]. The cells that have potential medical applications, especially in organ regeneration [13–17], and importantly posess no ethical issues concerning their employment are amniotic stem cells. They are mixture of stem cells that can be obtained from the amniotic fluid [18–20] and the amniotic membrane [21]. They represent a novel class of PSCs with intermediate characteristics between embryonic and ASCs, as they are able to differentiate into lineages representative of all three germ layers but do not form tumours when injected *in vivo* [22]. They can develop into various tissue types including skin, cartilage, cardiac tissue, nerves, muscle and bone [23–25]. In 2006, Kazutoshi Takahashi and Shinya Yamanaka established for the first time murine ES-like cell lines from mouse embryonic fibroblasts (MEFs) and skin fibroblasts by simply expressing four transcription factor genes encoding Oct4, Sox2, Klf4 and c-Myc [26]. They called these somatic cell-derived cell lines iPSCs. iPSCs exhibit similar morphology and growth properties as ESCs and express ESC-specific genes. The discovery that somatic cells can be reprogrammed into iPS cells has already had major effects on research in stem cell biology and regenerative medicine, but many obstacles remained and need to be resolved to take full advantage of this technology in research and therapy [27]. Therefore, the current clinical protocols are based on the use of autologous MSCs as the cell population that is safe and easy to obtain.

2.2. Sources of human MSCs

Extensive research of adult MSCs started in 1970 when Freidenstein et al. discovered these cells in bone marrow tissue [28]. Later, the presence of MSC-like population was discovered in a wide range of adult tissues, including trabecular bone [29], synovium [30], adipose tissues [31], skeletal muscle [32], periosteum [33], dermis [34], blood [35, 36] deciduous teeth [37], amniotic fluid [38] and umbilical cord blood [39]. Bone marrow-derived mesenchymal stromal cells (BM-MSCs) have become one of the main cell sources for bone tissue engineering [40, 41]. Isolation of MSCs from bone marrow requires invasive procedures that can be quite painful. Bone marrow aspirate could be obtained from the iliac crest, tibia or femur. Typically, the frequency of MSCs in whole bone marrow of adults is between 5×10^{-4} and 10^{-5}, which corresponds to yield of a hundred MSCs per milliliter of marrow. Even though BM-MSCs are rare, they are readily separated from the hematopoietic stem cells in culture by their preferential attachment to the plastic surface [42] and can be easily expanded *ex vivo*. The presence of MSC in adipose tissue has gained considerable attention because of the ease of accessibility of adipose tissue and its abundance in the body. Adipose tissue-derived mesenchymal stem cells (AD-MSCs) were first identified in 2001 by Zuk et al. A major advantage of AD-MSCs is their relative abundance as well as their faster proliferation rate compared to BM- MSCs, which allows more rapid expansion to obtain clinically relevant cell numbers [43, 44]. AD-MSCs have similar osteogenic potential to BM- MSCs with the added advantage of being highly abundant. For example, as many as 1×10^7 AD-MSCs can routinely be isolated from 300 ml of lipoaspirate, with purity greater than 95% [45, 46]. Comparative analysis of human BM-MSCs and AD-MSCs by Li et al. revealed that AD-MSCs have biological advantages in the proliferative capacity, secreted proteins (basic fibroblast growth factor, interferon-γ and insulin-like growth factor-1) and immunomodulatory effects, but BM-MSCs have advantages in osteogenic and chondrogenic differentiation potential and secreted proteins (stem cell-derived factor-1 and hepatocyte growth factor) [47]. These biological advantages should be considered systematically when choosing the MSC source for specific clinical application. Nevertheless, the utilization of human AD-MSCs in scaffolds for bone tissue engineering has been heralded as the alternative strategy of the twenty-first century to replace or restore the function of traumatized, damaged or lost bone.

MSC-like cells can be derived from the umbilical cord from a newborn baby which contains two arteries and a vein covered with mucus connective tissue rich in hyaluronic acid, referred to as a Wharton's jelly [48]. The blood from the umbilical cord is a rich source for pluripotent cells named as umbilical cord blood derived MSCs (UCB-MSCs). These cells are quite similar to bone marrow-derived MSCs and have osteogenic potential in an optimized culture [49]. Many investigations have thus far been conducted on bone engineering by using these cells and various scaffolds [50].

Several stem cell types in dental tissue have been reported including dental pulp stem cells (DPSCs), stem cells from human exfoliated deciduous teeth (SHED), stem cells of the apical papilla (SCAP), periodontal ligament stem cells (PDLSCs) and dental follicle progenitor cells (DFPCs) [37, 51]. Since DPSCs can be easily isolated by enzymatic digestion of pulp tissue, many studies have been conducted regarding bone engineering with these cells and appropriate 3D scaffolds [52, 53].

2.3. Phenotypic characterization of MSCs

Phenotypic characterization of MSCs is usually carried out using immunocytochemical detection or fluorescence-activated cell sorting (FACS) analysis of cell surface molecule expression [54, 55]. Methods of immunodepletion using such techniques as magnet-activated cell sorting (MACS) have also been used in the negative selection of MSCs [56]. However, the lack of specific markers renders the characterization of MSCs difficult and sometimes ambiguous, especially because many of these epitopes are shared between hematopoietic and mesenchymal stem cells. It is interesting that MSCs from different species do not express the same markers. The use of multiple markers such as cell surface cluster of differentiation (CD) markers, ECM proteins, cell adhesion molecules, integrins, cytokines genetic and proteomic fingerprinting can help identify MSCs. The most commonly used markers to identify MSCs are CD markers. Positive MSC markers include: Stro-1, SH2 (CD105), SH3 (CD73), SH4, CD29, CD44, CD54, CD90, CD133, CD166 and p75LNGFR, whereas negative markers are CD11, Cd14, CD19, Cd31, CD34, Cd45, CD79 and HLA-DR [57]. The International Society for Cellular therapy has provided minimum criteria for defining MSCs. Acceptable MSCs meet the minimum requirements of CD73, CD90 and CD105 positive and CD14, CD34, CD45 and HLA-DR negative expression [58].

2.4. Nonimmunogenic properties and immunosuppressive nature of MSCs

Previous studies have shown that yield of MSCs is affected by age and health of a donor. The trend is that yield is decreased with donor age. Patients with degenerative diseases, such as osteoporosis and osteoarthritis, tend to have lower MSC yield although they would benefit the most from MSC-based therapies. The alternative is the use of allogeneic MSCs because they have low immunogenic potential and immunosuppressive properties. Immunologic phenotypes of hMSCs are: positive expression for major histocompatibility complex (MHC) class I molecules, minimal expression for MHC class II and do not express the co-stimulatory molecules CD40, CD40 ligand, CD80 and CD86 [59–62]. MSCs do not fully activate T cells owing to the absence of CD80 and CD86 in their membrane. Apart from not being recognized as alloantigens, MSCs are able to suppress the activation and proliferation of different cells of the host immune system [59, 63–66]. Interleukin-10, transforming growth factor beta (TGF-β), hematopoietic growth factor (HGF), prostaglandin E2 (PGE_2), indoleamine 2,3-dioxygenase (IDO) and nitric oxide (NO) were some of the soluble molecules associated with the immunosuppressive effect of MSCs [67–69]. Another important soluble molecule involved in the immunoregulation of MSCs is HLA-G5, a non-classical human leukocyte antigen (HLA) class I protein that protects the fetus against rejection from the maternal immune system [70]. The HLA-G5 isoform released by MSCs can suppress allogeneic T cell proliferation and can also induce the expansion of $CD4^{+}CD25^{high}FOXP3^{+}$ regulatory T cells (Tregs). With regard to innate immunity, HLA-G5 is able to inhibit the lysis of MSCs mediated by NK cells, as well as the secretion of IFN-γ by these cells [71].

2.5. Tumor formation risk in MSCs application

In general, it is believed that MSCs can be safely cultured *in vitro* without risk of spontaneous malignant transformation [72], but there have been no reports of human trials demonstrating the formation of tumors with culture-expanded MSCs [73]. Concerns have been raised about the safety of MSCs for clinical use as there have been some reports of sarcoma formation by cultured murine MSCs *in vitro* and *in vivo* [74, 75]. The mechanism by which MSCs are transformed into malignant cells is known to be related to chromosomal abnormalities, including structural and numeric aberrations, and increases with higher passage numbers. Rubio et al. showed that although MSCs can be managed safely during the standard *ex vivo* expansion period (6–8 weeks), human MSCs can undergo spontaneous transformation following long-term *in vitro* culture (4–5 months), and the transformed cells lead to the formation of tumors in mice [76].

2.6. Osteogenic differentiation of MSCs

Various *in vitro* protocols have been developed to induce hMSCs to differentiate into mesodermal lineages, such as osteoblasts, chondrocytes, adipocytes, as well as transdifferentiate into tissue cells derived from different germ layers, such as neuronal cells or insulin-producing cells [55, 77, 78]. Osteogenic differentiation is a highly programmed process consisting of many stages, including proliferation, differentiation, matrix deposition, mineralization and matrix maturation. The general protocol for *in vitro* bone differentiation of MSCs involves incubation of the cell monolayer in a culture medium containing DEX, β-glycerophosphate and ascorbic acid for a period of 2–3 weeks (**Figure 1**) [79]. DEX is a synthetic glucocorticoid that stimulates MSC proliferation and is essential for osteogenic differentiation [80, 81]. Although the mechanisms underlying DEX's effects are not well known, it has been speculated that DEX upregulates the beta catenin-like molecule TAZ, which results in upregulation of Runx2-related transcription factor and osteogenic differentiation [82]. The optimal concentration of this reagent for MSC bone differentiation is approximately 10 nM, which corresponds to physiologic concentrations [83]. Organic phosphate released after enzymatic hydrolysis of beta glycerol phosphate plays an important role in matrix mineralization. This free phosphate is usually applied in 5–10 mM concentrations for MSC bone differentiation. Ascorbic acid is a cofactor in the hydroxylation of prolines and lysine moiety of collagen molecules and is an abundant protein in the ECM. This reagent is used in 50–500 μM concentrations [84]. When MSCs are cultured in osteogenic media, they express the same markers as bone-forming osteoblasts that are responsible for laying down the matrix and mineral during new bone formation *in vivo*. The osteogenic differentiation of MSCs *in vitro* has been divided into three stages. The first stage (days 1–4) is the proliferation stage where a peak in the number of cells is seen. This is followed by early cell differentiation (from days 5 to 14), which is characterized by the transcription and protein expression of alkaline phosphatase (ALP). After this initial peak of ALP, its level starts to decline. Also found at an early stage is the expression of a collagen type I matrix onto which the mineral is deposited. The final stage (from days 14 to 28) results in a high expression of osteocalcin and osteopontin, followed by calcium and phosphate deposition [4, 85].

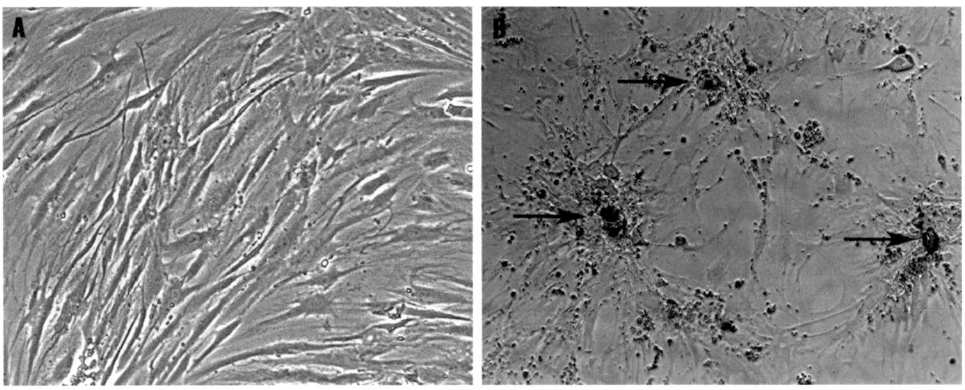

Figure 1. Monolayer of mesenchymal stem cells derived from human bone marrow before (A) and after 3 weeks of (B) differentiation. Arrows mark bone-forming nodules.

In addition to osteogenic supplements, there are other substances that act as biochemical signals capable of triggering cellular processes like growth, proliferation or differentiation. The most common growth factors in bone tissue engineering are listed below.

Bone morphogenetic proteins (*BMPs*) are a family of cytokines that stimulates the proliferation of chondrocytes and osteoblasts and increases extracellular matrix production. BMPs induce the differentiation of MSCs into osteoblasts. BMPs allow not only skeletal tissue formation during embryogenesis, growth, and adulthood but also bone healing process. In newborns' skeletons, BMPs can be found in the collagen fibers of the bone matrix and also in cells located in the periosteum and the bone marrow. After a fracture, BMPs' growth factors diffuse from bone matrix and activate osteoprogenitor cells which, in turn, produce more BMPs [86].

Fibroblast growth factors (*FGFs*) stimulate the proliferation of mesenchymal cells, osteoblasts and chondrocytes. FGFs enhance the growth of different tissues due to their angiogenic

http://dx.doi.org/10.5772/62546

properties. FGF-2 or bFGF is the most studied cytokine of this family for bone regeneration applications [87].

Insulin-like growth factors (IGFs) promote the proliferation of osteoblasts and chondrocytes and induce matrix secretion from both cell types [87]. IGFs stimulate collagen synthesis and mineralization of bone tissue [88].

Platelet-rich plasma (PRP) is another known source of various growth factors, namely, platelet-derived growth factor, transforming growth factor-β and vascular endothelial growth factor. The applicability of PRP for the repair of bony defects is well established [89] and several investigators have advocated the use of this product in combination with MSCs [90].

3. Scaffolds in bone engineering

3.1. Scaffold properties

The evolution of bone implant devices has resulted in an increase in knowledge about the microenvironment where the replacement will occur, which results in changes in requirements and properties of the biomaterials used. This evolution can be measured by defining three different generations. However, these generations are not chronological but technological since there is currently active research and development for each. First-generation bone graft substitutes require the biomaterial to match the physical properties of the tissue to be replaced, while maintaining inertness with the tissue microenvironment. These include metals such as stainless steel, titanium and alloys; ceramics such as alumina and zirconia; and polymers such as silicone rubber, polypropylene and polymethylmethacrylate. Second-generation bone graft substitutes are made biodegradable with the aim that the rate of degradation matches the healing rate of the injured bone tissue. These biomaterials are based on the use of synthetic or natural polymers that can provide a controlled chemical breakdown under physiological conditions into inert products that can be resorbed by the body. Examples of the synthetic polymers include polylactide, poly(ε-caprolactone) and polyglycolide; and collagen, chitosan and hyaluronic acid for natural ones. The mechanical and osteoconductive properties of these polymers can be improved by forming composites with bioactive ceramics. Third-generation bone graft substitutes try to get closer to the autograft standard by using biomaterials capable of inducing specific cellular responses at the molecular level, by integrating the bioactivity and biodegradability of second-generation devices. This type of bone graft is based on the concept of bone tissue engineering, which focused on creating a device that enhances bone repair and regeneration by incorporating bone progenitor cells or/and bioactive signals (e.g., growth factors, small molecules) to stimulate cells into a scaffold made of various natural or synthetic biomaterials or their combination and with sufficient vascularization to allow access to nutrients to support this process. Nowadays, many groups worldwide seek to develop scaffolds with osteoinductive properties that would enhance bone healing. These scaffolds have to accomplish certain requirements and have to be:

Biocompatible—cells must populate the scaffold, adhere and proliferate. They should be able to migrate as well as differentiate. Overall, cell function should not be compromised. The scaffolds should enable unobstructed transport of nutrients, gases, signaling molecules, proteins and waste products in, out and within the scaffold.

Biodegradable—the scaffold should be replaced with host/donor cells (tissues). Therefore, scaffolds must be biodegradable and byproducts must not be toxic. Ideal scaffold degradation should mirror the rate of new tissue formation.

Biofunctional—the scaffold should meet as many as possible functional requirements of the replaced tissue. Good scaffold should have specific mechanical properties and architecture, similar to properties of the replaced bone tissue. Properties like elasticity, permeability, compressibility, viscoelastic behavior, tensile strength and failure strain [91] should be similar and should give shape to the tissue that is regenerated on it [92]. It is very important to have strong, but at the same time, porous bone grafts. The pores should be big enough to allow smooth cell migration and proliferation besides vascularization and small enough to enable cell-to-cell communication and critical cell repopulation of the pores. Pores are crucial in a process of degradation. Their size should allow and promote scaffold degradation.

The main disadvantage of scaffolds is the lack of vascularization. Inspired by the nature of bone, different scaffolds have been studied extensively, and the main challenge is to precisely balance a desired structural strength and porosity. To design bone scaffolds, materials should have the desired biological properties for a specific application and should not be immunogenic causing inflammatory response. The long-term goal is the development of the scaffold that can be applied in a clinical setting. Manufacturing technology should follow good manufacturing practice (GMP) procedures. Ultimately, the main goal is to develop scaffold that fulfills all previously mentioned requirements and has slow-release properties of bioactive molecule. Multiple factors (signaling peptides, adhesion peptides, growth factors, plasmid DNA, antibodies, microRNAs, etc.) can be incorporated into scaffolds to promote osteoblast migration, to manipulate tissue formation and to effectively enhance bone regeneration [93]. For instance, bone morphogenic protein 2 (BMP-2) was photo-crosslinked into biodegradable diblock copolymers PEG-PLA and was slowly released as the polymer degrades [94]. Another approach is to covalently bind the adhesion peptide like well-known arginine-glycine-aspartate ligand or chemotactic factor like platelet-derived growth factors (PDGFs), to attract osteoblast and promote osteogenesis [95, 96] or incorporate angiogenic (FGFs [97]) and anti-angiogenic factors to control scaffold vascularization [98]. MicroRNAs can post-transcriptionally regulate gene expression and alter bone regeneration [99]. There are many problems to that approach, and the major one is controlled release of bioactive substance together with its rapid dilution. To reduce the risk of BMP dilution following release from the scaffold, monoclonal anti-BMP antibodies are encapsulated within the scaffold [100].

3.2. Scaffold types

With respect to source of biomaterials, scaffolds can be divided into two main groups: the ones made from natural and the ones made from synthetic materials. The natural biomaterials are obtained from natural sources and processed to make desired scaffolds. A few decades ago, researchers have discovered that decalcified bone matrix (DBM) possesses inherent osteoinductive properties (http://www.ncbi.nlm.nih.gov/pubmed/4870495), and DBM was used in the treatment of clinical orthopedic situations which has shown favorable results [101, 102]. Decellularized ECM (mammalian extracellular matrix) scaffolds recovered from allografts (tissue from individuals of same species) and xenografts (tissue from individuals of different species) have a desired three-dimensional porous structure and can be repopulated by host bone-forming cells. ECM is a complex of different glycosaminoglycans, glycoproteins and huge number of different small proteins. The cells can easily attach, grow and differentiate with excellent viability. Decellularization and treatments such as freeze-drying, irradiation and washing with acid minimize their immunogenicity, but some epitopes can still be recognized by the host. These treatments prevent any infection to be transferred from the tissue, but can affect their mechanical and biological properties [97]. Most commonly used biological materials for bone tissue engineering are chitosan, collagen, hyaluronic acid, alginate, elastin, cellulose, fibrin, gelatin, etc. Chitosan is a hydrophilic, linear polysaccharide (suh, matthew, application of chitosan-based) obtained by alkaline deacetylation of chitin from shrimp and other crustacean shells. It has many beneficial properties, such as biocompatibility (no inflammatory or allergic reaction, (chatelet, damour, influence of the degree), biodegradability (it is naturally degraded by hydrolytic enzymes such as lysozyme) and no toxicity [103]. Since collagen is the most abundant protein in various tissues including bone, scaffolds made of collagen are very attractive for biomedical applications. Collagen is composed from two $\alpha 1$ chains and one $\alpha 2$ chain wrapped together by hydrogen and covalent bonds to form right-handed triple helix. These fibers spontaneously pack together to form long thin fibrils of similar structure. Collagen is an attractive material for a scaffold synthesis because its mechanical properties can be altered by crosslinking, either with different chemicals (glutaraldehyde, formaldehyde, etc.) or with physical treatments (UV irradiation, heating, etc.) [104–106]. Hyaluronic acid is a simple linear polysaccharide composed of a repeating disaccharide, and it is hydrophilic, nonimmunogenic, and easy to modify and produce. It is easily replaced by extracellular matrix produced by host cells due to hyalurodinase degradation. These materials have a huge biological activity; they promote cell adhesion as well as cell growth. They are biodegradable, allowing host cells to replace the scaffold with their own extracellular matrix. The main drawbacks are their poor mechanical properties limiting their use as bone grafts and the reproducibility of their synthesis. Immunogenicity, limited physical and mechanical stability as well as limited resource of biomaterials have encouraged researches to develop composites using synthetic materials.

Typically, two individual groups of synthetic biomaterials are used in the fabrication of bone grafts: ceramics and synthetic polymers. Ceramics polymers (inorganic oxides and salts), such are hydroxyapatite (HA), β-tricalcium phosphate (β-TCP) and biphasic calcium phosphate (BCP) are mechanically stiff and have very low elasticity, making them suitable only for bone tissue grafts. Ceramics perfectly imitate natural bone structure, and cell interaction with ceramics promotes proliferation as well as differentiation of osteoblasts [107].

Synthetic polymers, such as polystyrene, polyglycolic acid (PGA) and poly-l-lactic acid (PLLA) acid, have the rewarding and satisfying properties because their architecture can be adjusted and changed by the composition of the polymer as well as by altering the synthesis method. However, cell might have difficulties to attach and proliferate on their surface, so there is always the risk of rejection due to reduced bioactivity. Degradation of synthetic polymers becomes the major issue because most of them are degraded by hydrolysis, causing lower local pH and cell necrosis [108].

Since ceramics have excellent osteoinductive properties but low mechanical strength, and synthetic polymers exhibit poor osteoinductivity but better mechanical strength and degradability, in the past decade researches have been trying to develop the scaffolds made of ceramic and polymer composites. Most commonly used 3D composites are made of synthetic polymers such as poly(lactic) acid (PLA), PGA, poly(ε-caprolactone) (PCL), poly(lactic-co-glycolide) (PLGA), poly(propylene fumarate) (PPF) and natural polymers such as collagen type I and chitosan. These composites have rigid sponge-like structures often containing HA (133-138 from three-dimensional alexander). Hydroxyapatite increases attachment of mesenchymal stem cells, differentiation to osteoprogenitors and promotes cell survival [109, 110].

3.3. The ideal scaffold for bone tissue engineering

The ideal scaffold is difficult to obtain and should be biocompatible, bioresorbable, osteoconductive (must allow bone cells to adhere, proliferate and secrete extracellular matrix), osteinductive (with the ability to induce new bone formation), osteogenic (should act as MSCs and osteoblasts reservoir), structurally similar to bone enabling formation of strong bonds with surrounding bone tissue, as well as it should be easy to use and cost-effective. New approach includes development of methods to isolate and transplant bone tissue-forming cells, bioactive matrix materials that act as tissue scaffolds mimicking what happens in nature, and delivery of bioactive molecules within scaffolds. In the past two decades, many 3D systems have been

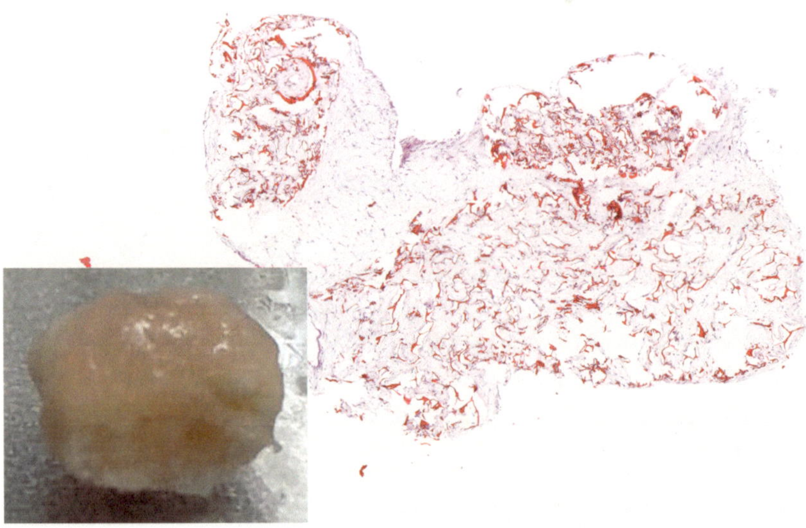

Figure 2. Bone graft grown on scaffold made of chitosan and hyaluronic acid. Section of graft stained with hemalaun/eosin staining shows equal cell distribution, formation of extracellular matrix and scaffold residues.

http://dx.doi.org/10.5772/62546

studied and some have been commercialized for clinical application. The main advantage of this system is that cells grown in 3D environment that is more representative to natural bone tissue. Final goal is to produce a "living" scaffold providing mechanical support, bioactive signal as well as cells with osteogenic potential. Researchers have developed bioreactors to mimic physiological conditions. The main advantage is that this system enables controlled manipulation of all variables. In contrast to classic static *in vitro* cultures, bioreactors allow to apply mechanical stimuli that are very important in osteogenic differentiation [111]. Many different bioreactors to promote good osteogenesis (Koller reactors [112]), spinner flask bioreactors, [113] have been investigated. Recently developed perfusion bioreactors have shown high efficiency in uniformed cell seeding on a scaffold, enhanced proliferation, great supply of oxygen and nutrients throughout the scaffold as well as enhanced osteogenic differentiation because the pump forces the medium to flow through the scaffold (**Figure 2**) [114–117].

4. Systems for 3D cultivation of bone tissue

Ex vivo tissue-engineering (TE) strategies for *de novo* generation of bone tissue enclose the combined use of autologous bone-forming cells and three-dimensional scaffold materials serving as structural support for the cells [118]. Bioreactors are used as a tool for studying and mimicking *in vivo* conditions in an *in vitro* environment for the growth of tissue substitutes and represent the device used to develop biological processes by closely monitoring and controlling the environment [119]. Parameters that must be controlled and appropriately adjusted in order to perform controlled and successful experiments are:

- Temperature
- pH
- Oxygen diffusion
- Nutrient transport
- Waste removal

Tissue-engineering bioreactors can be used to aid the *in vitro* development of new tissue by providing biochemical and physical regulatory signals to cells, encouraging them to undergo differentiation and produce extracellular matrix prior to *in vivo* implantation [120].

This 3D cell expansion on a scaffold poses several challenges. The first challenge is the **transport of nutrients** to cells and **removal of waste** metabolites from the interior of the scaffold. In 2D cell culture diffusion provides nutrients and oxygen to all cells as well as waste removal, but in 3D constructs diffusion is insufficient [121]. That represents an important issue in tissue engineering, limiting the tissue growth due to insufficient nutrient transport [122]. To overcome this problem, scientists developed more complex bioreactor systems 3D tissue culture to improve the media flow and transport of nutrients to cells which contribute to balanced development of tissue [118]. Dynamic bioreactor culture systems are essential for *in* *vitro* cultivation and maturation of tissue-engineering bone grafts, in particular for larger bone grafts where the core of the scaffold is more than 200 μm from the surface. Bioreactors improve the mass transport of nutrients and overcome the diffusion limitation of traditional static culture [123]. Bioreactors bring several advantages into the culture of functional tissues. They do not only increase mass transport inside three-dimensional structures but also reduce the handling steps, hence reducing contamination potential.

Fluid shear stress caused by mixing or perfusion the medium is also very important for bone tissue engineering because it exposes the cells to mechanical stimulation. *In vivo*, mechanical loading increase production of prostaglandins, alkaline phosphatase, collagen type I, along with osteoblast proliferation and mineralization [124]. Mechanical loading of the skeleton causes interstitial fluid flow through lacunar and canalicular space of bones. The cells lining these spaces are then influenced by the mechanical stimulation provided by the fluid flow, differentiating or proliferating accordingly [125, 126]. Based on this knowledge, it is clear that the recapitulation of these mechanisms *in vitro* is essential for the growth and the regenerative properties of human osteoprogenitor cells seeded onto scaffolds [127]. *In vitro*, mechanical stimulation can encourage cells to produce extracellular matrix (ECM) in a shorter time period and in a more homogeneous manner than in static culture [128]. A benefit of ECM production is the increase in mechanical steadiness of the scaffold and tissue graft. Another important advantage of bioreactors is **induced cellular differentiation**. Mechanical stimuli can be used to encourage stem cells down a particular path and hence provide the cell phenotype required [129].

As well as providing mechanical stimulation, bioreactors can also be used to improve **cellular spatial distribution**. A heterogeneous cell distribution is a major problem in developing three-dimensional tissue or organ *in vitro* [130]. Scaffolds in larger size range are easily fabricated, but problems arise with culturing cells on these scaffolds. As the size of the scaffold increases, diffusion of cells to the center becomes more difficult. Static culture conditions result in scaffolds with few cells in the center [131]. Thus, bioreactors can be used in tissue-engineering applications to overcome problems associated with traditional static culture conditions, improve cellular distribution and accelerate construct maturation [132] while applying biophysical signals to constructs to improve tissue formation *in vitro* prior to *in vivo* implantation [120].

The ultimate design of a tissue engineering bioreactor system must: (i) ensure a controlled and rapid cell growth; (ii) facilitate uniform cell distribution; (iii) provide and maintain the physiological requirements of the cell (nutrients, oxygen, growth factors); (iv) increase mass transport both by diffusion and convection using mixing medium systems (v) expose cells to physical stimuli; and (vi) enable reproducibility, control, monitoring and automation. For this purpose, different dynamic culture systems have been developed. These systems improve nutrient delivery to the cells and generate shear stress that promotes cell differentiation into osteoblastic phenotype. Bioreactors for bone engineering applications are broadly classified into few main categories, including rotating wall vessel, spinner flask, perfusion bioreactor and compression systems. In addition to these, combinations of different types of bioreactors have been explored in order to better mimic the bone physiological environment *in vitro* and

http://dx.doi.org/10.5772/62546

all these systems for tissue culture are used to achieve a homogeneous cell growth within the scaffold [120].

4.1. Rotating wall vessel bioreactor

Cells that grow *in vitro*—outside the body in 2D layers do not behave in the same way as cells grown *in vivo*—inside the body. *In vivo* cells grow three-dimensionally and form tissues that have modified their structure to perform a specific function and secrete extracellular matrix. Two-dimensional growth represented a limit to the scientists who wanted to understand mechanisms that govern cell behavior and tissue formation. In the 1970s, a small NASA group of scientists began to think about space as a possible answer. The group believed if cells could be grown without the Earth's gravity influence, they would not settle to the bottom of the culturing container, instead they would be suspended in the medium and therefore might compound and form tissue that more closely resembles the tissue in the body [133]. The rotating-wall vessel (RWV), developed by NASA, was originally designed to protect cell cultures from high shear forces generated during the launch and landing of the space shuttle. When the device was tested on the Earth for cells in suspension, cells aggregated and formed structures similar to tissues. These observations led to the possibility that the bioreactors might be used to study co-cultures of multiple cell types and their association, proliferation and differentiation during the early steps of tissue formation [134].

The RWV bioreactor provides a low turbulence culture environment which promotes the formation of large, three-dimensional cell clusters. Due to their high level of cellular organization and specialization, samples constructed in this bioreactor more closely resembled the original tumor or tissue found in the body. Cartilage, bone marrow, heart muscle, skeletal muscle, pancreatic islet cells, liver and kidney are just a few of the normal tissues cultured in rotating bioreactors [133].

The RWV bioreactor (**Figure 3A**) consists of a cylindrical growth chamber with a gas exchange membrane. The solid-body rotation is accomplished by a vessel rotating horizontally around its axis, randomizing the gravitational forces acting on the cell surface. The culture chamber is completely filled with medium and is oxygenated through a silicone rubber membrane by an air pump that draws incubator air through the filter. As the vessel rotates, the liquid inside accelerates until the entire fluid mass is rotating at the same angular rate as the wall. Thus, this environment eliminates most of the disruptive shear forces associated with a conventional bioreactor, scaffolds and cells obey simple kinematics and are uniformly suspended in the culture medium with minimum shear forces. In this environment, cells aggregate and undergo three-dimensional growth to form tissue-like structures. As aggregates grow during culture, the speed of vessel rotation is increased to contrary gravitational sedimentation [134].

Cultures using an RWV bioreactor proved useful for growing tissues, such as bone. Many studies showed enhanced proliferation, distribution and differentiation of osteoprogenitor cells on scaffolds when cultured in a free fall manner in RWV-based bioreactor systems [135]. Until today, many designs of rotating bioreactor systems have been developed for dynamic 3D bone tissue engineering. One of them is RWV bioreactor with the scaffolds attached to the external wall by use of stainless steel clamps. External and internal cylinders were driven by

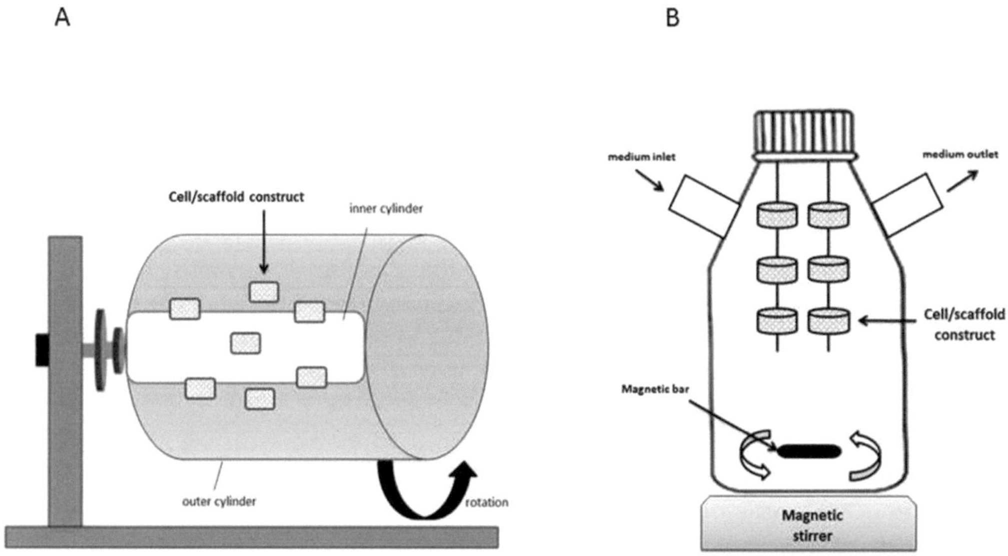

Figure 3. Design of rotating vessel (A) and spinner flask (B) bioreactor systems.

step motors and compared to the cultivation in static culture. The use of RWV resulted in better cell proliferation and differentiation. The second one is a rotating bed bioreactor (RBB). In an RBB, constructs are attached directly on the axis and moved between gas and liquid phases in an alternating manner. One major benefit of the system besides the positive effect in terms of proliferation and differentiation is the compatibility with good manufacturing practices (GMP) standards. Disadvantage of RWV system is the collision of scaffolds with the bioreactor wall, which may damage scaffolds and disrupt seeded cells. This can be omitted by the use of the RBB concept. Another major disadvantage of the rotating system is that mineralization is limited to the outer part of the scaffold. Internal nutrient transport limitations could not be eliminated by rotation-based bioreactor systems [118]. Rotating wall vessels are limited to the small-sized constructs due to insufficient transport inside the scaffold. Additionally, because of the low range of values of shear stress, these systems may not be efficient in promoting robust osteogenic differentiation. On the other hand, rotating wall vessels allow the accompanying culture of several cell/scaffold constructs. These systems could be adopted to engineer thin bone substitutes for the reconstruction of flat bones or as bone patches for restorative applications of the skeletal system [3].

4.2. Spinner flask bioreactor

A simple bioreactor system based on media mixing is the spinner flask (**Figure 3B**). Spinner flasks are composed of a glass media reservoir with side arms that can be opened to remove scaffolds and media and also to allow gas exchange. The flask has a stir bar mechanism that stirs the media in the flask. They are often used in bone tissue engineering because of the ability to increase expression of early osteoblastic marker alkaline phosphatase, late osteoblastic marker osteocalcin and calcium deposition as compared to static culture and rotating wall bioreactors. This effect is the result of convective transport of nutrients to the surface of the scaffold in contrast to the purely diffusional transport in static culture. It also increases the concentration of oxygen throughout the scaffold [136].

Scaffolds are hanging attached to vertical needles from the top of the vessel and are submerged in the medium. The top of the vessel is usually used for gas exchange and medium oxygenation. Mixing of the medium is maintained by stir bar mechanism at the bottom of the vessel. The convective forces generated during stirring moderate the nutrient concentration gradients at the surface of the scaffold and produce turbulences that enhance mass transport according to the center of the samples [3].

Commonly, spinner flasks are around 120 ml in volume (up to 8 liters), are run at 50–80 rpm and 50% of the medium used in them is replaced every 2 days [137]. An important advantage of the spinner flask design is its maintenance of well-mixed environment within the flask. However, spinner flasks are not always an ideal solution, since the constant mixing motion causes turbulent flow within the capsule and the associated high shear stress. Spinner flasks have been modified form their original design to reduce the turbulent flow. Current designs induce small waves during mixing instead of the rough, turbulent flow induced from traditional spinner flasks. Spinner flasks are intended for small-scale production and do not appear to be used as much as other types. They are primarily used for the seeding of cells in 3D scaffolds until they are ready for more large-scale cell culture procedures [119].

4.3. Perfusion bioreactor

Spinner flasks and rotating wall bioreactors do not effectively perfuse media through the center of the scaffold. Bioreactors that use a pump system to perfuse media directly through a scaffold are known as perfusion bioreactors [136]. In perfusion bioreactors, scaffolds are placed in the perfusion chamber (**Figure 4A**) in a press-fit manner so that the medium is forced to pass through the center of the samples [3]. Flow perfusion bioreactors have been shown to provide more homogeneous cell distribution throughout scaffolds. This has resulted in greater cellularity throughout the scaffold in comparison to static controls, suggesting the better nutrient exchange [120].

These bioreactors have an advantage over the others because they provide a uniform mixing of the media, enabling better control of the environment and the physical stimulation of the cells in the bone tissue [121]. They are very effective for the culture of mesenchymal stem cells and have been shown to induce osteogenesis. This is attributed to the ability of the perfusion system to increase the transport of oxygen and nutrient through the scaffold and expose the cells to the mechanical stimulation [137]. The optimization of the perfusion bioreactor protocols for tissue engineering must ensure balance between the transport of substances and waste metabolites and hold newly synthesized tissue within the scaffold, taking care of the fluid flow rate which goes through the pores [120]. Many different perfusion bioreactor systems have been developed, but most systems are based on the similar basic design—media reservoir, pump, tubing circuit and scaffold chamber. The scaffold is sealed within the chamber so media cannot flow around it. Thus, media flows directly through the pores of the scaffold [136]. Scaffolds should have interconnected pores and should have between 70 and 99% porosity in

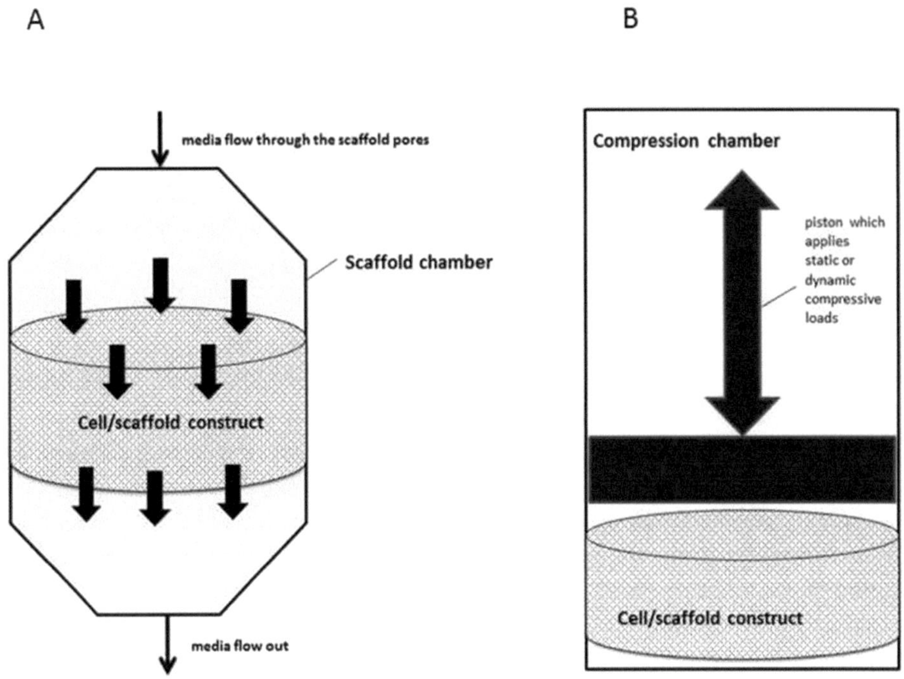

Figure 4. Design of the scaffold chambers in perfusion (A) and compression (B) bioreactor systems.

order to facilitate direct perfusion. In most cases, the major difference between the systems is the design of the perfusion chamber because it is the key element to ensure deep perfusion of the scaffold center [121]. Despite these difficulties, many perfusion bioreactor systems have been developed and tested for bone tissue-engineering purposes [136]. The pump produces a force that travels through the tubing circuit and perfuse the media through the scaffold pores in a continuous or noncontiguous way [120]. This force represents the perfusion flow rate applying mechanical stimulation in the form of shear stress to cells in the scaffold. This mechanical stimulation proved to be a powerful tool to stimulate osteogenic differentiation, and data show that cell-matrix and cell-cell junction molecules are capable of converting mechanical stimuli into biochemical signals.

One of the most important parameters when optimizing a bioreactor is the flow rate. It depends on the composition, porosity and geometry of the scaffold. The pump is capable of precisely and consistently pumping flow rates from 0.01 to 6.0 ml/min through each chamber [138]. Still, there is a big variation of values and there are not many studies that compare a significant range of flow rates. It appears that the increase in flow rate leads to an increase in the deposition of mineralized matrix. Very low flow rates such as 0.01 ml/min have been reported to lead to higher cell viability, but this does not seem an optimal flow rate for bone tissue engineering as it might be too low to actually accomplish an adequate distribution of nutrients, oxygen and removal of waste products. It is also necessary to bear in mind that lower values of flow rate will provide lower values of shear stress, which might facilitate cell attachment and spreading, hence leading to higher values of cell viability. Despite the wide variation of the flow rates tested, it seems that the optimal values would range from 0.2 to 1 ml/min, depending obviously on the system being used. This is the range of values that seems to have a more positive effect on osteoblastic differentiation, ECM deposition and distribution [121]. Perfusion bioreactor is so far the only system that produces such a force, making it ideal for growing large bone grafts *ex vivo* [139].

4.4. Compression bioreactors and combined systems

Compression bioreactors (**Figure 4B**) were intended to mimic the bone physiological *in vitro* environment, characterized by repeated mechanical stimulation required for functional bone regeneration. Many studies provide evidence that mechanical loading, when combined with flow perfusion, can play a main role in promoting survival and functional osteogenic differentiation of the cells within the scaffold. Short-term mechanical stimulation enhanced the expression of several genes encoding for factors involved in osteogenesis, including *RUNX2, osteopontin, integrin-β1, TGFβR1, SMAD5, annexin-V* and *PDGFα* [3]. These experiments demonstrate that even short mechanical stimuli can be sufficient to activate the osteogenic differentiation pathways in human mesenchymal stem cells. Compression bioreactors systems consist of a motor, a system providing linear motion and a compression chamber in which one or more clips apply static or dynamic compressive loads directly to the scaffold [3]. The bioreactor chamber holds the scaffold in place and ensures hermetic sealing as well as force transmission onto the cell-seeded scaffold. It consists of medium flow distributors, a flexible force transmitting disk and the intended space for scaffold placement. The power transmission rack includes a plunger, a pre-load screw and a cam-shaft. The chamber is placed on the clip and fixed via tightening of the pre-load screw. The camshaft moves the clip in order to apply a sinusoidal compression pattern onto the bioreactor chamber [140]. The system can be controlled by a signal generator, and load response can be measured by using linear variable differential transformers and load cell, respectively. In contrast to static culture, mass transfer is considerably improved in compression bioreactor culture since compression leads to the fluid flow through the scaffold [141]. The compression bioreactors provide a promising tool for bone fracture research and for *in vitro* estimate of alternative fracture treatments based on engineered tissue grafts, allowing the reduction of animal experiments.

5. Conclusion

Bone defects that are due to trauma or pathological and physiological bone resorption represent a global health problem. The need for bone regeneration is one of the central issues in regenerative medicine. Tissue engineering is becoming a useful addition to medical therapies for repairing and restoring the function of bone tissue. Bone constructs elaborated with tissue-engineering principles are a promising substitute for autologous bone graft and have long been considered the golden standard for repair of large bone defects. Mesenchymal stem cells from adult tissues are the most suitable cell source for bone tissue engineering. Although the application of MSCs as cellular material facilitates the construct fabrication, more work needs to be done to fully determine the clinical potential, efficacy and safety of stem cell-based treatments. There is a constant need in the development of new scaffolds that have optimal characteristics, and are affordable as well as easy for manipulation. Bioreactor dynamic setting enables better culture conditions and mechanical stimuli for improved bone tissue growth. In spite of the existing problems, advances in the field are enormous and therapy using scaffolds, healing signals and stem cells together should be able to solve the current limitations in managing bone injuries.

Acknowledgements

This project has received funding from the European Union's Seventh Program for research, technological development and demonstration under grant agreement No. 278807, BIO-COMET. This publication was supported from the European Union's Horizon 2020 research and innovation programme under grant agreement project BioChip, No. 681103.

Author details

Inga Marijanovic[1], Maja Antunovic[1], Igor Matic[1], Marina Panek[2] and Alan Ivkovic[2*]

*Address all correspondence to: alan.ivkovic@gmail.com

1 Faculty of Science, University of Zagreb, Zagreb, Croatia

2 School of Medicine, University of Zagreb, Zagreb, Croatia

References

[1] Ivkovic A, Marijanovic I, Hudetz D, Porter RM, Pecina M, Evans CH. Regenerative medicine and tissue engineering in orthopaedic surgery. Front Biosci. 2011;3:923–44.

[2] de Peppo GM, Marolt D. State of the art in stem cell research: human embryonic stem cells, induced pluripotent stem cells, and transdifferentiation. J blood Transfus. 2012;2012: Article ID 317632.

[3] Sladkova M, de Peppo G. Bioreactor Systems for Human Bone Tissue Engineering. Processes. 2014;2(2):494–525.

[4] Panek M, Marijanovic I, Ivkovic A. Stem cells in bone regeneration. Period Biol. 2015;117(1):175–82.

[5] Melissa K Carpenter. Characterization and culture of human embryonic stem cells. Nat Biotechnol. 2005;23(6):699–708.

[6] Bonab MM, Alimoghaddam K, Talebian F, Ghaffari SH, Ghavamzadeh A, Nikbin B. Aging of mesenchymal stem cell in vitro. BMC Cell Biol. 2006;7:14.

[7] Stenderup K. Aging is associated with decreased maximal life span and accelerated senescence of bone marrow stromal cells. Bone. 2003;33(6):919–26.

[8] De Wert G, Mummery C. Human embryonic stem cells: research, ethics and policy. Human Reprod. 2003;672–82.

[9] Hentze H, Soong PL, Wang ST, Phillips BW, Putti TC, Dunn NR. Teratoma formation by human embryonic stem cells: Evaluation of essential parameters for future safety studies. Stem Cell Res. 2009;2(3):198–210.

[10] Prokhorova TA, Harkness LM, Frandsen U, Ditzel N, Schrøder HD, Burns JS, et al. Teratoma formation by human embryonic stem cells is site dependent and enhanced by the presence of Matrigel. Stem Cells Dev. 2009;18(1):47–54.

[11] Taapken SM, Nisler BS, Newton MA, Sampsell-Barron TL, Leonhard KA, Mc Intire EM, et al. Karotypic abnormalities in human induced pluripotent stem cells and embryonic stem cells. Nat Biotechnol. 2011;29(4):313–4.

[12] Arvidson K, Abdallah BM, Applegate LA, Baldini N, Cenni E, Gomez-Barrena E, et al. Bone regeneration and stem cells. J Cell Mol Med 2011;1:718–46.

[13] Abdi R, Fiorina P, Adra CN, Atkinson M, Sayegh MH. Immunomodulation by mesenchymal stem cells: a potential therapeutic strategy for type 1 diabetes. Diabetes. 2008;57(7):1759–67.

[14] Fuchs JR, Kaviani A, Oh JT, La Van D, Udagawa T, Jennings RW, et al. Diaphragmatic reconstruction with autologous tendon engineered from mesenchymal amniocytes. J Pediatr Surg. 2004;39(6):834–8.

[15] Hauser P V, De Fazio R, Bruno S, Sdei S, Grange C, Bussolati B, et al. Stem cells derived from human amniotic fluid contribute to acute kidney injury recovery. Am J Pathol. 2010;177(4):2011–21.

[16] Kunisaki SM, Freedman DA, Fauza DO. Fetal tracheal reconstruction with cartilaginous grafts engineered from mesenchymal amniocytes. J Pediatr Surg. 2006;41(4):675–82.

[17] Le Blanc K, Frassoni F, Ball L, Locatelli F, Roelofs H, Lewis I, et al. Mesenchymal stem cells for treatment of steroid-resistant, severe, acute graft-versus-host disease: a phase II study. Lancet. 2008;371(9624):1579–86.

[18] Wadman M. Congress and Bush set to clash on stem cells again. Nature. 2007;445(7124): 134–5.

[19] Sessarego N, Parodi A, PodestàM, Benvenuto F, Mogni M, Raviolo V, et al. Multipotent mesenchymal stromal cells from amniotic fluid: solid perspectives for clinical application. Haematologica. 2008;93(3):339–46.

[20] Siegel N, Valli A, Fuchs C, Rosner M, Hengstschlaeger M. Induction of mesenchymal/epithelial marker expression in human amniotic fluid stem cells. Reprod Biomed Online. 2009;19(6):838–46.

[21] Kim EY, Lee KB, Kim MK. The potential of mesenchymal stem cells derived from amniotic membrane and amniotic fluid for neuronal regenerative therapy. BMB Rep. 2014;47(3):135–40.

[22] Cananzi M, Atala A, De Coppi P. Stem cells derived from amniotic fluid: new potentials in regenerative medicine. Reprod Biomed Online. 2009;18 Suppl 1:17–27.

[23] Antonucci I, Iezzi I, Morizio E, Mastrangelo F, Pantalone A, Mattioli-Belmonte M, et al. Isolation of osteogenic progenitors from human amniotic fluid using a single step culture protocol. BMC Biotechnol. 2009.

[24] Perin L, Sedrakyan S, Da Sacco S, De Filippo R. Characterization of human amniotic fluid stem cells and their pluripotential capability. Met Cell Biol 2008;85–99.

[25] Siegel N, Rosner M, Hanneder M, Freilinger A, Hengstschläger M. Human amniotic fluid stem cells: a new perspective. Amino Acids. 2008;35(2):291–3.

[26] Takahashi K, Yamanaka S. Induction of pluripotent stem cells from mouse embryonic and adult fibroblast cultures by defined factors. Cell. 2006;126(4):663–76.

[27] Saha K, Jaenisch R. Technical challenges in using human induced pluripotent stem cells to model disease. Cell Stem Cell. 2009;5(6):584–95.

[28] Friedenstein AJ, Chailakhjan RK, Lalykina KS. The development of fibroblast colonies in monolayer cultures of guinea-pig bone marrow and spleen cells. Cell Tissue Kinet. 1970;3(4):393–403.

[29] Nöth U, Osyczka AM, Tuli R, Hickok NJ, Danielson KG, Tuan RS. Multilineage mesenchymal differentiation potential of human trabecular bone-derived cells. J Orthop Res. 2002;20(5):1060–9.

[30] De Bari C, Dell'Accio F, Tylzanowski P, Luyten FP. Multipotent mesenchymal stem cells from adult human synovial membrane. Arthritis Rheum. 2001;44(8):1928–42.

[31] Zuk PA, Zhu M, Mizuno H, Huang J, Futrell JW, Katz AJ, et al. Multilineage cells from human adipose tissue: implications for cell-based therapies. Tissue Eng. 2001;7(2):211–28.

[32] Bosch P, Musgrave DS, Lee JY, Cummins J, Shuler F, Ghivizzani SC, et al. Osteoprogenitor cells within skeletal muscle. J Orthop Res. 2000;18(6):933–44.

[33] Nakahara H, Goldberg VM, Caplan AI. Culture-expanded human periosteal-derived cells exhibit osteochondral potential in vivo. J Orthop Res. 1991;9(4):465–76.

[34] Young HE, Steele TA, Bray RA, Hudson J, Floyd JA, Hawkins K, et al. Human reserve pluripotent mesenchymal stem cells are present in the connective tissues of skeletal muscle and dermis derived from fetal, adult, and geriatric donors. Anat Rec. 2001;264(1):51–62.

[35] Zvaifler NJ, Marinova-Mutafchieva L, Adams G, Edwards CJ, Moss J, Burger JA, et al. Mesenchymal precursor cells in the blood of normal individuals. Arthritis Res. 2000;2(6):477–88.

[36] He Q, Wan C, Li G. Concise review: multipotent mesenchymal stromal cells in blood. Stem Cells. 2007;25(1):69–77.

[37] Huang GT-J, Gronthos S, Shi S. Mesenchymal stem cells derived from dental tissues vs. those from other sources: their biology and role in regenerative medicine. J Dent Res. 2009;88(9):792–806.

[38] Baghaban Eslaminejad M, Jahangir S, Aghdami N. Mesenchymal stem cells from murine amniotic fluid as a model for preclinical investigation. Arch Iran Med. 2011;14(2):96–103.

[39] Karahuseyinoglu S, Cinar O, Kilic E, Kara F, Akay GG, Demiralp DO, et al. Biology of stem cells in human umbilical cord stroma: in situ and in vitro surveys. Stem Cells. 2007;25(2):319–31.

[40] Bianco P, Riminucci M, Gronthos S, Robey PG. Bone marrow stromal stem cells: nature, biology, and potential applications. Stem Cells. 2001;19(3):180–92.

[41] Zou Z, Zhang Y, Hao L, Wang F, Liu D, Su Y, et al. More insight into mesenchymal stem cells and their effects inside the body. Expert Opin Biol Ther. 2010;10(2):215–30.

[42] Prockop DJ. Marrow stromal cells as stem cells for nonhematopoietic tissues. Science (80-) 1997;276(5309):71–4.

[43] Cowan CM, Shi Y-Y, Aalami OO, Chou Y-F, Mari C, Thomas R, et al. Adipose-derived adult stromal cells heal critical-size mouse calvarial defects. Nat Biotechnol. 2004;22(5): 560–7.

[44] Nakagami H, Morishita R, Maeda K, Kikuchi Y, Ogihara T, Kaneda Y. Adipose tissue-derived stromal cells as a novel option for regenerative cell therapy. J Atheroscler Thromb. 2006;13(2):77–81.

[45] Boquest AC, Shahdadfar A, Brinchmann JE, Collas P. Isolation of stromal stem cells from human adipose tissue. Methods Mol Biol. 2006;325(4):35–46.

[46] Strem BM, Hicok KC, Zhu M, Wulur I, Alfonso Z, Schreiber RE, et al. Multipotential differentiation of adipose tissue-derived stem cells. Keio J Med. 2005;54(0022-9717 (Print)):132–41.

[47] Li C, Wu X, Tong J, Yang X, Zhao J, Zheng Q, et al. Comparative analysis of human mesenchymal stem cells from bone marrow and adipose tissue under xeno-free conditions for cell therapy. Stem Cell Res Ther. 2015;6:55.

[48] Hilfiker A, Kasper C, Hass R, Haverich A. Mesenchymal stem cells and progenitor cells in connective tissue engineering and regenerative medicine: Is there a future for transplantation? In: Langenbeck's Archives of Surgery. 2011. pp. 489–97.

[49] Hutson EL, Boyer S, Genever PG. Rapid isolation, expansion, and differentiation of osteoprogenitors from full-term umbilical cord blood. Tissue Eng. 2005;11(9/10):1407–20.

[50] Diao Y, Ma Q, Cui F, Zhong Y. Human umbilical cord mesenchymal stem cells: osteogenesis in vivo as seed cells for bone tissue engineering. J Biomed Mater Res A. 2009;91(1):123–31.

[51] Nakamura S, Yamada Y, Katagiri W, Sugito T, Ito K, Ueda M. Stem cell proliferation pathways comparison between human exfoliated deciduous teeth and dental pulp stem cells by gene expression profile from promising dental pulp. J Endod. 2009;35(11): 1536–42.

[52] Laino G, Carinci F, Graziano A, D'Aquino R, Lanza V, De Rosa A, et al. In vitro bone production using stem cells derived from human dental pulp. J Craniofac Surg. 2006;17(3):511–5.

[53] D'Aquino R, Papaccio G, Laino G, Graziano A. Dental pulp stem cells: a promising tool for bone regeneration. Stem Cell Rev. 2008;4(1):21–6.

[54] Caplan A, Minguell JJ, Erices A, Conget P, Roufosse CA, Direkze NC, et al. Mesenchymal stem cells. J Orthop Res. 1991;36(4):507–20.

[55] Pittenger MF. Multilineage potential of adult human mesenchymal stem cells. Science (80-). 1999;284(5411):143–7.

[56] Tondreau T, Lagneaux L, Dejeneffe M, Delforge A, Massy M, Mortier C, et al. Isolation of BM mesenchymal stem cells by plastic adhesion or negative selection: phenotype, proliferation kinetics and differentiation potential. Cytotherapy. 2004;6(4):372–9.

[57] Deans RJ, Moseley AB. Mesenchymal stem cells: biology and potential clinical uses. Exp Hematol. 2000;28(8):875–84.

[58] Dominici M, Le Blanc K, Mueller I, Slaper-Cortenbach I, Marini F, Krause D, et al. Minimal criteria for defining multipotent mesenchymal stromal cells. The International Society for Cellular Therapy position statement. Cytotherapy. 2006;8(4):315–7.

[59] Tse WT, Pendleton JD, Beyer WM, Egalka MC, Guinan EC. Suppression of allogeneic T-cell proliferation by human marrow stromal cells: implications in transplantation. Transplantation. 2003;75(3):389–97.

[60] Nicola M Di, Carlo-Stella C, Magni M, Milanesi M, Longoni PD, Matteucci P, et al. Human bone marrow stromal cells suppress T-lymphocyte proliferation induced by cellular or nonspecific mitogenic stimuli. Blood. 2002;99(10):3838–43.

[61] Klyushnenkova E, Mosca JD, Zernetkina V, Majumdar MK, Beggs KJ, Simonetti DW, et al. T cell responses to allogeneic human mesenchymal stem cells: immunogenicity, tolerance, and suppression. J Biomed Sci. 2005;12(1):47–57.

[62] Ryan JM, Barry FP, Murphy JM, Mahon BP. Mesenchymal stem cells avoid allogeneic rejection. J Inflamm (Lond). 2005;23(6):8.

[63] Corcione A, Benvenuto F, Ferretti E, Giunti D, Cappiello V, Cazzanti F, et al. Human mesenchymal stem cells modulate B-cell functions. Blood. 2006;107(1):367–72.

[64] Spaggiari GM, Capobianco A, Abdelrazik H, Becchetti F, Mingari MC, Moretta L. Mesenchymal stem cells inhibit natural killer-cell proliferation, cytotoxicity, and cytokine production: Role of indoleamine 2,3-dioxygenase and prostaglandin E2. Blood. 2008;111(3):1327–33.

[65] Asari S, Itakura S, Ferreri K, Liu C-P, Kuroda Y, Kandeel F, et al. Mesenchymal stem cells suppress B-cell terminal differentiation. Exp Hematol. 2009;37(5):604–15.

[66] Jiang XX, Zhang Y, Liu B, Zhang SX, Wu Y, Yu XD, et al. Human mesenchymal stem cells inhibit differentiation and function of monocyte-derived dendritic cells. Blood. 2005;105(10):4120–6.

[67] Meisel R, Zibert A, Laryea M, Göbel U, Däubener W, Dilloo D. Human bone marrow stromal cells inhibit allogeneic T-cell responses by indoleamine 2,3-dioxygenase-mediated tryptophan degradation. Blood. 2004;103(12):4619–21.

[68] Sato K, Ozaki K, Oh I, Meguro A, Hatanaka K, Nagai T, et al. Nitric oxide plays a critical role in suppression of T-cell proliferation by mesenchymal stem cells. Blood. 2007;109(1):228–34.

[69] Patel SA, Meyer JR, Greco SJ, Corcoran KE, Bryan M, Rameshwar P. Mesenchymal stem cells protect breast cancer cells through regulatory T cells: role of mesenchymal stem cell-derived TGF. J Immunol. 2010;184(10):5885–94.

[70] Hunt JS, Petroff MG, Morales P, Sedlmayr P, Geraghty DE, Ober C. HLA-G in reproduction: studies on the maternal-fetal interface. Hum Immunol. 2000;61(11):1113–7.

[71] Selmani Z, Naji A, Zidi I, Favier B, Gaiffe E, Obert L, et al. Human leukocyte antigen-G5 secretion by human mesenchymal stem cells is required to suppress T lymphocyte and natural killer function and to induce CD4+CD25high FOXP3+ regulatory T cells. Stem Cells. 2008;26(1):212–22.

[72] Bernardo ME, Zaffaroni N, Novara F, Cometa AM, Avanzini MA, Moretta A, et al. Human bone marrow-derived mesenchymal stem cells do not undergo transformation

after long-term in vitro culture and do not exhibit telomere maintenance mechanisms. Cancer Res. 2007;67(19):9142–9.

[73] Uccelli A, Moretta L, Pistoia V. Mesenchymal stem cells in health and disease. Nat Rev Immunol. 2008;8(9):726–36.

[74] Miura M, Miura Y, Padilla-Nash HM, Molinolo AA, Fu B, Patel V, et al. Accumulated chromosomal instability in murine bone marrow mesenchymal stem cells leads to malignant transformation. Stem Cells. 2006;24(4):1095–103.

[75] Zhou YF, Bosch-Marce M, Okuyama H, Krishnamachary B, Kimura H, Zhang L, et al. Spontaneous transformation of cultured mouse bone marrow-derived stromal cells. Cancer Res. 2006;66(22):10849–54.

[76] Rubio D, Garcia-Castro J, Martin MC, De La Fuente R, Cigudosa JC, Lloyd AC, et al. Spontaneous human adult stem cell transformation. Cancer Res. 2005;65(8):3035–9.

[77] Woodbury D, Schwarz EJ, Prockop DJ, Black IB. Adult rat and human bone marrow stromal cells differentiate into neurons. J Neurosci Res. 2000;61(4):364–70.

[78] Lee K-D, Kuo TK-C, Whang-Peng J, Chung Y-F, Lin C-T, Chou S-H, et al. In vitro hepatic differentiation of human mesenchymal stem cells. Hepatology. 2004;40(6):1275–84.

[79] Eslaminejad MB, Taghiyar L. Study of the structure of canine mesenchymal stem cell osteogenic culture. J Vet Med Ser C Anat Histol Embryol. 2010;39(5):446–55.

[80] Bellows CG, Heersche JNM, Aubin JE. Determination of the capacity for proliferation and differentiation of osteoprogenitor cells in the presence and absence of dexamethasone. Dev Biol. 1990;140(1):132–8.

[81] Leboy PS, Beresford JN, Devlin C, Owen ME. Dexamethasone induction of osteoblast m RNAs in rat marrow stromal cell cultures. J Cell Physiol. 1991;146(3):370–8.

[82] Yamachika E, Iida S. Bone regeneration from mesenchymal stem cells (MSCs) and compact bone-derived MSCs as an animal model. Jpn Dent Sci Rev. 2013;49(1):35–44.

[83] Walsh S, Jordan GR, Jefferiss C, Stewart K, Beresford JN. High concentrations of dexamethasone suppress the proliferation but not the differentiation or further maturation of human osteoblast precursors in vitro: relevance to glucocorticoid-induced osteoporosis. Rheumatology. 2001;40(1):74–83.

[84] Vater C, Kasten P, Stiehler M. Culture media for the differentiation of mesenchymal stromal cells. Acta Biomater. 2011;7(2):463–77.

[85] Matic I, Antunovic M, Brkic S, Josipovic P, Caput Mihalic K, Karlak I, et al. Expression of OCT-4 and SOX-2 in bone marrow-derived human mesenchymal stem cells during osteogenic differentiation. Open Access Maced J Med Sci. 2016;1–8.

[86] Kirker-Head CA. Potential applications and delivery strategies for bone morphogenetic proteins. Adv Drug Deliv Rev. 2000;43(1):65–92.

[87] Bai Y, Yin G, Huang Z, Liao X, Chen X, Yao Y, et al. Localized delivery of growth factors for angiogenesis and bone formation in tissue engineering. Int Immunopharmacol. 2013;16(2):214–23.

[88] Mc Carthy TL, Centrella M, Canalis E. Insulin-like growth factor (IGF) and bone. Connect Tissue Res. 2009;20(1–4):277–82.

[89] Hallman M, Thor A. Bone substitutes and growth factors as an alternative/complement to autogenous bone for grafting in implant dentistry. Periodontol 2000. 2008;47(1):172–92.

[90] Ito K, Yamada Y, Naiki T, Ueda M. Simultaneous implant placement and bone regeneration around dental implants using tissue-engineered bone with fibrin glue, mesenchymal stem cells and platelet-rich plasma. Clin Oral Implants Res. 2006;17(5):579–86.

[91] Drury JL, Mooney DJ. Hydrogels for tissue engineering: scaffold design variables and applications. Biomaterials. 2003;24(24):4337–51.

[92] Chen Y, Zhou S, Li Q. Microstructure design of biodegradable scaffold and its effect on tissue regeneration. Biomaterials. 2011;32(22):5003–14.

[93] Suzuki Y, Tanihara M, Suzuki K, Saitou A, Sufan W, Nishimura Y. Alginate hydrogel linked with synthetic oligopeptide derived from BMP-2 allows ectopic osteoinduction in vivo. J Biomed Mater Res. 2000;50(3):405–9.

[94] Saito N, Okada T, Horiuchi H, Murakami N, Takahashi J, Nawata M, et al. A biodegradable polymer as a cytokine delivery system for inducing bone formation. Nat Biotechnol. 2001;19:332–5.

[95] Alsberg E, Anderson KW, Albeiruti a, Franceschi RT, Mooney DJ. Cell-interactive alginate hydrogels for bone tissue engineering. J Dent Res. 2001;80(11):2025–9.

[96] Kaigler D, Avila G, Wisner-Lynch L, Nevins ML, Nevins M, Rasperini G, et al. Platelet-derived growth factor applications in periodontal and peri-implant bone regeneration. Expert Opin Biol Ther. 2011;11(3):375–85.

[97] Velasco MA, Narváez-Tovar CA, Garzón-Alvarado DA. Design, materials, and mechanobiology of biodegradable scaffolds for bone tissue engineering. Biomed Res Int. 2015;2015:21.

[98] Hutmacher DW. Scaffolds in tissue engineering bone and cartilage. Biomaterials. 2000;21(24):2529–43.

[99] Li J, Baker BA, Mou X, Ren N, Qiu J, Boughton RI, et al. Biopolymer/calcium phosphate scaffolds for bone tissue engineering. Adv Healthc Mater. 2014;3(4):469–84.

[100] Moshaverinia A, Ansari S, Chen C, Xu X, Akiyama K, Snead ML, et al. Co-encapsulation of anti-BMP2 monoclonal antibody and mesenchymal stem cells in alginate microspheres for bone tissue engineering. Biomaterials. 2013;34(28):6572–9.

[101] Russell J, Block J. Clinical utility of demineralized bone matrix for osseous defects, arthrodesis, and reconstruction: impact of processing techniques and study methodology. Orthopedics. 1999;22(5):524–31.

[102] Tiedeman JJ, Garvin KL, Kile TA, Connolly JF. The role of a composite demineralized bone matrix and bone marrow in the treatment of osseous defects. Orthopedics. 1995;18(12):1153–8.

[103] Rodriguez-Vazquez M, Vega-Ruiz B, Ramos-Zuniga R, Saldana-Koppel DA, Quinones-Olvera LF. Chitosan and its potential use as a scaffold for tissue engineering in regenerative medicine. Biomed Res Int. 2015;2015:1–15.

[104] Lee CR, Grodzinsky AJ, Spector M. The effects of cross-linking of collagen-glycosaminoglycan scaffolds on compressive stiffness, chondrocyte-mediated contraction, proliferation and biosynthesis. Biomaterials. 2001;22(23):3145–54.

[105] Park SN, Park JC, Kim HO, Song MJ, Suh H. Characterization of porous collagen/hyaluronic acid scaffold modified by 1-ethyl-3-(3-dimethylaminopropyl)carbodiimide cross-linking. Biomaterials. 2002;23(4):1205–12.

[106] Schoof H, Apel J, Heschel I, Rau G. Control of pore structure and size in freeze-dried collagen sponges. J Biomed Mater Res. 2001;58(4):352–7.

[107] Ambrosio AM, Sahota JS, Khan Y, Laurencin CT. A novel amorphous calcium phosphate polymer ceramic for bone repair: I. Synthesis and characterization. J Biomed Mater Res. 2001;58:295–301.

[108] Liu HL, Liu SJ, Chen QY. Excess molar enthalpies for ternary mixtures of (methanol or ethanol plus water plus tributyl phosphate) at T=298.15 K. J Therm Anal Calorim. 2012;107(2):837–41.

[109] Ciapetti G, Granchi D, Devescovi V, Baglio SR, Leonardi E, Martini D, et al. Enhancing osteoconduction of PLLA-based nanocomposite scaffolds for bone regeneration using different biomimetic signals to MSCs. Int J Mol Sci. 2012;13(2):2439–58.

[110] Chou YF, Huang W, Dunn JCY, Miller TA, Wu BM. The effect of biomimetic apatite structure on osteoblast viability, proliferation, and gene expression. Biomaterials. 2005;26(3):285–95.

[111] Mauney JR, Sjostorm S, Blumberg J, Horan R, O'Leary JP, Vunjak-Novakovic G, et al. Mechanical stimulation promotes osteogenic differentiation of human bone marrow stromal cells on 3-D partially demineralized bone scaffolds in vitro. Calcif Tissue Int. 2004;74(5):458–68.

[112] Koller MR, Emerson SG, Palsson BO. Large-scale expansion of human stem and progenitor cells from bone marrow mononuclear cells in continuous perfusion cultures. Blood. 1993;82(2):378–84.

[113] Meinel L, Karageorgiou V, Fajardo R, Snyder B, Shinde-Patil V, Zichner L, et al. Bone tissue engineering using human mesenchymal stem cells: effects of scaffold material and medium flow. Ann Biomed Eng. 2004;32(1):112–22.

[114] Fritton SP, Weinbaum S. Fluid and solute transport in bone: flow-induced mechano-transduction. Annu Rev Fluid Mech. 2009;41(1):347–74.

[115] Bancroft GN, Sikavitsas VI, Mikos AG. Design of a flow perfusion bioreactor system for bone tissue-engineering applications. Tissue Eng. 2003;9(3):549–54.

[116] Holtorf HL, Jansen JA, Mikos AG. Modulation of cell differentiation in bone tissue engineering constructs cultured in a bioreactor. Adv Exp Med Biol. 2006;585:225–41.

[117] Temple JP, Yeager K, Bhumiratana S, Vunjak-Novakovic G, Grayson WL. Bioreactor cultivation of anatomically shaped human bone grafts. Methods Mol Biol. 2014;1202:57–78.

[118] Rauh J, Milan F, Günther K-P, Stiehler M. Bioreactor systems for bone tissue engineering. Tissue Eng Part B Rev. 2011;17(4):263–80.

[119] Van Blitterswijk C, Thomsen P, Lindahl A, Hubbell J, Williams DF, Cancedda R, et al. Bioreactors for tissue engineering. In: Tissue Engineering. 2008; pp. 483–506.

[120] Subia B, Kundu J, Kundu S. Biomaterial scaffold fabrication techniques for potential tissue engineering applications. In: Eberli D, editor. Tissue Engineering. In Tech; 2010; (3):141–59.

[121] Gaspar DA, Gomide V, Monteiro FJ. The role of perfusion bioreactors in bone tissue engineering. Biomatter. 2012;167–75.

[122] Yu X, Botchwey EA, Levine EM, Pollack SR, Laurencin CT. Bioreactor-based bone tissue engineering: the influence of dynamic flow on osteoblast phenotypic expression and matrix mineralization. Proc Natl Acad Sci U S A. 2004;101(31):11203–8.

[123] Zhang Z-Y, Teoh SH, Teo EY, Khoon Chong MS, Shin CW, Tien FT, et al. A comparison of bioreactors for culture of fetal mesenchymal stem cells for bone tissue engineering. Biomaterials. 2010;31(33):8684–95.

[124] Kuznetsov SA, Cherman N, Robey PG. In vivo bone formation by progeny of human embryonic stem cells. Stem Cells Dev. 2011;20(2):269–87.

[125] Levi B, Hyun JS, Montoro DT, Lo DD, Chan CKF, Hu S, et al. In vivo directed differentiation of pluripotent stem cells for skeletal regeneration. Proc Natl Acad Sci U S A. 2012;109(50):20379–84.

[126] Marolt D, Campos IM, Bhumiratana S, Koren A, Petridis P, Zhang G, et al. Engineering bone tissue from human embryonic stem cells. Proc Natl Acad Sci U S A. 2012;109(22): 8705–9.

[127] Salter E, Goh B, Hung B, Hutton D, Ghone N, Grayson WL. Bone tissue engineering bioreactors: a role in the clinic? Tissue Eng Part B Rev. 2012;18(1):62–75.

[128] Carver SE, Heath CA. Semi-continuous perfusion system for delivering intermittent physiological pressure to regenerating cartilage. Tissue Eng. 1999;5(1):1–11.

[129] Altman GH, Horan RL, Martin I, Farhadi J, Stark PRH, Volloch V, et al. Cell differentiation by mechanical stress. FASEB J. 2002;16(2):270–2.

[130] Goldstein AS, Juarez TM, Helmke CD, Gustin MC, Mikos AG. Effect of convection on osteoblastic cell growth and function in biodegradable polymer foam scaffolds. Biomaterials. 2001;22(11):1279–88.

[131] Cartmell SH, Porter BD, García AJ, Guldberg RE. Effects of medium perfusion rate on cell-seeded three-dimensional bone constructs in vitro. Tissue Eng. 2003;9(6):1197–203.

[132] Freed LE, Guilak F, Guo XE, Gray ML, Tranquillo R, Holmes JW, et al. Advanced tools for tissue engineering: scaffolds, bioreactors, and signaling. Tissue Eng. 2006;12(12): 3285–305.

[133] NASA/Marshall Space Flight Center: Free Download & Streaming: Internet Archive. Bioreactor rotating wall vessel.

[134] Granet C, Laroche N, Vico L, Alexandre C, Lafage-Proust MH. Rotating-wall vessels, promising bioreactors for osteoblastic cell culture: comparison with other 3D conditions. Med Biol Eng Comput. 1998;36(4):513–9.

[135] Nishi M, Matsumoto R, Dong J, Uemura T. Engineered bone tissue associated with vascularization utilizing a rotating wall vessel bioreactor. J Biomed Mater Res - Part A. 2013;101 A(2):421–7.

[136] Yeatts AB, Fisher JP. Bone tissue engineering bioreactors: dynamic culture and the influence of shear stress. Bone. 2011. 171–81.

[137] Yeatts AB, Choquette DT, Fisher JP. Bioreactors to influence stem cell fate: augmentation of mesenchymal stem cell signaling pathways via dynamic culture systems. Biochim Biophys Acta. 2013;1830(2):2470–80.

[138] Dahlin RL, Meretoja V V., Ni M, Kasper FK, Mikos AG. Design of a high-throughput flow perfusion bioreactor system for tissue engineering. Tissue Eng Part C Methods. 2012;18(10):817–20.

[139] Mikos. Flow perfusion culture of mesenchymal stem cells for bone tissue engineering. Stem Book. Harvard Stem Cell Institute; 2008; pp. 1–18.

[140] Hoffmann W. Novel perfused compression bioreactor system as an in vitro model to investigate fracture healing. Front Bioeng Biotechnol. 2015;3:10.

[141] Chua CK, Yeong WY. Bioprinting: Principles and Applications. World Scientific Publishing Co. Pte. Ltd.; 2015.

Chapter 12

Regenerative Medicine: A New Paradigm in Bone Regeneration

Orlando Chaparro and Itali Linero

Additional information is available at the end of the chapter

http://dx.doi.org/10.5772/62523

Abstract

Bone defects are the cause of functional disability and the restoration of skeletal function remains an important challenge on orthopedics, neurosurgery and oral and maxillofacial surgery. Because of the limitations of the currently used techniques for the reconstruction of bone defects and the difficulties for the implementation of new therapeutic strategies, a new paradigm in the field of reconstructive surgery has arisen, leading to tissue engineering and regenerative medicine. Mesenchymal stem cells (MSC) have emerged as a promising alternative for the treatment of bone lesions. It was postulated that the therapeutic action was the result of proliferation and differentiation of MSCs, replacing injured tissue. However, recent studies have shown that MSCs secrete a number of trophic factors that have a strong effect during repair and tissue regeneration. This represents a shift from a paradigm centered on MSC proliferation and differentiation to a new paradigm in which the MSCs exert their beneficial effect by the secretion of paracrine factors that induce endogenous repair mechanisms. This chapter will bring together basic and clinical aspects, focused on novel findings on MSC paracrine effect and the development of new therapeutic strategies based on growth factors, cytokines and signaling molecules involved in bone regeneration.

Keywords: mesenchymal stem cells, paracrine effect, bone regeneration, growth factors, cytokines

1. Introduction

The regeneration of bone tissue remains an important challenge in the field of orthopedic and maxillofacial surgery. Bone defects produced by trauma, tumors, infectious diseases, biochemical disorders, congenital disorders or abnormal skeletal development are the major causes of functional disability, and esthetic and psychological trauma for patients.

One of the goals of treating a bone defect is to restore the normal morphology and function of the affected structure. Specific surgical techniques such as distraction osteogenesis, implantation of biomaterials (bone substitutes) and implants of bone grafting have been developed to reach bone regeneration [1, 2]. Demand for bone grafts is considerable and represents the second most common procedure after blood transplants, with more than 2.2 million bone grafts performed annually worldwide in orthopedics and dentistry [3].

Despite advances in bone regeneration and the availability of many treatments, most clinicians and researchers continue to come to the same conclusion: autologous bone grafting remains the "gold standard," compared to other reconstructive procedures [4–9]. Bone from the same patient lacks immunogenicity and contains all the elements necessary to effectively induce tissue regeneration. It has osteoprogenitor cells which go directly to the implant site, cytokines and extracellular matrix [5], providing the three classic elements of an ideal bone graft: osteogenesis, osteoconduction and osteoinduction [5–7, 9, 10]. However, autologous bone grafts have several important limitations, including high risk of morbidity in the donor site [5, 6, 11], with disadvantages in terms of costs, time of surgical procedure, discomfort for the patient and possible complications.

Additionally, many times the volume of tissue available for the procedure is not sufficient to fill or cover a defect, given the limited availability of autologous tissue [4, 10], and the quality of the autograft is highly variable and is influenced by age and metabolic abnormalities of the patient [7]. To overcome these limitations, a variety of exogenous substitutes, including allografts, xenografts and alloplastic materials, have been introduced into clinical practice in the past three decades [4]. However, these substitutes have less osteogenic and osteoinductive properties [6, 12] and a greater possibility of transmission of infectious diseases [6, 8], restricting their use [8].

In order to successfully overcome the shortcomings of current approaches for bone regeneration, tissue engineering emerged as a discipline that provides the necessary tools for bone regeneration and restoration. The presence of cell populations that orchestrate the release of growth factors, the maintenance of a stable matrix and the stimulation of angiogenesis are key factors to successful regeneration of bone tissue, because they play a decisive role in the healing process [13, 14]. The technologies developed recently based on tissue engineering, such as gene therapy, stem cell therapy and the application of osteoinductive growth factors, looking for the control of the dynamics of these elements to enable more predictable bone regeneration surge as a significant promise in clinical practice [15].

Cell-based therapy for the regeneration of bone tissue has been extensively investigated. Several cell types have been used as alternatives for the reconstruction of bone tissue, including osteoblasts, embryonic stem cells, periostium derived-progenitor cells (a specialized cell type that covers bone surfaces and have the potential to differentiate into multiple mesenchymal tissues, including bone) and mesenchymal stem cells, also known as multipotential stromal cells (MSC) [16].

MSC has become one of the best alternatives in cell therapy and specifically in bone regeneration. MSCs can be isolated from virtually all vascularized tissue and they are able to differentiate into various mesenchymal tissues such as bone, cartilage, muscle, tendon, adipose tissue and hematopoiesis-supporting stroma. However, a growing number of recent reports in the literature have revealed that even if a therapeutic effect can be documented, the implanted MSC cells do not differentiate and do not survive for a long time [17, 18].

The use of MSCs in the treatment of musculoskeletal injuries was initially based on their ability to differentiate into various cell types [1, 7, 8]. The rationale was that after implantation or MSC injection, the cells would be able to colonize the injured site and differentiate into the appropriate lineages. This mechanism has now been challenged by a new paradigm to extend it to an alternative mechanism called **paracrine effect**, where MSCs secrete biologically active molecules which have beneficial effects on the injured tissues [9] by inhibiting fibrosis, apoptosis and inflammation [10, 11] and promoting angiogenesis and tissue regeneration [19–21].

2. Physiological process of bone regeneration

For the development of new therapeutic tools for restoring bone defects exceeding the critical size, it is necessary to look at the prototype model of physiological bone regeneration. This process, involving a coordinated interaction of cells, growth factors and extracellular matrix, consists of multiple and well-orchestrated stages that start immediately after the injury occurs, with a local inflammatory response followed by the mobilization of hematopoietic and mesenchymal stem cells to the site of injury to form new vascular networks, soft tissue matrix, cartilage and/or bone and finally inducing mature bone formation [22–24]. All four components involved in the site of injury, including cortical bone, periosteum, bone marrow and external soft tissue, contribute to a different extent in the healing process, depending on various parameters such as growth factors, hormones and nutrients, pH, oxygen tension, the electrical environment and mechanical stability [25].

Immediately after bone trauma, damage of the local vasculature at the site of injury is responsible for producing a blood clot or hematoma [24, 26, 27]. This hematoma is a localized collection of blood products, including platelets, leukocytes, macrophages, fibrin, soluble growth factors and cytokines, which in turn provides a matrix that allows the migration of inflammatory cells, endothelial cells and fibroblasts [24] (**Figure 1**).

This first stage of fracture healing is the beginning of the so-called **inflammatory phase**, which begins within the first 12 to 14 hours, has its peak during the first 24 hours and is completed around 7 days after the injury. It is characterized by a destructive phase, with a local acute inflammatory response and hypoxia. The first cells to arrive at the site of injury are neutrophils, and subsequently macrophages and lymphocytes. Macrophages not only phagocyte necrotic tissue but also release a number of growth factors and cytokines that initiate the healing process of bone wound [26] (**Figure 1**).

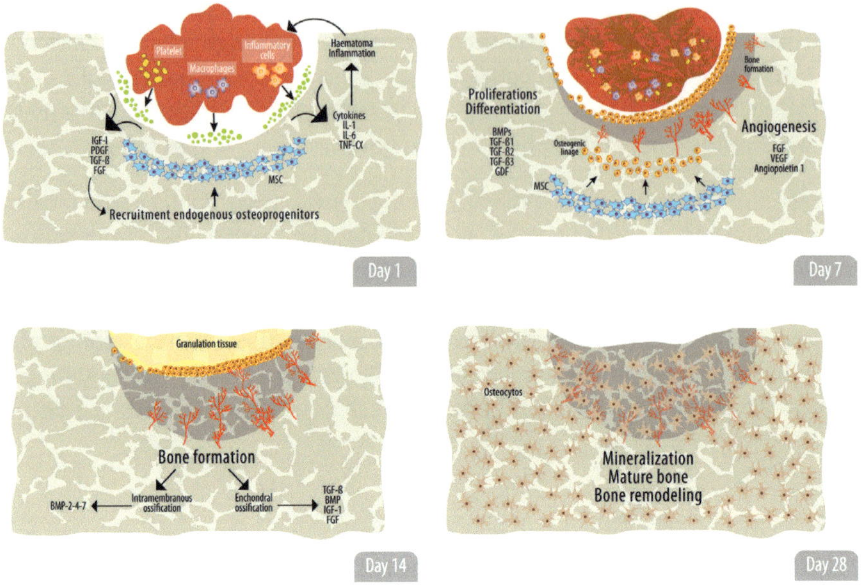

Figure 1. Temporal progression of bone healing. The healing response to bone injury is characterized by overlapping biological processes: immediately after bone injury, hematoma formation and inflammatory response permits the release of pro-inflammatory cytokines and growth factors that initiate the process of wound healing. Between days 1–7, MSCs proliferate and differentiate into the osteogenic or chondrogenic lineages and increase the production of blood vessels from pre-existing vessels. New bone formation occurs through intramembranous or endochondral ossification that is finally mineralized, forming a mature bone that is continuously remodeled through the rest of his life.

The factors secreted by platelets, macrophages and bone cells include transforming growth factor beta (TGF-β), vascular endothelial growth factor (VEGF), platelet-derived growth factor (PDGF), interleukins 1 and 6 (IL-1 and IL-6), tumor necrosis growth factor alpha (TNF-α), bone morphogenetic proteins (BMPs) [26, 27], fibroblast growth factor (FGF) and insulin-like growth factors I and II (IGF-I and IGF-II) [26]. These factors stimulate the migration of multipotent stem cells, probably originated from the periosteum, bone marrow, blood vessels and the surrounding soft tissue and induce the differentiation of cells to different mesenchymal cell types including angioblasts, fibroblasts, chondroblasts and osteoblasts [26].

During the following days, the **construction phase** starts. This phase is characterized by the formation of new blood vessels [17], and the thrombus reorganization into granulation tissue, which is then condensed in a soft callus providing an osteoid and/or cartilage scaffold, which acts as a stabilization structure and a template for subsequent mineralization [26] (**Figure 1**).

Depending on the type of bone, the type of bone lesion, the morphology and structure of the tissue and the fixation method, bone healing can take two forms: primary healing, where osteoblasts secrete an osteoid matrix for future mineralization (intramembranous ossification); and secondary healing, which occurs through the formation of a cartilage matrix produced by chondrocytes, which is then replaced by an osteoid matrix with subsequent mineralization (endochondral ossification) [24–27]. Most common growth factors related to bone healing, osteoinduction and osteoconduction are: PDGF, BMPs [15, 28, 29], IGFs [28, 30], TGF-β [15, 28], FGF [24, 29] and VEGF [15, 24, 29].

Local vascularization at the site of injury has been identified as one of the most important parameters that influence the healing process [14, 31, 32]. Bone formation can only proceed successfully if the tissue is adequately vascularized [15]; therefore, angiogenesis is a key component in bone repair. The new blood vessels carry oxygen and nutrients to the metabolically active callus, allowing gas exchange and the output of waste products and serve as a route for inflammatory cells, and cartilage and bone precursor cells [33, 34], and also provide the gateway of systemically circulating factors that can modify the bone healing process [34]. Vascularization is needed for both the formation of intramembranous and endochondral bone. During the formation of endochondral bone, cartilage avascular environment is invaded by blood vessels that allow the osteoblastic, chondroblastic and progenitor cells, to deposit new bone on the surface of the islands of cartilage. During intramembranous ossification, vascularization is also needed to allow the arrival of osteoblast precursor cells [34].

Angiogenesis and migration of vascular endothelial cells are stimulated by pro-angiogenic factors such as VEGF, BMPs, TGF-β, FGF and angiopoietins (especially angiopoyectina I and II) [26].

Finally, over the course of months to years, the third stage, the **remodeling phase** of bone healing occurs, whose main objective is to reshape the bone in order to restore its original structure and strength. During this phase, osteoclasts reabsorb recently formed bone tissue, due to the stimulation of growth factors and cytokines that promote osteoclastogenesis as TNF-α, TGF and BMPs. Osteoblasts deposit more osteoid and calcium phosphate in the newly regenerated bone, increasing the density of mineralized matrix. Therefore, the transverse diameter of the bone decreases but the density of internal structure increases, closer and closer to the architecture of the intact bone. As this stage keeps going, cellularity is gradually reduced and bone density is enhanced [26].

3. Biological factors in bone regeneration

During the process of bone regeneration, the release of growth factors occurs as a series of highly time-space regulated biological events. These soluble molecules are able to regulate signaling cascades that specifically influence cellular responses such as differentiation and proliferation [28].

Biological signaling molecules function effectively by a limited window of time to get a proper result in the target cell. Therefore, it is necessary to have a precise understanding of the temporal pathways for natural bone regeneration. Biological signaling agents can be classified into the following categories: pro-inflammatory cytokines, growth and differentiation factors and angiogenic factors. Pro-inflammatory cytokines are activated immediately after bone injury and establish and maintain the acidic and hypoxic environment for the initial destruction phase. Growth and differentiation factors function during the constructive and destructive phases, while angiogenic factors are focal points for the revascularization of the wounded area [25, 26, 35] (**Table 1**).

Signaling Molecules	Expression Pattern	Source	Target cells	function
Cytokines (IL-1,IL-6, TNF-α)	Increased levels from days 1 to 3 and during bone remodeling	Macrophages Inflammatory cells Cells of mesenchymal origin	Mesenchymal and inflammatory cells	Chemotactic effect on other inflammatory cells Stimulation of extracellular matrix synthesis, angiogenesis, recruitment of endogenous fibrogenic cells to the injury site and at later stages bone resorption
TGF-β	Expressed from very early stages throughout fracture healing	Degranulating platelets Inflammatory cells endothelium, extracellular matrix, chondrocytes, osteoblasts	MSCs, osteoprogenitor cells, osteoblasts, chondrocytes	Potent mitogenic and chemotactic for bone-forming cells, chemotactic for macrophages
PDGF	Released at very early stages of fracture healing	Degranulating platelets, macrophages, monocytes (during the granulation stage) and endothelial cells, osteoblasts (at later stages)	Mesenchymal and inflammatory cells, osteoblasts	Mitogenic for mesenchymal cells and osteoblasts, chemotactic for inflammatory and mesenchymal cells
BMPs	Various temporal expression patterns	Osteoprogenitors and mesenchymal cells, osteoblasts, bone extracellular matrix and chondrocytes	Mesenchymal and osteoprogenitor cells, osteoblasts	Differentiation of undifferentiated mesenchymal cells into chondrocytes and osteoblasts and osteoprogenitors into osteoblasts
FGFs	Expressed from the early stages until osteoblasts formation	Monocytes, macrophages, mesenchymal cells, osteoblasts, chondrocytes	Mesenchymal and epithelial cells, osteoblasts and chondrocytes	Angiogenic and mitogenic for mesenchymal and epithelial cells, osteoblasts, chondrocytes α-FGF mainly effects chondrocyte proliferation β-FGF (more potent) involved in chondrocytes maturation and bone resorption
IGFs	Expressed throughout fracture healing and endochondral ossification	Bone matrix, endothelial and mesenchymal cells (in granulation stage) and osteoblasts and non-hypertrophic chondrocytes (in bone and cartilage formation)	MSCs, endothelial cells, osteoblasts, chondrocytes	IGF-I: mesenchymal and osteoprogenitor cells recruitment and proliferation IGF-II: cell proliferation and protein synthesis

Signaling Molecules	Expression Pattern	Source	Target cells	function
VEGFs	Expressed during endochondral and bone formation	Bone matrix, endothelial and mesenchymal cells	Endothelial progenitor cells	Potent stimulators of endothelial cell proliferation
Angiopoietin (I and II)	Expressed from the early stages throughout fracture healing	Extravascular tissue cells	Endothelial progenitor cells	Formation of larger vessel structures, development of co-lateral branches from existing vessels

Essential signaling molecules in bone regeneration: their time of expression, source, target cells and their major functions (Adapted with the permission from Dimitriou et al. [25]. Copyright© 2005).

Table 1. Biological factors in bone regeneration.

In the next section, we will list some of the common molecules associated with the bone regeneration process, and describe their biological significance.

3.1. Transforming growth factor-beta (TGF-β) superfamily

Members of the TGF- β are the most widely studied growth factors in recent years. This family includes, among others, five isoforms of TGF-β (1–5), bone morphogenetic proteins (BMPs) and growth differentiation factors (GDFs), which participate in a complex series of molecular events that lead to mesenchymal precursors during bone morphogenesis [25, 29, 33, 36]. They originate from high molecular weight precursors and are activated by proteolytic enzymes. They act on serine/threonine kinase membrane receptor on target cells. This ligand-receptor interaction activates intracellular signaling pathways which ultimately affects gene expression in the nucleus [25].

3.1.1. Bone morphogenetic proteins (BMPs)

The BMPs are a unique family of proteins within the TGF-β superfamily that play an essential role in regulating the formation, maintenance and bone repair [30]. To date, about 20 different proteins have been termed BMPs, but not all of them have osteogenic potential [37]. Among the BMPs with osteogenic potential we have, BMPs-2, -3 (osteogenin), -4, -6, -7 (also known as osteogenic protein-1 [OP-1]), -12 (also known as growth/differentiation factor 7 [GDF-7]) and -14 (also known as GDF-5, or cartilage-derived morphogenetic protein-1 [CDMP-1]). These proteins have been evaluated for healing and bone regeneration in clinical and preclinical models showing enhanced and accelerated bone formation [30]. In bone tissue, BMPs are produced by osteoprogenitor cells, osteoblasts, chondrocytes and platelets. Their regulatory effects depend on the target cell, stage of differentiation, local concentration, as well as interactions with other secreted proteins. BMPs induce a sequential cascade of events leading to chondrogenesis, osteogenesis, controlled angiogenesis and extracellular matrix synthesis [37]. Large number of preclinical studies has shown that BMPs are capable of inducing bone formation at ectopic sites and induce critical size defects healing [29]. It has been shown that BMPs 2, 4 and 7 play an important role in determining, migration, condensation, proliferation and apoptosis of skeletal cells. It has also been reported that BMP-4 and BMP-7 are responsible for inducing the cells of the neural crest, while BMP-2 is involved in the condensation of mesenchymal cells appearing before formation of immature bone structures during both endochondral and intramembranous ossification [33]. BMP-4 is predominantly active from days 1–5 after injury, with a peak closer to day 5. The BMP-2 is active during the bone regeneration process, culminating the bone remodeling to lamellar and haversian bone tissue, while BMP-7 is active after 14 days [23]. Target cells of BMPs include MSC, bone marrow cells, osteoblasts, myoblasts, prefibroblast and neuronal cells. The general effects on osteoblasts and cells of the periosteum involve an increase in the activity of DNA synthesis and transcription of genes involved in the synthesis of bone matrix proteins [23].

Scientific evidence of the role of BMPs in bone regeneration is overwhelming. There are a number of publications confirming that the delivery of BMP at the site of injury promotes bone regeneration in animal and human models [38–40].

BMP-2 and BMP-7 have been extensively evaluated in clinical studies of nonunion, bone defects, open tibial fractures and spinal fusion, demonstrating their efficacy in the acceleration of bone regeneration and healing of fractures [29]. In order to be used in the clinical practice, a local and controlled delivery of BMPs is required; so, it is important to consider its short half-life time. Various delivery systems have been developed to overcome this limitation [37]. Currently, there are several forms of the human recombinant proteins commercially available. For example, for rh-BMP2: InductOs® (United Kingdom) and InFUSE (United States), (Medtronic Sofamor Danek, Inc., Minneapolis, MN), which are supplied in a bovine collagen sponge allowing slow release over time, and for rhBMP-7, Osigraft® (United Kingdom) and OP-1™ (United States) (Stryker Biotech, Hop-kinton, MA), in a bovine collagen granular form [34, 36, 37].

3.1.2. Transforming growth factor-beta (TGF-β)

The five isoforms of TGF-β regulate cellular functions such as proliferation, apoptosis, differentiation and cell migration. TGF-β is produced by osteoblasts and chondrocytes, and is stored in the bone matrix [25, 41]. TGF-β is also released by platelets and TGF-β1 indeed, was the first member of the family to be described in human platelets, as a 25 kDa protein with a possible role in the healing process [42]. During the initial phase of inflammation resulting from a bone injury, platelets release TGF-β and therefore this factor seems to be involved in the initial callus formation stage [25, 41].

TGF-β is a multifunctional, secreted protein, with different functions in the cell, such as control of cell growth and proliferation, differentiation and apoptosis. TGF-β induces the proliferation of MSCs, pre-osteoblasts, osteoblasts and chondrocytes and stimulates the extracellular production of proteins such as collagen, proteoglycans, osteopontin, osteonectin and alkaline phosphatase [25, 41]. It is also a potent chemotactic agent for MSCs. During chondrogenesis and endochondral bone formation, it induces the synthesis of BMP by osteoprogenitor cells, and it inhibits the activation and promotes osteoclast apoptosis [41].

3.2. Platelet-derived growth factors (PDGF)

This polypeptide growth factor has potent chemotactic and mitogenic stimulatory effects on MSCs [30], plays an important role in the differentiation of pre-osteoblasts to osteoblasts [43] with the ability to promote angiogenesis during wound healing [30]. The PDGF family includes four isoforms: PDGF-A, PDGF-B, the more recently discovered PDGF-C and PDGF-D [44]. PDGF-A and B form homodimers (AA or BB) and a heterodimer (AB) [30]. PDGF-AB and PDGF-BB are variants circulating in alpha platelet granules and are released when platelets bind to the site of injury. The PDGF-BB variant has an active role in mitogenesis and chemotaxis of cells in the injured area [15] and plays a key role in bone regeneration [23]. After bone injury, PDGF is released by macrophages and platelets and acts as a potent chemo-attractant and mitogenic factor for cells of mesenchymal lineage, recruit fibroblasts, endothelial cells, osteoblasts and cells of the immune system. PDGF is active during the first 72 hours after injury, and as a promoter of angiogenesis plays a role in revascularization of bone defects [23].

3.3. Fibroblast growth factor (FGF)

They constitute a family of structurally related polypeptides with a potent mitogenic effect on osteoprogenitor cells [29]. They are humoral factors originally identified by their ability to stimulate cell proliferation [33]. During bone healing, they can be secreted by monocytes, macrophages, mesenchymal cells, osteoblasts and chondrocytes in the early stages of bone fractures healing [33]. Members of the FGF family are present at the site of the wound for up to three weeks and its main activity is to stimulate endothelial cell migration and subsequent angiogenesis and mesenchymal cell mitogenesis [25, 34]. α-FGF mainly affects chondrocyte proliferation and is probably important for chondrocyte maturation, while β-FGF is expressed by osteoblasts and is generally more potent than α-FGF [45].

3.4. Vascular endothelial growth factor (VEGF)

Two separate pathways are involved in the regulation of angiogenesis during bone healing: a VEGF dependent pathway and the angiopoietin-dependent pathway [31]. VEGF is a potent angiogenic [29, 43] and vasculogenic [23] factor that not only increases the differentiation and proliferation of endothelial cells but also increases the tubular formation and mobilization and recruitment of endothelial progenitor cells [34]. VEGF is increased in response to hypoxia, ischemia and during healing of bone tissue [15, 34]. It has been shown that VEGF works synergistically with BMPs. VEGF by itself does not promote bone regeneration, but rather acts in coordination with BMPs to increase the recruitment of MSCs to the defect site and induce active differentiation of osteoblasts [46]. VEGF is expressed predominantly 14 to 21 days after the injury; and therefore, it is a candidate for early in situ application to promote mineralization and bone regeneration remodeling [23].

3.5. Insulin-like growth factors (IGF)

IGF-1 and -2 play a critical role in stimulation of organogenesis and growth during the first stages of embryogenesis as well as in regulating the functions of specific tissues and organs in later stages of development [47]. The sources of IGF-1 and IGF-2 are the bone matrix, endothelial cells, osteoblasts and chondrocytes [25]. IGF-1 promotes bone matrix formation (type I collagen and non-collagenous matrix proteins) by fully differentiated osteoblasts and is more potent than IGF-2 [45]. IGF-2 acts at a later stage of endochondral bone formation and stimulates type I collagen production, cartilage matrix synthesis and cellular proliferation [25].

4. Regenerative therapies

Clinical failure of bone tissue is defined as a discontinuity of the integrity of bone resulting from trauma, congenital malformation or surgical recession. Particularly, bone deficiency "critical size" is the bone defect that cannot regenerate spontaneously during the lifespan of the patient and, therefore, requires a surgical intervention for recovery [23].

The processes that drive the biology and biomechanics of bone regeneration remain largely unknown. During regeneration of bone tissue, many highly complex interactions between multiple cell types are mediated by soluble and insoluble factors and they have not been sufficiently characterized. The challenge for tissue engineering and regenerative medicine is to rebuild the regenerative healing process of bone tissue and then join the components to produce osteoangiogenic and, therefore, osteoregenerative therapies that fulfill the biomechanical parameters for the healing of a bone defect that exceeds the critical size.

We must remember that the bone has an inherent capacity for regeneration, so it is important to not only design therapies that do not interfere with the natural regenerative processes but also complement them and work synergistically with the endogenous bone healing process.

Regenerative therapy of bone tissue should include the three essential elements of bone regeneration: osteogenesis, osteoinduction and osteoconduction. Osteogenesis refers to the ability to produce new bone by bone-forming cells. Osteoinduction is the process whereby the presence of biological mediators stimulates the recruitment of mesenchymal stem cells to the wound site and their subsequent differentiation into mature bone cells, and osteoconduction is the physical property of providing a matrix facilitating the invasion of blood vessels and the new bone formation [48, 49].

Based on these fundamental principles, the main goal of regenerative medicine in clinical treatment is to reduce surgical morbidity by applying biological signals or cellular components that allow the reconstruction and restoration of lost tissue without autologous tissue transfer.

4.1. Mesenchymal stem cells-based therapy

Bone cell-based therapies seek to create viable tissue equivalents, providing live and metabolically active cells to repair the site of injury by continuous synthesis of bone matrix [50].

Mesenchymal stem cells are the center of a multitude of clinical studies currently underway (http://clinicaltrials.gov) [51]. Scientific evidence shows that they are one of the best choices in cell therapy, because of their ease of access and isolation, great potential of expansion in culture, immunosuppressive properties, paracrine effect and ability to migrate to injured tissues [52]. Moreover, their great therapeutic potential has been documented in the repair and regeneration of injured tissues in nearly every organ of the body, including the heart [53], immune system [54], liver [55], kidneys [56] and bone and cartilage tissue [57].

Mesenchymal stem cells are defined as pluripotent cells capable of self-renewal and differentiation into various specialized types of mesenchymal cells, such as osteoblasts, chondrocytes, adipocytes, myocytes, fibroblasts [52, 58–61]. MSCs are a group cells that have been isolated from virtually every vascularized tissue [62]. MSCs are a group cells that have been isolated from virtually every vascularized tissue [52]; however, recent reports have documented that they can also be isolated from other sources as umbilical cord [62], peripheral blood [63], adipose tissue [64–67], hair follicle [68], periodontal ligament [69–72], gingival tissue [73] and dental pulp [74, 75], among others.

MSCs, for its ability to differentiate to multiple lineages, specifically, their osteogenic potential and their immunomodulatory, anti-inflammatory and anti-apoptotic properties, have become a major tool in cell therapy for the regenerative treatment of pathologies affecting functionally bone tissue [76–79]. In vitro analyzes show that MSCs induced by osteogenic differentiation medium increase the expression of osteogenic differentiation markers such as alkaline phosphatase, osteocalcin, osteopontin, bone sialoprotein and calcium deposits in the extracellular matrix. The progress in the study of the biology of bone tissue and the isolation and in vitro cultivation of MSCs opened the possibility of studying the molecular and biological mechanisms of bone regeneration, making significant progress, as evidenced by the more two thousand publications of experimental reports on the application of MSCs in bone defects in animal models promoting bone regeneration, and the more than five hundred clinical trials currently registered on the NIH clinical trials website (http://clinicaltrials.gov) [51].

4.1.1. MSCs mechanism of action

The mechanisms through which MSCs enhance the bone tissue repair process are complex, since they can participate in the three phases of bone healing: inflammation, proliferation and remodeling [80]. The in vivo identity and location of MSC have been difficult to establish. However, various reports, especially the work of Crisan et al., presented evidence of a relationship between MSCs and perivascular pericytes. Irrespective of their tissue origin, perivascular cells exhibit osteogenic, chondrogenic and adipogenic potentials and express MSC markers [81]. Based on these reports, Caplan suggests that all MSCs are pericytes, which would explain the presence of MSC in all vascularized tissues. When an injury disrupts the normal architecture of the blood vessels, pericytes are activated giving rise to MSCs that then contribute to tissue repair by secreting trophic factors that can control the endogenous inflammatory reaction, promote angiogenesis and stimulate the proliferation and differentiation of progenitor cells [82] (**Figure 2**).

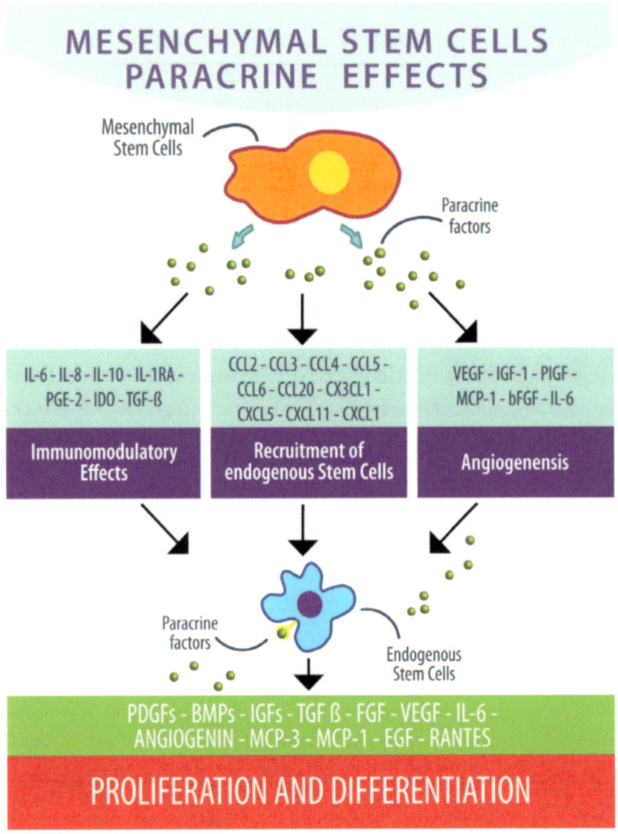

Figure 2. Schematic model of the MSCs' paracrine effect on tissue regeneration.

As mentioned before, a growing number of recent reports in the literature have revealed that even if a therapeutic effect can be observed, the implanted MSC cells do not differentiate and do not survive for a long time. For example, in an animal model of acute myocardial infarction, it was established that the MSCs implanted do not survive, and only 4.4% of grafted MSC could be found 1–2 weeks after transplantation [17], and MSC transplantation in a model of spinal cord injury in rats revealed that MSCs implanted disappeared from the host after 1–2 weeks [18]. It has been also reported that human adipose tissue-derived MSCs effectively induce bone regeneration in rabbit jaws, but they do not differentiate and do not survive more than 12 days in the site of implantation [21]. Recent reports have demonstrated that many of the therapeutic effects of MSCs can be mediated by the secretion of trophic factors, opening the possibility that direct administration of these mediators may replace the use of the cells in some instances [57]. This implies a shift from a paradigm centered on cell differentiation to a new vision where the MSCs can have a therapeutic effect even if they are not grafted or differentiated into specific tissue cells, which significantly increases the options of MSC therapeutic applications. According to this concept, Caplan has proposed that the most important feature of the MSC which determines its therapeutic potential is not their stemness

http://dx.doi.org/10.5772/62523

but the ability to secrete a large number of trophic factors, and he has proposed that their name to be changed to medicinal signaling cells, keeping the same MSC acronym [83].

Caplan also proposes a model whereby MSCs exert their therapeutic action at the site of the injury by two different activities: from the front of the cells, away from the area of injury, MSCs create a curtain, by the production of bioactive molecules that control local inflammation and prevent autoimmune reactions. From the back of the MSC, they produce molecules that: (1) stop scar formation, (2) inhibit cell apoptosis due to ischemia, (3) stimulate the formation and stabilization of blood vessels and (4) secrete trophic factors that induce the replication of endogenous tissue progenitors [84] (**Figure 3**).

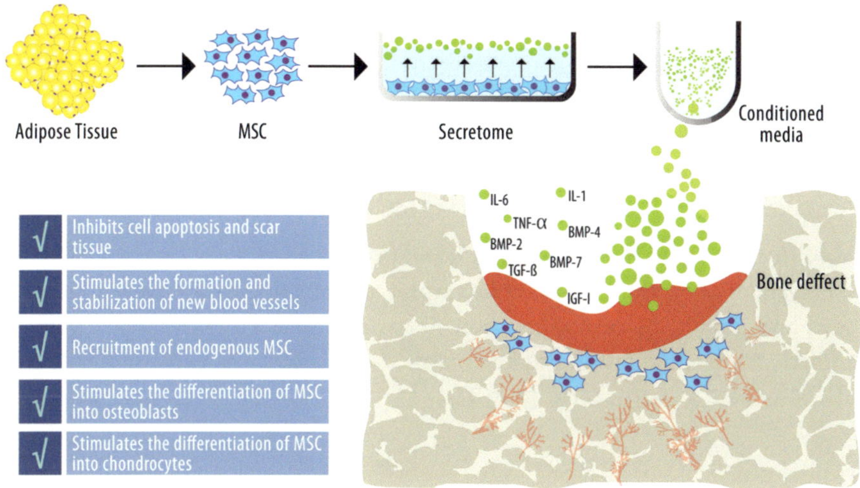

Figure 3. Schematic diagram illustrating the concept of application of MSC conditioned media in bone injuries. The MSC secretome, containing chemokines and growth factors, promote the recruitment of endogenous osteogenic cells and stimulate their migration to injured sites, inducing their differentiation and bone formation.

4.2. Secretome as a therapeutic strategy: conditioned media

The broad spectrum of factors secreted by the different types of MSCs is generally referred as MSC secretome. Recent data demonstrate that MSC secretome factors, collected as conditioned media (CM), are sufficient to exert the MSC therapeutic effects.

Previous studies have reported many growth factors and cytokines derived from the CM of various stem cells [19–21, 85–89], which could be responsible for the paracrine protective effects of stem cells against several diseases. Consequently, the use of stem cells CM instead of direct implantation of stem cells may be a feasible approach to overcome the limitations of current cell-based therapy. In addition, because CM is not a cell, but a conjugate of many growth factors, the administration of CM has no ethics concerns related with cell therapies.

However, secretomic signatures of the various types of MSC are not completely known, and the qualitative and quantitative characterization of MSC secretomes and their functions in secretome-mediated repair will contribute to the development of new regenerative therapies that will not require cell transplants [90].

Recently, the great potential of tissue engineering and regenerative medicine strategies for bone augmentation has been demonstrated, and the feasibility of using CM from MSC as an osteoinductive agent for future clinical use is becoming more evident. CM from bone marrow-MSC increased the migration and proliferation of MSCs, vascularization and the early bone regeneration in rabbit sinus model, showing CM as a promising novel therapeutic agent to promote bone regeneration after maxillary sinus floor elevation [91]. It has been shown that CM can have stronger effects than MSCs, accelerating the mobilization of endogenous endothelial and MSC cells for bone regeneration in rat calvarial bone defect model [92]. Intravenous administration of MSC-CM provided the protection of osteoblasts and osteoclasts, induced angiogenesis, anti-apoptotic and anti-inflammatory effects in a rat bisphosphonate-related osteonecrosis of the jaw-like model [93]. It has also been reported that the use of MSC-CM may be an alternative therapy for periodontal tissue regeneration [94]. CM from human MSC accelerates the formation of new bone callus, shortening the time period required for distraction osteogenesis treatment in a mouse model by recruiting endogenous mouse bone marrow stem cells (mBMSCs) and EC/EPCs via MCP-1/-3 and IL-3/-6 signaling [95].

We have also reported that human Ad-MSCs and their CM induce bone regeneration in a jaw rabbit model, and that morphometric, radiographic and histological analysis demonstrate that the amount and quality of neoformed bone, repaired area, bone density, arrangement of collagen fibers, maturation and inorganic matrix calcification are very similar between Ad-MSC and CM-treated groups [21] (**Figure 3**).

5. Perspectives

All the scientific evidence on the paracrine effect of MSC provide the opportunity to exploit the therapeutic potential of MSC-CM and opens up scenarios for the identification of new candidate molecules for tissue repair via proteomic analysis of the MSC secretome. MSC-CM delivers osteoinductive growth factors and cytokines that modulate the behavior of endogenous cells contributing to the formation of new tissue. Furthermore, the use of MC allows us to avoid some of the limiting factors associated with the clinical application of stem cells, such as the risk of tumorigenesis and transmission of infectious diseases [80], immunological incompatibility, costs and waiting time for cell ex vivo expansion [80].

The use of MSC-CM as a novel therapeutic strategy has several practical advantages. CM storage and transportation procedures are not as complex as they are for MSC. CM production can be less expensive, enabling access to disadvantaged populations and reducing costs for health systems.

Despite the advantages of its use, CM application may not always supersede the use of MSC, and it is possible that for some type of disorders MSC could be a more effective alternative. The number of known molecules mediating the paracrine effect of MSC grows every day, and significantly increases the potential range of their therapeutic applications.

Author details

Orlando Chaparro* and Itali Linero

*Address all correspondence to: ochaparrog@unal.edu.co

Universidad Nacional de Colombia, Facultad de Medicina - Facultad de Odontología Biología de Células Madre, Ciudad Universitaria, Bogotá, Colombia

References

[1] Lane JM, Tomin E, Bostrom MP. Biosynthetic bone grafting. Clin Orthop Relat Res. 1999;(367 Suppl):S107-17.

[2] Meinel L, Hofmann S, Betz O, Fajardo R, Merkle HP, Langer R, et al. Osteogenesis by human mesenchymal stem cells cultured on silk biomaterials: comparison of adenovirus mediated gene transfer and protein delivery of BMP-2. Biomaterials. 2006;27(28): 4993-5002.

[3] Lewandrowski KU, Gresser JD, Wise DL, Trantol DJ. Bioresorbable bone graft substitutes of different osteoconductivities: a histologic evaluation of osteointegration of poly(propylene glycol-co-fumaric acid)-based cement implants in rats. Biomaterials. 2000;21(8):757-64.

[4] Pagni G, Kaigler D, Rasperini G, Avila-Ortiz G, Bartel R, Giannobile WV. Bone repair cells for craniofacial regeneration. Adv Drug Deliv Rev. 2012;64(12):1310-9.

[5] Pape HC, Evans A, Kobbe P. Autologous bone graft: properties and techniques. J Orthopaed Trauma. 2010;24(Suppl 1):S36-40.

[6] Roden RDJr. Principles of bone grafting. Oral Maxillofac Surg Clin North Am. 2010;22(3):295-300, v.

[7] Skovrlj B, Guzman JZ, Al Maaieh M, Cho SK, Iatridis JC, Qureshi SA. Cellular bone matrices: viable stem cell-containing bone graft substitutes. Spine J. 2014;14(11): 2763-72.

[8] Vo TN, Kasper FK, Mikos AG. Strategies for controlled delivery of growth factors and cells for bone regeneration. Adv Drug Deliv Rev. 2012;64(12):1292-309.

[9] Zimmermann G, Moghaddam A. Allograft bone matrix versus synthetic bone graft substitutes. Injury. 2011;42(Suppl 2):S16-21.

[10] Zouhary KJ. Bone graft harvesting from distant sites: concepts and techniques. Oral Maxillofac Surg Clin North Am. 2010;22(3):301-16, v.

[11] Cancedda R, Giannoni P, Mastrogiacomo M. A tissue engineering approach to bone repair in large animal models and in clinical practice. Biomaterials. 2007;28(29):4240-50.

[12] Shibuya N, Jupiter DC. Bone graft substitute: allograft and xenograft. Clin Podiatr Med Surg. 2015;32(1):21-34.

[13] Taba MJr., Jin Q, Sugai JV, Giannobile WV. Current concepts in periodontal bioengineering. Orthod Craniofac Res. 2005;8(4):292-302.

[14] Giannoudis PV, Einhorn TA, Schmidmaier G, Marsh D. The diamond concept--open questions. Injury. 2008;39(Suppl 2):S5-8.

[15] Khojasteh A, Behnia H, Naghdi N, Esmaeelinejad M, Alikhassy Z, Stevens M. Effects of different growth factors and carriers on bone regeneration: a systematic review. Oral Surg Oral Med Oral Pathol Oral Radiol. 2013;116(6):e405-23.

[16] Mesimaki K, Lindroos B, Tornwall J, Mauno J, Lindqvist C, Kontio R, et al. Novel maxillary reconstruction with ectopic bone formation by GMP adipose stem cells. Int J Oral Maxillofac Surg. 2009;38(3):201-9.

[17] Nakamura Y, Wang X, Xu C, Asakura A, Yoshiyama M, From AH, et al. Xenotransplantation of long-term-cultured swine bone marrow-derived mesenchymal stem cells. Stem Cells. 2007;25(3):612-20.

[18] Ide C, Nakai Y, Nakano N, Seo TB, Yamada Y, Endo K, et al. Bone marrow stromal cell transplantation for treatment of sub-acute spinal cord injury in the rat. Brain Res. 2010;1332:32-47.

[19] Perin EC, Silva GV. Autologous cell-based therapy for ischemic heart disease: clinical evidence, proposed mechanisms of action, and current limitations. Catheter Cardiovasc Interv 2009;73(3):281-8.

[20] Yoon SH, Kim SK, Kim JF. Secretory production of recombinant proteins in *Escherichia coli*. Recent Pat Biotechnol. 2010;4(1):23-9.

[21] Linero I, Chaparro O. Paracrine effect of mesenchymal stem cells derived from human adipose tissue in bone regeneration. PLo S One. 2014;9(9):e107001.

[22] Ratanavaraporn J, Furuya H, Tabata Y. Local suppression of pro-inflammatory cytokines and the effects in BMP-2-induced bone regeneration. Biomaterials. 2012;33(1):304-16.

[23] Shrivats AR, Mc Dermott MC, Hollinger JO. Bone tissue engineering: state of the union. Drug Discov Today. 2014;19(6):781-6.

[24] Shrivats AR, Alvarez P, Schutte L, Hollinger JO. Bone Regeneration. In: Lanza R, Vacanti J, Langer R, editors. Principles of Tissue Engineering. 4th ed. San Diego: Elseiver; 2014. p. 1201-1221. DOI: 10.1016/B978-0-12-398358-9.00055-0

[25] Dimitriou R, Tsiridis E, Giannoudis PV. Current concepts of molecular aspects of bone healing. Injury. 2005;36(12):1392-404.

[26] Oryan A, Alidadi S, Moshiri A. Current concerns regarding healing of bone defects. Hard Tissue 2013;2(2):1-12.

[27] Lindahl A, Brittberg M, Gibbs D, Dawson JI, Kanczler J, Black C, Tare R, Oreffo ROC. Cartilage and bone regeneration. In: Van Blitterswijk CA, De Boer J, editors. Tissue Engineering. 2nd ed. San Diego: Elseiver; 2015. p. 529-582. DOI: 10.1016/B978-0-12-420145-3.00016-X

[28] Fernandez-Yague MA, Abbah SA, Mc Namara L, Zeugolis DI, Pandit A, Biggs MJ. Biomimetic approaches in bone tissue engineering: Integrating biological and physicomechanical strategies. Adv Drug Deliv Rev. 2014;84:1-29. DOI:10.1016/j.addr.2014.09.005

[29] Nauth A, Ristevski B, Li R, Schemitsch EH. Growth factors and bone regeneration: how much bone can we expect? Injury. 2011;42(6):574-9.

[30] Lee J, Stavropoulos A, Susin C, Wikesjo UM. Periodontal regeneration: focus on growth and differentiation factors. Dent Clin North Am. 2010;54(1):93-111.

[31] Keramaris NC, Calori GM, Nikolaou VS, Schemitsch EH, Giannoudis PV. Fracture vascularity and bone healing: a systematic review of the role of VEGF. Injury. 2008;39(Suppl 2):S45-57.

[32] Sun X, Kang Y, Bao J, Zhang Y, Yang Y, Zhou X. Modeling vascularized bone regeneration within a porous biodegradable CaP scaffold loaded with growth factors. Biomaterials. 2013;34(21):4971-81.

[33] Ji W, Wang H, van den Beucken JJ, Yang F, Walboomers XF, Leeuwenburgh S, et al. Local delivery of small and large biomolecules in craniomaxillofacial bone. Adv Drug Deliv Rev. 2012;64(12):1152-64.

[34] Hankenson KD, Dishowitz M, Gray C, Schenker M. Angiogenesis in bone regeneration. Injury. 2011;42(6):556-61.

[35] Gerstenfeld LC, Cullinane DM, Barnes GL, Graves DT, Einhorn TA. Fracture healing as a post-natal developmental process: molecular, spatial, and temporal aspects of its regulation. J Cell Biochem. 2003;88(5):873-84.

[36] Seo BB, Choi H, Koh JT, Song SC. Sustained BMP-2 delivery and injectable bone regeneration using thermosensitive polymeric nanoparticle hydrogel bearing dual interactions with BMP-2. J Control Release. 2015;209:67-76. DOI: 10.1016/j.jconrel.2015.04.023

[37] Lissenberg-Thunnissen SN, de Gorter DJ, Sier CF, Schipper IB. Use and efficacy of bone morphogenetic proteins in fracture healing. Int Orthopaed. 2011;35(9):1271-80.

[38] Jones AL, Bucholz RW, Bosse MJ, Mirza SK, Lyon TR, Webb LX, et al. Recombinant human BMP-2 and allograft compared with autogenous bone graft for reconstruction

of diaphyseal tibial fractures with cortical defects. A randomized, controlled trial. J Bone Joint Surg Am. 2006;88(7):1431-41.

[39] Kanakaris NK, Calori GM, Verdonk R, Burssens P, De Biase P, Capanna R, et al. Application of BMP-7 to tibial non-unions: a 3-year multicenter experience. Injury. 2008;39(Suppl 2):S83-90.

[40] Zimmermann G, Wagner C, Schmeckenbecher K, Wentzensen A, Moghaddam A. Treatment of tibial shaft non-unions: bone morphogenetic proteins versus autologous bone graft. Injury. 2009;40(Suppl 3):S50-3.

[41] Tsiridis E, Upadhyay N, Giannoudis P. Molecular aspects of fracture healing: which are the important molecules? Injury. 2007;38(Suppl 1):S11-25.

[42] Assoian RK, Komoriya A, Meyers CA, Miller DM, Sporn MB. Transforming growth factor-beta in human platelets. Identification of a major storage site, purification, and characterization. J Biol Chem. 1983;258(11):7155-60.

[43] Khojasteh A, Behnia H, Dashti SG, Stevens M. Current trends in mesenchymal stem cell application in bone augmentation: a review of the literature. J Oral Maxillofac Surg. 2011;70(4):972-82.

[44] Bergsten E, Uutela M, Li X, Pietras K, Ostman A, Heldin CH, et al. PDGF-D is a specific, protease-activated ligand for the PDGF beta-receptor. Nat Cell Biol. 2001;3(5):512-6.

[45] Lieberman JR, Daluiski A, Einhorn TA. The role of growth factors in the repair of bone. Biology and clinical applications. J Bone Joint Surg Am. 2002;84-A(6):1032-44.

[46] Schilephake H. Bone growth factors in maxillofacial skeletal reconstruction. Int J Oral Maxillofac Surg. 2002;31(5):469-84.

[47] Butler AA, LeRoith D. Minireview: tissue-specific versus generalized gene targeting of the igf1 and igf1r genes and their roles in insulin-like growth factor physiology. Endocrinology. 2001;142(5):1685-8.

[48] Giannoudis PV, Dinopoulos H, Tsiridis E. Bone substitutes: an update. Injury. 2005;36(Suppl 3):S20-7.

[49] Kalfas IH. Principles of bone healing. Neurosurg Focus. 2001;10(4):E1.

[50] Drosse I, Volkmer E, Capanna R, De Biase P, Mutschler W, Schieker M. Tissue engineering for bone defect healing: an update on a multi-component approach. Injury. 2008;39(Suppl 2):S9-20.

[51] clinicaltrials.gov. http://www.clinicaltrials.gov: http://www.clinicaltrials.gov/ct2/results?term=mesenchymal+stem+cells&Search=Search; 2016 [cited 2016 January].

[52] Salem HK, Thiemermann C. Mesenchymal stromal cells: current understanding and clinical status. Stem Cells. 2010;28(3):585-96.

[53] Badimon L, Onate B, Vilahur G. Adipose-derived mesenchymal stem cells and their reparative potential in ischemic heart disease. Revis Esp Cardiol. 2015;68(7):599-611.

[54] Coulson-Thomas VJ, Coulson-Thomas YM, Gesteira TF, Kao WW. Extrinsic and intrinsic mechanisms by which mesenchymal stem cells suppress the immune system. Ocul Surf. 2016;1-14. DOI:10.1016/j.jtos.2015.11.004

[55] Christ B, Bruckner S, Winkler S. The therapeutic promise of mesenchymal stem cells for liver restoration. Trends Mol Med. 2015;21(11):673-86.

[56] Hu J, Zhang L, Wang N, Ding R, Cui S, Zhu F, et al. Mesenchymal stem cells attenuate ischemic acute kidney injury by inducing regulatory T cells through splenocyte interactions. Kidney Int. 2013;84(3):521-31.

[57] Prockop DJ, Kota DJ, Bazhanov N, Reger RL. Evolving paradigms for repair of tissues by adult stem/progenitor cells (MSCs). J Cell Mol Med. 2010;14(9):2190-9.

[58] Caplan AI, Bruder SP. Mesenchymal stem cells: building blocks for molecular medicine in the 21st century. Trends Mol Med. 2001;7(6):259-64.

[59] Caplan AI, Dennis JE. Mesenchymal stem cells as trophic mediators. J Cell Biochem. 2006;98(5):1076-84.

[60] Asahara T, Kawamoto A. Endothelial progenitor cells for postnatal vasculogenesis. Am J Physiol Cell Physiol. 2004;287(3):C572-9.

[61] Clarke D, Frisen J. Differentiation potential of adult stem cells. Curr Opin Genet Dev. 2001;11(5):575-80.

[62] Hendijani F, Haghjooy Javanmard S, Sadeghi-Aliabadi H. Human Wharton's jelly mesenchymal stem cell secretome display antiproliferative effect on leukemia cell line and produce additive cytotoxic effect in combination with doxorubicin. Tissue Cell. 2015;47(3):229-34.

[63] Roufosse CA, Direkze NC, Otto WR, Wright NA. Circulating mesenchymal stem cells. Int J Biochem Cell Biol. 2004;36(4):585-97.

[64] Dicker A, Le Blanc K, Astrom G, van Harmelen V, Gotherstrom C, Blomqvist L, et al. Functional studies of mesenchymal stem cells derived from adult human adipose tissue. Exp Cell Res. 2005;308(2):283-90.

[65] Levi B, Longaker MT. Osteogenic differentiation of adipose-derived stromal cells in mouse and human: in vitro and in vivo methods. J Craniofac Surg. 2010;22(2):388-91.

[66] Levi B, Nelson ER, Brown K, James AW, Xu D, Dunlevie R, et al. Differences in osteogenic differentiation of adipose-derived stromal cells from murine, canine, and human sources in vitro and in vivo. Plast Reconstr Surg. 2010;128(2):373-86.

[67] Badimon L, Onate B, Vilahur G. Adipose-derived mesenchymal stem cells and their reparative potential in ischemic heart disease. Rev Esp Cardiol. 2015;68:599–611. DOI: 10.1016/j.rec.2015.02.025

[68] Shih DT, Lee DC, Chen SC, Tsai RY, Huang CT, Tsai CC, et al. Isolation and characterization of neurogenic mesenchymal stem cells in human scalp tissue. Stem Cells. 2005;23(7):1012-20.

[69] Lin NH, Gronthos S, Mark Bartold P. Stem cells and future periodontal regeneration. Periodontol 2000. 2009;51:239-51.

[70] Ishikawa I, Iwata T, Washio K, Okano T, Nagasawa T, Iwasaki K, et al. Cell sheet engineering and other novel cell-based approaches to periodontal regeneration. Periodontol 2000. 2009;51:220-38.

[71] Kawanabe N, Murata S, Murakami K, Ishihara Y, Hayano S, Kurosaka H, et al. Isolation of multipotent stem cells in human periodontal ligament using stage-specific embryonic antigen-4. Differentiation. 2010;79(2):74-83.

[72] Yang Y, Rossi FM, Putnins EE. Periodontal regeneration using engineered bone marrow mesenchymal stromal cells. Biomaterials. 2010;31(33):8574-82.

[73] Mitrano TI, Grob MS, Carrion F, Nova-Lamperti E, Luz PA, Fierro FS, et al. Culture and characterization of mesenchymal stem cells from human gingival tissue. J Periodontol. 2010;81(6):917-25.

[74] Yamada Y, Fujimoto A, Ito A, Yoshimi R, Ueda M. Cluster analysis and gene expression profiles: a cDNA microarray system-based comparison between human dental pulp stem cells (hDPSCs) and human mesenchymal stem cells (hMSCs) for tissue engineering cell therapy. Biomaterials. 2006;27(20):3766-81.

[75] Chen B, Sun HH, Wang HG, Kong H, Chen FM, Yu Q. The effects of human platelet lysate on dental pulp stem cells derived from impacted human third molars. Biomaterials. 2012;33(20):5023-35.

[76] Chamberlain G, Fox J, Ashton B, Middleton J. Concise review: mesenchymal stem cells: their phenotype, differentiation capacity, immunological features, and potential for homing. Stem Cells. 2007;25(11):2739-49.

[77] Phinney DG, Prockop DJ. Concise review: mesenchymal stem/multipotent stromal cells: the state of transdifferentiation and modes of tissue repair: current views. Stem Cells. 2007;25(11):2896-902.

[78] Slater BJ, Kwan MD, Gupta DM, Panetta NJ, Longaker MT. Mesenchymal cells for skeletal tissue engineering. Expert Opin Biol Ther. 2008;8(7):885-93.

[79] Ankrum J, Karp JM. Mesenchymal stem cell therapy: two steps forward, one step back. Trends Mol Med. 2010;16(5):203-9.

[80] Wang Q, Jin Y, Deng X, Liu H, Pang H, Shi P, et al. Second-harmonic generation microscopy for assessment of mesenchymal stem cell-seeded acellular dermal matrix in wound-healing. Biomaterials. 2015;53:659-68.

[81] Crisan M, Yap S, Casteilla L, Chen CW, Corselli M, Park TS, et al. A perivascular origin for mesenchymal stem cells in multiple human organs. Cell Stem Cell. 2008;3(3):301-13.

[82] Caplan AI. All MSCs are pericytes? Cell Stem Cell. 2008;3(3):229-30.

[83] Caplan AI, Correa D. The MSC: an injury drugstore. Cell Stem Cell. 2011;9(1):11-5.

[84] Caplan AI, Sorrell JM. The MSC curtain that stops the immune system. Immunol Lett. 2015;168:136-139. DOI: 10.1016/j.imlet.2015.06.005

[85] Kinnaird T, Stabile E, Burnett MS, Shou M, Lee CW, Barr S, et al. Local delivery of marrow-derived stromal cells augments collateral perfusion through paracrine mechanisms. Circulation. 2004;109(12):1543-9.

[86] Succar P, Breen EJ, Kuah D, Herbert BR. Alterations in the secretome of clinically relevant preparations of adipose-derived mesenchymal stem cells cocultured with hyaluronan. Stem Cells Int. 2015;2015:421253.

[87] Kwon HM, Hur SM, Park KY, Kim CK, Kim YM, Kim HS, et al. Multiple paracrine factors secreted by mesenchymal stem cells contribute to angiogenesis. Vascul Pharmacol. 2014;63(1):19-28.

[88] Tran C, Damaser MS. Stem cells as drug delivery methods: application of stem cell secretome for regeneration. Adv Drug Deliv Rev. 2015;82-83:1-11.

[89] Blaber SP, Webster RA, Hill CJ, Breen EJ, Kuah D, Vesey G, et al. Analysis of in vitro secretion profiles from adipose-derived cell populations. J Transl Med. 2012;10:172.

[90] Kim JM, Kim J, Kim YH, Kim KT, Ryu SH, Lee TG, et al. Comparative secretome analysis of human bone marrow-derived mesenchymal stem cells during osteogenesis. J Cell Physiol. 2013;228(1):216-24.

[91] Katagiri W, Osugi M, Kinoshita K, Hibi H. Conditioned medium from mesenchymal stem cells enhances early bone regeneration after maxillary sinus floor elevation in rabbits. Implant Dent. 2015;24(6):657-63.

[92] Osugi M, Katagiri W, Yoshimi R, Inukai T, Hibi H, Ueda M. Conditioned media from mesenchymal stem cells enhanced bone regeneration in rat calvarial bone defects. Tissue Eng Part A. 2012;18(13-14):1479-89.

[93] Ogata K, Katagiri W, Osugi M, Kawai T, Sugimura Y, Hibi H, et al. Evaluation of the therapeutic effects of conditioned media from mesenchymal stem cells in a rat bisphosphonate-related osteonecrosis of the jaw-like model. Bone. 2015;74:95-105.

[94] Kawai T, Katagiri W, Osugi M, Sugimura Y, Hibi H, Ueda M. Secretomes from bone marrow-derived mesenchymal stromal cells enhance periodontal tissue regeneration. Cytotherapy. 2015;17(4):369-81.

[95] Ando Y, Matsubara K, Ishikawa J, Fujio M, Shohara R, Hibi H, et al. Stem cell-conditioned medium accelerates distraction osteogenesis through multiple regenerative mechanisms. Bone. 2014;61:82-90.

Chapter 13

Doped Bioactive Glass Materials in Bone Regeneration

Samit Kumar Nandi, Arnab Mahato,
Biswanath Kundu and Prasenjit Mukherjee

Additional information is available at the end of the chapter

http://dx.doi.org/10.5772/63266

Abstract

In the arena of orthopaedic surgery, autograft is considered to be the gold standard for correction of fracture repair or other bone pathologies. But, it has some limitations such as donor site morbidity and shortage of supply, which evolved the use of allograft that also has some disadvantages such as immunogenic response to the host, low osteogenicity as well as possibilities of disease transmission. Despite the benefits of autografts and allografts, the limitations of each have necessitated the pursuit of alternatives biomaterials that has the ability to initiate osteogenesis, and the graft should closely mimic the natural bone along with regeneration of fibroblasts. A variety of artificial materials such as demineralised bone matrix, coralline hydroxyapatite and calcium phosphate-based ceramics such as hydroxyapatite (HA), β-tricalcium phosphate (β-TCP) and bioactive glass have been used over the decades to fill bone defects almost without associated soft tissue development. Most of them were having only the properties of osteointegration and osteoconduction. Only bioactive glass possesses osteogenic property that stimulates proliferation and differentiation of osteoprogenitor cells and in some cases influencing the fibroblastic properties. But, this material has also some disadvantages such as short-term and low mechanical strength along with decreased fracture resistance; but, this was further minimised by ion doping that positively enhanced new bone formation. There are many metal ions such as magnesium (Mg), strontium (Sr), manganese (Mn), iron (Fe), zinc (Zn), silver (Ag) and some rare earths that have been doped successfully into bioactive glass to enhance their mechanical and biological properties. In some of the cases, mesoporous bioactive glass materials with or without such doping have also been employed (with homogeneous distribution of pores in the size ranging between 2 and 50 nm). These biomaterials can be served as scaffold for bone regeneration with adequate mechanical properties to restore bone defects and facilitate healing process by regeneration of soft tissues as well. This chapter encompasses the use of bioactive glass in bulk and mesoporous form with doped therapeutic ions, their role in bone tissue regeneration, use as delivery of growth factors as well as coating material for orthopaedic implants.

1. Introduction

Bone tissue repair and regeneration have made considerable strides in the modern era. An in-depth perceptive of the underlying principles has been achieved, new methods and materials developed and a multidisciplinary approach was used to accomplish successful bone tissue regeneration. Many scaffold systems have been planned for hard tissue engineering. Novelty has been worked out in terms of scaffold design, material selection, inclusion of drugs and growth factors, mechanical stability and bone regeneration competence. Nevertheless, autografts are still considered as 'gold standard' for bone tissue repair; equivalent osteogenic or osteoinductive performance is not obtained by the synthetic bone graft substitutes. Due to limitations of autografts in sufficient quantities to meet the overall medical demand for orthopaedic implants, allografts and xenografts are alternatives sources to overcome such problems, but are having the risks of disease transmission and immune rejection. As a result, synthetic bone graft substitutes are the rational choice to meet the huge demand for orthopaedic implants, even though its inherent limitations in terms of strength, osteoconduction, osteoinduction, osseointegration and biodegradation. Accordingly, modern research area has been focussed on development of new biomaterials, modification of mechanical and structural features, improvement of biocompatibility, osteoinductivity and to incorporate growth factors and stem cells onto scaffolds to encourage bone regeneration.

Bone tissue regeneration strategies intend to use synthetic temporary templates to assist the natural healing of bone defects. Bone extracellular matrix (ECM) containing collagen fibrous structure, with mineralised calcium phosphate, is secreted from osteoblasts [1, 2]. For effective bone regeneration in non-load-bearing defects require a biomaterial scaffold that might have a three-dimensional (3D) fibrous structure mimicking the ECM [3–5] and can be easily placed into position during surgery. The scaffolds are also required to be biocompatible (should not elicit an inflammatory response nor exhibit immunogenicity or cytotoxicity), bioactive (bond with bone), bioresorbable, allow new bone formation at an acceptable rate, be economical to make and allow easy fabrication into the final preforms [6–8]. The scaffolds must be easily sterilisable to prevent infection especially for bulk degradable scaffolds [9]. Additionally, the mechanical properties of the scaffold must be optimal to prevent structural failure during handling and patient's normal activities. Furthermore, controllable interconnected porosity is of paramount necessity for cells to grow into the scaffold and to support angiogenesis. The scaffolds should also have porosity of 90% with pore diameter of at least 100 μm for proper cell penetration and vascularisation of the ingrown tissue [10–12].

A number of inorganic and organic materials are being used as bone substitutes that include calcium phosphate ceramics, phosphates of magnesium, sulphate, carbonate and silicate of calcium and collagen with positive cell-material interactions. Inert inorganic materials, such as alumina, zirconia, titanium alloy and cobalt-chromium alloy, are also used in hard tissue applications, but lack resorbability and absence of osseointegration at the bone-implant interface. Positive interaction with cells was established using synthetic biodegradable polymers, such as polylactic-co-glycolic acid (PLGA), polycaprolactone (PCL) and polyethylene glycol (PEG) [13, 14]. The degradation products of these materials have no detrimental effects in body system. Furthermore, degradation rate, hydrophilicity and mechanical strength can be controlled by changing the chemical composition. Many natural biopolymers are also available and are very suitable bone substitutes in terms of cell-material interactions. Large polymers of very high molecular weight such as chitosan, alginate, cellulose, gelatin, collagen, keratin and hyaluronic acid also exhibit favourable cell-material interactions. Additional biocompatibility to a structurally stable scaffold is the selection criteria for bone substitute materials currently in vogue [15, 16].

In bone tissue engineering, commonly used materials are ceramic and glass due to their superior biocompatibility. Poor mechanical strength and stability are the major deficits rendering them unsuitable as porous scaffolds. In addition, processing defects such as irregularly shaped pores, surface defects and residual stress, all reduce the mechanical strength of the scaffold systems. These limitations compelled the researchers to find out the solutions for the improvement of biological performance of these materials by combinations of various strategies to augment cell-material interactions and stimulation of cells to ensure rapid but controlled bone regeneration. One of the alternate strategies is metallic ion doping for improving biological performance enhancement.

The aim of this chapter is to summarise the recent advancement of metallic ion dopants in addition to bioactive glass scaffold and their studies in orthopaedic surgical challenges. Our discussion broadly covers innovations in materials development and fine tuning together with structural and functional improvisations.

2. Bioactive glass materials

"Bioactive" glass can be defined by its name itself, which include "Bioactive", means *One that elicits a specific biological response at the interface of the material which results in the formation of a bond between the tissues and the material*, and "glass", often defined as *solid that possesses a non-crystalline (that is, amorphous) structure at the atomic scale and that exhibits a glass transition when heated towards the liquid state* [17]. In short, bioactive glass has been designed to elicit a particular biological reaction at the interface of the material, which stimulates cell proliferation, gene response and the formation of a bond between living tissues and the material [17–20]. Its surface develops a biologically active apatite layer (HCA), which initiates bonding with bone. The apatite phase formed chemically and structurally mimics the mineral phase of bone [21]. Among other essential qualities of bioactive glass are that they should be non-mutagenic, non-carcinogenic and non-antigenic so that they do not have any adverse effect on the cells [22]. With these typical properties, bioactive glasses are reported to be capable of more bone regeneration than other bioactive ceramics available. However, in the case of bioactive glass there are many areas to improve as it has not yet reached its true potential.

The invention of bioactive glass was not by accident, in contrary it was being invented through a series of curious set of events. The first bioactive glass as an alternative to nearly inert implant materials was invented by Prof. Larry Hench at the University of Florida in 1969. A US army colonel, returned from Vietnam war, asked him if material could be developed that could survive the aggressive environment of human body. All available materials at that time, such as metals and polymers, were designed to be bio-inert, which were found to trigger fibrous encapsulation after implantation rather than forming a stable interface or bond with the tissues [23]. The melt-derived bioactive glass invented by professor L. Hench was composed of 46.1 mol% SiO_2, 24.4 mol% Na_2O, 26.9 mol% CaO and 2.6 mol% P_2O_5, later termed as 45S5 and Bioglass®, which forms a bond with bone strong enough so that it could not be removed without breaking the bone [24]. It is now almost 50 years since the discovery of bonding of bioactive glass with living bone and over time many advances have been made in this field, understanding the mechanism of bone bonding, and respectively modifying the properties of bioactive glass by adjustment of the composition [25–28]. The most interesting aspect of bioactive glass is the high adaptiveness to the biological environment and the tuneable properties, by which the rate of bonding with bone can be controlled, thus the fabrication of patient-specific implants is possible. Today, new bioactive glasses can be made specifically for different types of clinical applications, in different forms such as fibres, microspheres and to show required bioactivity at when implanted.

2.1. Synthesis

According to process method used, bioactive glasses can be classified into two different categories: (1) melt derived, (2) sol-gel derived. In these fabrication techniques, melting method is traditional [27, 29–32]; however, the latter appealed the scientists in the last two decades [33, 34]. The synthesis route of bioactive glass has eminent effect on the specific surface area as well as degradability of the material.

2.2. Melt derived

The first bioactive glass itself made by Professor Larry Hench in the 1970s was made through melt-quenched method. The idea behind the invention was to make an implant material which can form a hydroxyapatite (HA) layer on its surface when implanted, which can develop a living bond with the host [35]. As the main aim was to mimic bone and bone contains hydroxyapatite [$Ca_5(PO_4)_3OH$], Ca^+ and PO_4^{3-} were taken as a component of glass. The other main components of glass Si^{4+} and Na^{2+} can also be found in human body. Among the compositions Hench and co-workers made, 45S5 were found to bond with rat femur. The selection of the components of this glass, named as Bioglass®, was ideal. The low silica content compared to the previous soda-lime-silicate glasses forms a layer of silica and amorphous calcium phosphate on the surface of the implant. Since then the research on bioactive glass somehow concentrated mostly compositions similar to 45S5 bioactive glass.

Most of those bioactive glasses were produced by melting raw materials at an elevated temperature because it is a simple, low-cost technique and does not take much time to complete. It typically involves raw materials selection, weighing, mixing of components in appropriate proportion and removal of impurities to get a homogeneous melt. The reactivity of a glass in aqueous solutions is strongly dependent on the composition of the glass and thus the choice of composition is very important. Because the limited range of glass composition shows bioactivity, the glass composition should be chosen in a way so that it can be melted and formed into required shapes with available methods. The raw materials can be divided into five different categories according to their role: glass former, flux, modifier, colourant and fining agent. Glass formers are the most important components of glass as they form the matrix of the glass structure. Silica (SiO_2), boric acid (B_2O_3) and phosphoric acid (P_2O_5) are the most common type of glass former normally present in oxide glass. In between these silica is widely used; however, the melting temperature of silica is too high (1600–1725°C) and so different types of flux such as Na_2O and PbO can be used to decrease the melting temperature of the mixture. The addition of flux sometime degrades the properties of glass, which can be overcame by introducing different property modifier or intermediates such as boron, sodium, magnesium, titanium and calcium. Colourants are used to control the colour in the final product. Finally, fining agents such as arsenic, antimony oxides, potassium and sodium nitrates are added to raw materials to remove bubbles from the melt. During melting of the raw materials inside the furnace, they react with each other and carbon dioxide and Water-vapour emission takes place, which causes the formation of bubbles. To raise the bubbles up to the upper surface of the melt, low viscosity is maintained. Batch particle size and their mixing in proper proportion are other factors that provide homogeneity in glass structure. Glass forming is an intermediate stage in between glass melting and annealing. The stages of glass synthesis are illustrated schematically in **Figure 1**.

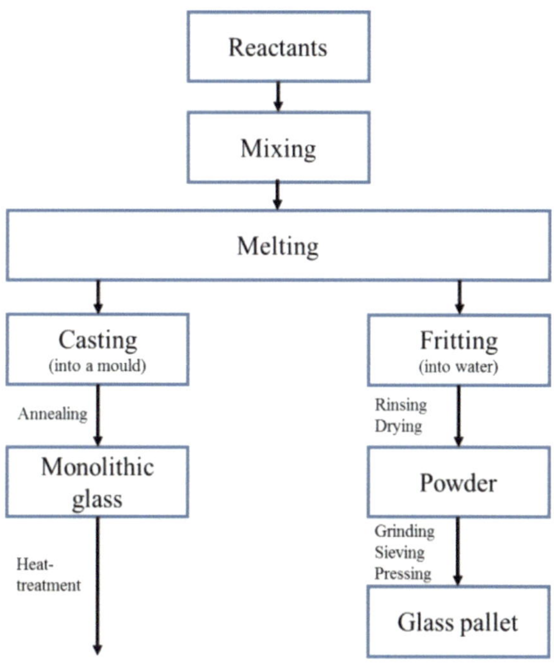

Figure 1. Schematic representation of melt-derived glass synthesis.

Practically appropriate amount (mole/weight fraction) of initial ingredients is mixed, followed by grinding, to break agglomerated particles. In order to obtain more uniform powder, the mixture of ingredients is ground in ball mill using acetone (water can also be used unless some ingredient is hygroscopic). After drying the mixture in air, the powder can be transferred in platinum crucible and melted in a high-temperature furnace. Generally, around 500°C, the gaseous substances (moisture and gas) come out of the composition. Hence, it is better to calcine the mixture at 500°C for at least 2 h. Before taking out the melt, it must be confirmed that the glass mixture is held at the melting temperature for at least an hour to achieve homogeneous, bubble-free molten materials. Then, the molten glass can be quenched in liquid such as water, liquid nitrogen, etc. Granules of different sizes formed collectively known as frits can be collected and milled to get glass powder. Desirable size and shapes can be made by pouring the molten mixture into moulds of particular shapes. In the case of preparation of glass with particular shape, the poured glass is annealed slightly below the glass transition temperature of the corresponding glass for 12 h in air in pit furnace.

2.2.1. *Important factors*

Important factors to remember while melting a glass are viscosity, thermal expansion and crystallisation characteristics. Low viscosity helps the melt to be bubble free and homogeneous and also facilitates easy elimination from the platinum pot. It is a crucial factor in determining the best possible procedure for a particular composition. Viscosity values at high temperatures can be linked with melt-forming processes and low-temperature values indicate the suitability of the glass, whether for sintering into porous bodies or coating on metal implants. The approximate viscosity values for a bioactive-glass-forming process are given in **Table 1**.

Processing	**Viscosity (η) (dPa s)**
Melting	$10\text{-}10^{2}$
Pressing	$10^{4}\text{-}10^{6}$
Drawing of continuous fibres	$10^{2.5}\text{-}10^{3.5}$
Sinter glass powder to porous body	$10^{8}\text{-}10^{9}$
Annealing	$10^{12}\text{-}10^{13}$

Table 1. Approximate viscosity values (dPa s) for bioactive-glass-forming process.

Bioactive glass coating provides better bone-implant connection when coated on metal prostheses [36–41]. According to the implantation area, lower surface reactivity may be preferred and in such cases glass composition with less bioactivity are favoured. Whatever be the case the thermal expansion of the glass must be compatible with the metal otherwise cracks may appear on the coating leading to peeling off of the coating.

Another important factor is that the melting temperature should be higher than liquidus temperature of the compositions. Recent development of bioactive glasses focuses on the change of chemical composition and different heat treatment condition [42, 43]. Aboud et al. analysed the effect of increasing temperature on the crystallisation behaviour and the phase formation order of different crystals of SiO_2–P_2O_5–Al_2O_3–MgO–Na_2O glasses [44]. The changes in microstructure, mechanical and chemical properties of this glass with different heat treatment conditions result in an important application in dental restoration [45]. Also, thermal treatments of bioactive glass tend to enable the glass to attain different elastic properties and a range of bioactivity, which could be helpful for making patient-specific implant [46].

2.3. Sol-gel derived

Sol-gel glasses are made by a chemical-based process at much lower temperatures than the traditional processing methods [47–51]. The method has been recently accepted by a number of research groups to make a new generation of bioactive glass and offers assurance for tailoring the composition to match the specific requirements. Recently, scientists have preferred the sol-gel method in order to increase the specific surface area, and thus, the surface reactivity and degradability of the material [52]. It also provides better control over homogeneity and purity [53].

A sol is a colloidal suspension of solid particles (with a diameter of 1–100 nm) in a liquid, where the colloids exhibit *Brownian motion*, a random walk driven by momentum imparted by collisions with molecules of the suspending medium. Gel can be described as a rigid network of covalently bonded silica comprised of interconnected pores [54, 55]. Three methods can be used to make sol-gel materials: gelation of colloidal particles, hypercritical drying or controlled hydrolysis and condensation of metal alkoxide precursors followed by drying at ambient pressure. All the three methods create a three-dimensional, interconnected network. Gels can be categorised into three types, such as alcogels, xerogels and aerogels [53]. Alcogels are generally alcohol based, whereas xerogels are formed from thermal removal of pore liquid. Gels with low density (80 kg m^{-3}) and large pore volumes (up to 98%) are called aerogels, which are the result of removal of pore liquid from the rigid network without collapsing it.

Preparation of gel glasses by a sol-gel method composed of seven steps. First, the alkoxide or organometallic precursors are mixed to form the low-viscosity sol, followed by hydrolysis of liquid alkoxide precursors with de-ionised water [56, 57]. Hydrolysis of silicon alkoxide forms silanol groups [$Si(OH)_4$], eventually interact with each other to make the Si-O-Si bond and increase the viscosity of the sol (**Figure 2**). This is the time where the sol can be applied as a coating, be pulled into fibre, electrospun, impregnated into a composite or formed into powders. During the process of gelation, the viscosity of the solution sharply increases [58]. The gelation time depends upon the concentration of the solvent, nature of the oxide group and the amount of water used for the hydrolysis [59, 60]. While aging of a gel for several hours at 25-80°C, decrease in porosity and increase in the strength can be observed due to polycondensation and reprecipitation of the gel network [61–63]. Aging process also affects the pore volume, surface area and density of the gel. The removal of pore liquid has different effect on arising stress for colloidal gels (pore size > 100 nm) and alkoxide-based gels with pore size 1-10 nm. Colloidal gels can be dried easily; however, in the case of alkoxide-based gels, large capillary stress may arise during drying. Hypercritical drying at elevated temperature and pressure, above the pore-liquid-solid critical point, avoids the solid-liquid interface and eliminates drying stress [17].

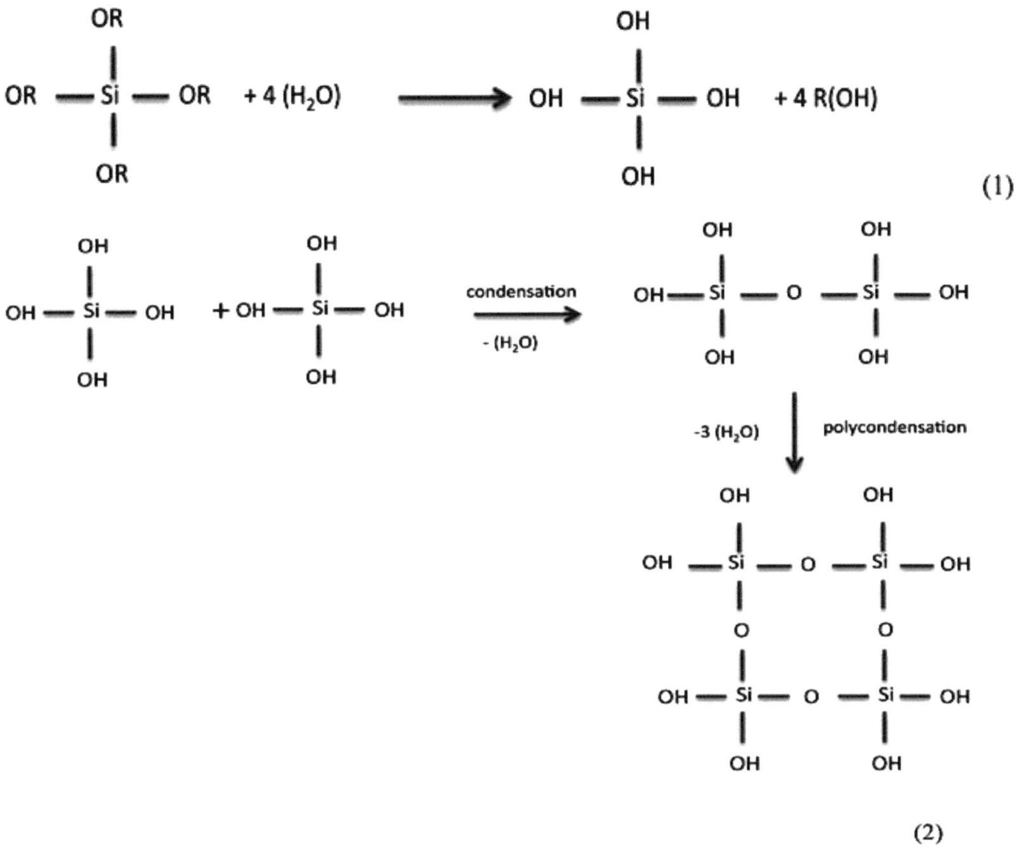

Figure 2. (1) Hydrolysis of $Si(OH)_4$; (2) formation of Si-O-Si bond.

In order to control the stability of the material, chemical stabilisation of the dried gel is required. Sintering of the gel at 500-900°C desorbs silanol groups from the surface and eliminates 3-Si rings from the gel. It also increases the density, strength and hardness of the gel. The sintering temperature of alkoxide-based gels is in the range of 900-1150°C depending upon composition. The schematic diagram of the sol-gel process is provided in **Figure 3**.

The physical differences between the two synthesis routes are that sol-gel glasses tend to have an inherent nanoporosity whereas melt-derived glasses are dense in nature [64]. The surface area of sol-gel glasses is also higher than melt-quenched glass, which results in greater dissolution rate, and hence higher cellular response. The hierarchical pore structure consisting of interconnected macropores (>100 μm) and nanopores is beneficial for interaction and stimulation with cells as it mimics the hierarchical structure of natural tissues. Also bioactive glasses in the form of nanoporous powders or monoliths or as nanoparticles can be made by changing the pH of the sol-gel process [65]. However, the sol-gel made scaffolds have lower strengths than melt-quenched glasses, and thus inappropriate to use in hard tissue engineering (**Figures 4** and **5**).

http://dx.doi.org/10.5772/63266

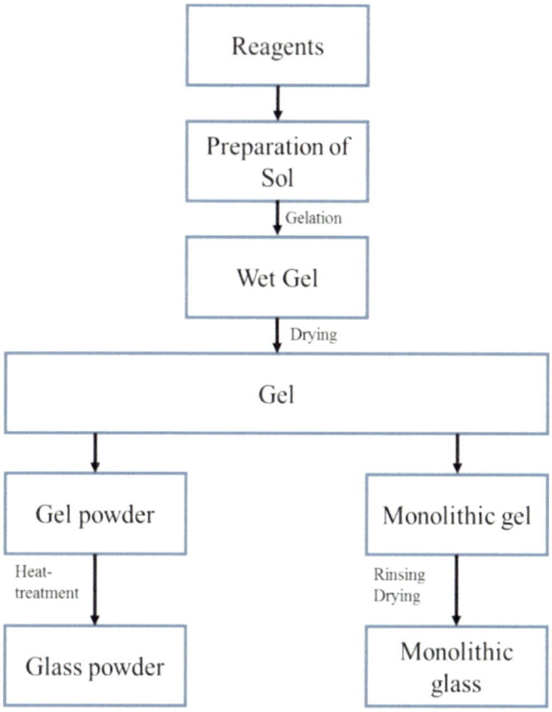

Figure 3. Schematic representation of sol-gel glass synthesis.

2.3.1. Important factor

The physical and chemical properties of sol-gel bioactive glass mainly depend upon silica and so the hydrolysis and condensation of silica plays an important role. The kinetics of hydrolysis and condensation of silica depend upon several factors such as pH, composition, temperature, precursor, catalysis and concentration of ions and the ratio of moles of water/moles of tetraethyl orthosilicate (TEOS). Iler divides the polymerisation of silica in between three pH ranges: <pH 2, pH 2-7 and >pH 7. pH 2 and pH 7 appear to be boundaries because at pH 2 the surface charge (PZC) and the electrical mobility of silica (isoelectric point, IEP) are zero, whereas above pH 7 the solubility and dissolution rates of silica are maximised leading to particle growth without gelation [65].

2.4. Composition of bioactive glasses and their effects on bioactivity

Since the report of bone-bonding properties of bioactive glass, silica has been used as the major component of glass composition and also most widely researched with changing its amount. Silicate glasses comprise an amorphous network structure based on SiO^{4-} tetrahedron, which are linked to each other at the oxygen centres. Silicate glasses have open structure of silica due to the presence of non-bridging oxygen ions attached with silicon. Addition of network modifiers such as Na^+, K^+, Ca^+ also causes the opening of silica network structures. These ions replace bridging oxygens of the network with non-bridging oxygens, hence opening of the glass structure. The number of modifier ion-oxygen bonds and non-bridging oxygen bonds determines several properties of the corresponding glass [66]. Detailed structural features of silicate glasses and their effect on different physical and chemical properties have been reported by various research groups [67–69]. In the case of bioactive silicate (SiO_2 less than 60 wt%) glasses, each silica tetrahedron contains more than 2.6 number of non-bridging oxygen ions, which is necessary in order to be bioactive [70].

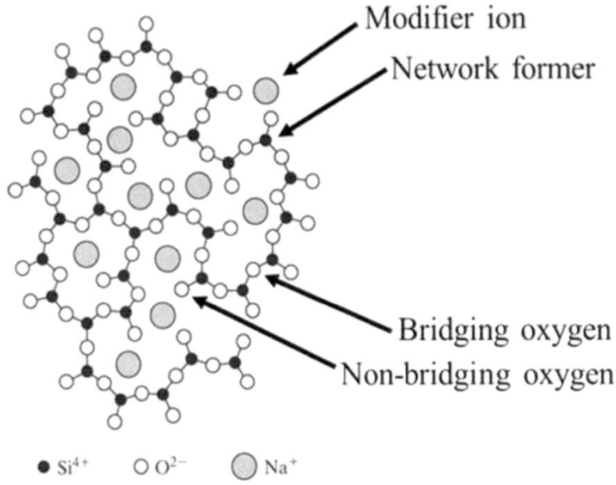

Figure 4. 2D presentation of random glass network modifiers and network formers [70].

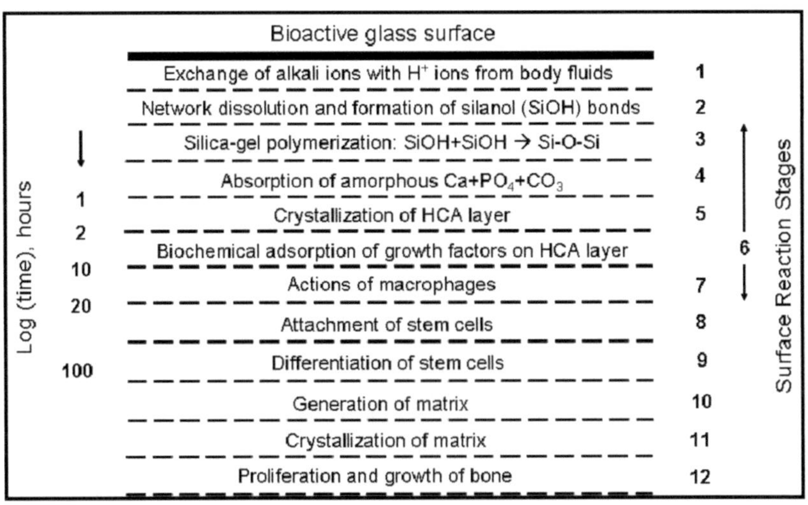

Figure 5. Sequence of interfacial reactions kinetics involved in forming a bond between bone and a bioactive glass [87].

The composition of bioactive glass is different from the traditional soda-lime-silica gasses that consist more than 65 wt% of silica. Basic components required for a glass to obtain bioactivity are SiO_2, Na_2O, CaO and P_2O_5, which can be distinguished in three main features according to Hench and Anderson [71]; the amount of SiO_2 should be in between 45 and 60 wt%, Na_2O and CaO content must be high and a high CaO/P_2O_5 ratio. Higher content of SiO_2 decrease the dissolution rate of the glass ions from the surface, leading to decrease of bioactivity. Very low content of silica also leads to totally dissolvable monomeric SiO^{4-} units. Silica content also plays an important role to form hydroxyapatite carbonate (HCA) upon contact with physiological fluids, thus leading to the chemical attachment to soft/hard tissues. As a result, the interfacial bonding strength with bone increases, and a stable bond with strength equivalent to or greater then bone forms. High CaO/P_2O_5 ratio tends to enable the release of ions from the surface of the material when soaked in body fluid, forming a surface layer of HCA in a very short time span. It also supports cell proliferation on the surface of the implant by maintaining the ion concentration [35]. Previously, Hench and co-workers assumed that a typical range (2–6 wt%) of P_2O_5 is required for a glass to be bioactive as it aid the formation of calcium phosphate phase on the surface, but later Hench and Andersson observed that bioactivity can be independent of P_2O_5 as phosphate ion is also available in physiological fluids.

In the last two decades, a number of different oxide systems have been studied to understand the effect on glass bioactivity and to increase its mechanical strength, still a complete understanding of the correlation between composition and bioactivity is insufficient but mechanical improvement can be possible. Different partial substitutions in the already approved glass compositions have been made, as CaO by 12.5 wt% CaF_2, SiO_2 by 5-15 wt% B_2O_3, but no significant effects were found. Even fluoride substitution reduced the bone bonding capability of the glass [72]. The substitution of MgO for CaO or K_2O for Na_2O showed slight increase in bioactivity. During 1990s glasses with alumina and boron oxide gained enormous interest. Sadly, the addition of small 3 wt% Al_2O_3 to the 45S5 formula was found to prevent bonding with bone. Andersson proved that substitution by Al_2O_3 (1-1.5 wt%) can reduce the bioactivity of glass because of its carcinogenicity [71]. Osaka et al. and Saranti et al. studied glasses with B_2O_3 content and found that the presence of boron has a positive impact on the bioactivity of the glass [73, 74]. In the case of only B_2O_3-substituted glass, the ratio between B_2O_3 and SiO_2 plays an important role in the rate of formation of calcium phosphate layer on the surface of the implant [75]. Later, de Arenes proposed to control the B_2O_3/Al_2O_3 ratio in B_2O_3 and Al_2O_3 containing glasses in order to show bioactivity [76]. In recent years, researchers tend to play with the composition of glass incorporating the ions that are abundant in human bone, such as Mg, Zn, Cu etc. [77–83]. Xia Li et al. found that by incorporating Mg, Zn or Cu in different amounts in place of Ca^{2+} can affect the bioactivity of the glass to different extent in a sequence of Cu < Mg < Zn [84]. Potassium substitution in place of Na^+ reduces the viscosity of silicate glasses and their susceptibility of crystallisation [85]. Even now, a lot of research is going on to find a relation between the composition of the glasses, which have more than four components and tissue connectivity through phase diagram, but relation between these two factors is yet to come. Some researchers such as Andersson et al. and Brink et al. predicted the *in vivo* reactivity of glasses with six or seven oxides as a function of their composition with phenomenological models suggested by regression analysis [71, 86].

2.5. Surface reaction kinetics

Chemical reactivity of a glass in contact with body fluid holds the key of the bone bonding properties of the glass. Due to the chemical reactions, a layer of hydroxycarbonate apatite forms on the surface to which bone can connect. When immersed in an aqueous solution, such as SBF (simulated body fluid) or PBS (phosphate-buffer solution), three general processes occur: leaching, dissolution and precipitation. Leaching can be characterised as release of ions, generally by exchange of alkali or alkaline earth metals ions with H^+ or H_3O^+ ions of the solution. Glass modifier ions leach very easily from the surface of the glass when immersed in an aqueous solution, as they are not part of the glass network. The ion exchange process leads to increase in the hydroxide ion concentration, i.e., the basicity of the solution increases to pH > 7. Network dissolution occurs simultaneously by breaking of the network forming silica bonds (-Si-O-Si-O-Si-) by the attack of hydroxyl ions (OH^-). It releases silica into the solution in the form of silicic acid ($Si(OH)_4$). In this step, glass composition plays an important role as the rate of silica dissolution depends very much on glass composition. Silica dissolution rate rapidly decreases if the weight percentage of SiO_2 goes beyond 60% because of the increase of bridging oxygen, which can hold the network very strongly. Hydrated silica then undergoes polycondensation with neighbouring silanols to form silica-rich layer. In the precipitation part, calcium and phosphate ions released from the glass together with those from solution to form a calcium-phosphate-rich layer on the glass surface. Slowly, it crystallises to form HCA by incorporating carbonate ions from solution. Generally, there are five reaction stages on the implant side of the interface with a bioactive glass [72].

Stage 1: Leaching and formation of silanols (SiOH).

Stage 2: Loss of soluble silica and formation of silanols.

Stage 3: Polycondensation of silanols to form a hydrated silica gel.

Stage 4: Formation of an amorphous calcium phosphate layer.

Stage 5: Crystallisation of a hydroxycarbonate apatite layer.

Hench et al. have been extensively described the reaction processes [25, 72, 87–89].

1. Rapid exchange of alkali or alkaline earth metal ions Na^+ or K^+ with H^+ or H_3O^+ from solution

$$\text{Si-O-Na}^+ + \text{OH} \rightarrow \text{Si-OH}^+ + \text{Na}^+ \text{(solution)} + \text{OH}^-.$$

2. -Si-O-Si-O-Si- bonds break through the action of hydroxyl ions and form Si-OH (silanols)

$$\text{Si-O-Si} + H_2O \rightarrow \text{Si-OH} + \text{OH-Si}.$$

3. Condensation of Si-OH groups near the glass surface: re-polymerisation of the silica rich layer

http://dx.doi.org/10.5772/63266

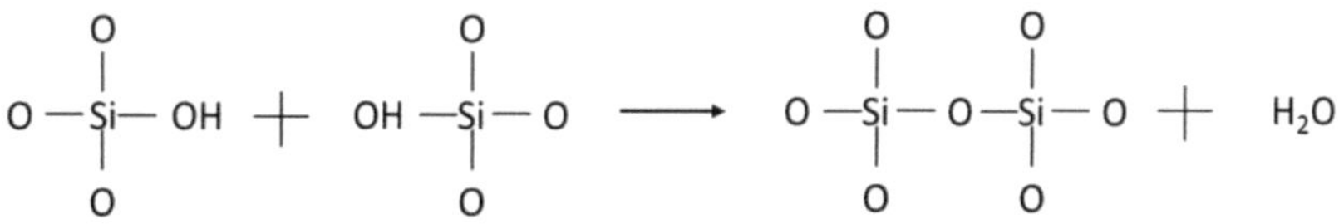

4. Migration of Ca^{+} and PO_4^{3-} groups to the surface through the SiO_2-rich layer forming a CaO-P_2O_5-rich film on top of the SiO_2-rich layer, followed by growth of the amorphous CaO-P_2O_5-rich film by incorporation of soluble calcium and phosphate ions from solution.

5. Incorporation of hydrolysis and carbonate from solution and crystallisation of the CaO-P_2O_5 film to HCA.

As these stages were proposed many years ago, they are proved through time by various types of characterisation techniques. ^{17}O nuclear magnetic resonance (NMR) confirmed the increase of bridging oxygen bonds during leaching, which indicates the repolymerisation of Si-OH groups in the silica-rich layer [90]. The formation of crystallise HCA layer on the surface was confirmed by surface-sensitive-small-angle X-ray diffraction (XRD) [91]. Calcium phosphate nucleate on the SI-OH groups as they have negative charge in solution and the separation of the SI-OH groups is thought to dictate the orientation of the apatite crystals, which grow with a preferred orientation in the 001 plane on Bioglass 45S5 [23, 92–95].

2.6. Bioactive glass *in vivo*

The bioactivity of glasses can only be investigated and confirmed after testing with living tissues. If a calcium phosphate layer can be found on a silica gel layer at the surface of the implants, the glass can be called bioactive. The extent of bioactivity of the glass is directly dependent on the ability of the glass to form calcium apatite layer. The above-mentioned five stages on the surface of bioactive glass do not depend on the presence of tissues. The sequence of *in-vivo* reactivity of bioactivity glass with tissues has been investigated by Hench and Andersson [37, 87, 96].

Stage 6: Adsorption of biological moieties in the SiO_2-hydroxycarbonate apatite layer

Stage 7: Action of macrophases

Stage 8: Attachment of stem cells

Stage 9: Differentiation of stem cells

Stage 10: Generation of matrix

Stage 11: Mineralisation of matrix

Through the 11 stages, a bioactive glass bonds with the bone. Gradually, the bioactive glass will be absorbed with increasing bone ingrowth.

45S5 Bioglass® was the first bioactive glass successfully investigated *in vivo* by many researchers [17]. After that another bioactive glass S53P4 was developed by Andersson and Karlsson and has been successfully used in clinical applications [97–99]. Later, glass 13-93 and glass 1-98 also showed good bioactivity *in vivo* [86, 100–102].

Extensive research in this field in recent years comes out with some limitations of the model of reaction kinetics proposed by Prof. Hench. Hench proposed that in the first stage of the reaction a rapid exchange of Na^+ ions released from the glass with the protons (H^+) of the solution occur, although in the modern era bioactive glass has been synthesised without sodium. Influence of the mole fraction of silica on the bioactivity is still not clear. Also, it was observed that if the implant is broken and the broken surfaces stay in contact with SBF, they tend to self-repair by fusing themselves through their apatite surface layers [103].

In the case of clinical trial, the main problem is to make patient-specific implants because every patient is different. To study the implant specificity and implant site adjustment *in vivo* animal model, studies can be compared if the same models are used. The first *in vivo* study was completed for Bioglass monoliths on the rat femurs, and after 6 weeks the interfacial shear strength of the bond between the glass and the cortical bone was equal or greater than the strength of the host bone [24, 104]. Bioglass 45S5 also degrades more rapidly than hydroxyapatite, and the degeneration was because of solution-mediated dissolution. The model of the study later named as Oonishi model was completed by drilling 6 mm diameter into the femoral condyle of rabbits. Bleeding was stopped before inserting the particles [105–107]. Recently, it was found that initially the bone grew into the particles that were on the outer periphery in contact with the host bone, but within 2 months of implantation bone also formed inside the isolated Bioglass particles. This study indicates that the Bioglass particles can trigger stem cell differentiation and convert it into osteoblasts [108]. Hands-on experience by various surgeons points out the advantage of making a putty-like material by mixing the particles with blood prior to implantation, which later encourages the development of Nova bone [109]. The explanation behind this advantage of putty-like material is either it can separate the particles to allow new bone to grow between them or the pH environment created was more suitable for bone ingrowth. Fujibayashi et al. used the Oonishi model to test phosphate-free glass particles and for one of his compositions almost similar amount of bone ingrowth to Bioglass was found. But with increasing SiO_2 content the bone ingrowth reduce rapidly [110]. Wheeler et al. compared Bioglass 45S5 with sol-gel glasses 77S and 58S using the Oonishi model and observed that up to 8 weeks the bone ingrowth was more in the case of Bioglass, but after 12 weeks the amounts were equivalent. The procedure of bone ingrowth, *viz.* formation of silica layer, apatite formation and finally bone formation via HCA was found to be same as Bioglass [111]. The initial slower rate can be result in the rapid release of calcium in the case of sol-gel glasses causing increase in pH at the site.

2.7. Bioactivity *in vitro*

Before going to *in vivo* trials, a glass material has to be passed *in vitro* tests. The *in vitro* test helps us both ethically and economically as they reduce the number of animals necessary for *in vivo* tests. Earlier *in vitro* test was performed by immersing the glass in either distilled water or tris-buffered solutions, but after development of SBF by Kokubo et al. it has become the most widely used solution for *in vitro* investigation. SBF contains all the essential inorganic components of human blood, and proportions are also almost similar to human blood plasma [112]. During *in vitro* studies, pH of the solution is buffered between 7.25 and 7.4 at 37°C.

	Na^+	K^+	Mg^{2+}	Ca^{2+}	Cl^-	HCO_3^-	HPO_4^{2-}	SO_4^{2-}
Plasma	142.0	5.0	1.5	2.5	103.0	27.0	1.0	0.5
SBF	142.0	5.0	1.5	2.5	147.8	4.2	1.0	0.5

Table 2. Ion concentrations of SBF and human blood plasma (mM) [112].

SBF is a supersaturated solution and hence precipitation of calcium phosphate can easily take place during preparation, storage and *in vitro* test. Many researchers have tried to correct the difference of ion concentrations of Cl^- and HCO_3^-. Oyane et al. made a revised SBF (r-SBF) in which the concentrations were matched, but the solution shows a strong tendency to precipitate calcium carbonate [113]. In 2004, Takadama proposed a modified SBF (n-SBF) in which only CL^- ion concentration was increased [114]. Several properties of bioactive glasses have been studied in SBF by observing the changes in weight and surface morphology of the glass and also observing the change of pH and ionic concentrations of the solution. Some research groups focussed on the physical and mechanical properties whereas some groups are interested in knowing chemical and bioactive properties of glass [115–118]. It was observed that the extent of bone ingrowth among glass particles increased according to their ability to form apatite in SBF. Thus, it can be said that the *in vivo* bioactivity of a glass can be assumed precisely from its nature in SBF.

Five typical reaction stages, as described in surface reaction kinetics part, occur when *in vitro* bioactivity test is performed. Initially, due to ion exchange of alkali or alkaline earth metal ions with H^+ ions of the SBF solution, pH of the solution increases. By the action of OH^- ions network, dissolution occurs with the formation of $Si(OH)_4$. The dependency of dissolution rate is more or less same as described before. The leaching and dissolution phenomenon is followed by a formation of silica-rich layer on the surface by polycondensation of neighbouring silanols, which ultimately form a calcium-phosphate-rich layer by incorporating Ca^+ and PO_4^{3-} ions. The layer increases by including soluble calcium and phosphates from the SBF, forming an amorphous CaP-rich layer. Finally, the CaP-rich layer crystallises to a hydroxycarbonate apatite structure.

With changes in composition, differences in sample dosage, shape and size, sample porosity and surface morphology also affect the bioactivity of a glass [117, 119–123]. Most studies of bioactive glasses have used samples in the form of discs or plates, however in accordance with their applications other forms are also of interest.

2.8. Mesoporous bioactive glass (MBG)

For treatment of bone defects resulting from trauma, infections, tumours or genetic malformations, bioactive glass scaffolds have been extensively studied. In the case of bone regeneration, combination of osteoconductive, osteostimulative and angiogenic factors with bioactive glass are proved to be useful [124–126]. This advantage of bioactive glass made it a subject of interest for almost 50 years and day by day according to rise in life expectancy, the field of its application is increasing. Extensive research in this topic comes out with a handful of modifications for the last two to three decades. Recently, it was found that kinetic deposition process of HCA on bioactive glass can be enhanced by increasing the surface area and pore volume [127]. Therefore, control over porosity, pore size and internal pore connectivity of bioactive glasses is essential to understand and design better bone forming biomaterials. A new field of application was started when surgeons found that in the case of bone reconstruction surgery, bacterial infection may cause osteomyelitis. Traditionally, techniques such as systemic antibiotic administration, surgical debridement, wound drainage and implant removal have limitations and may lead to additional surgical interventions for the patients [128]. Conventional drug delivery options, such as injection or taking a pill, increase the concentration of drug in blood up to peaks and then suddenly decline [129]. Hence, to improve drug delivery efficacy, continuous action, reduce toxicity and convenience to patients a lot of work has done. In addition, the procedure was also considered for treating malignant bone disease in which drug will be effectively released at the sites of bone disease from loaded biomaterials [130, 131]. Since the invention of first bioactive glass, in the last 40 years it has shown various attractive properties for bone tissue regeneration application by virtue of their osteoconductivity and degradability [124, 132, 133]. In 2004, Yu et al. for the first time prepared mesoporous bioactive glasses (MBG) by the sol-gel method using surfactants, which opened a new direction in the field of regenerative medicine [134]. The materials were composed of highly ordered mesopore channel structure with a pore size ranging from 5 to 20 nm. MBG has gained the interest of researchers very rapidly for its drug loading and release properties, which depend on the mesoporous structure of the materials. Due to its tuneable pore size, large specific surface area and pore volume, the materials can be used in bone-forming activity and can be loaded with osteogenic or therapeutic agents [125, 126, 128, 131, 135, 136].

2.8.1. Preparation of different types of mesoporous bioactive glasses and their in vitro bioactivity

Mesoporous bioactive glasses were emerged when the supramolecular chemistry of surfactants was incorporated into the bioactive glasses field. These materials have the composition of bioactive glasses but with designed mesoporosity and textural parameters. MBGs are generally prepared by combining non-ionic surfactants (triblock copolymers, CTAB, P123, F127, PEO, PU, etc.) into the reaction system, which are essential for obtaining well-ordered structures [134, 137]. The most well-known and accepted procedure of making mesoporous bioactive glass is evaporation-induced self-assembly (EISA) method [138]. The initial homogeneous mixture is obtained by dissolving precursors in a common medium such as ethanol-water mixed solvent system. The surfactants can act as micelles and are able to link with the hydrolysed precursors (e.g., TEOS and TEP) to form an ordered mesophase, where a constant ratio of network former and precursors and the surfactant was kept [139]. After that, following the process of sol-gel, gelling and drying takes place, and by the removal of surfactant through calcination finally gives MBG with a well-ordered mesoporous structure. The order of porosity of the material depends on surfactant chemistry (ionic, non-ionic, polymeric, etc.), surfactant concentration, organic/inorganic phase volume ratio, temperature and pH of the sol.

Recent studies on mesoporous bioactive glass show increasing use of MBG in different fields of tissue engineering and drug delivery. The types of MBG used in these fields may be particle, sphere, fibres or 3D scaffolds. The first MBG powders or particles were prepared by using P123 and F127 as a surfactant, with the composition of 80Si-15Ca-5P, 70Si-25Ca-5P and 60Si-35Ca-5P. Calcination at 700°C gives a highly ordered MBG powder. The bioactive characteristics of a scaffold can be assumed from their ability to form apatite layer on their surface *in vitro*. Zhu and Kaskel reported that the rate of apatite formation in the case of MBG is noticeably higher than its contemporary bioactive glass scaffolds [140]. Other than the mesoporous structure, the chemical composition of the mesoporous bioactive glass is the other factor to influence *in vitro* bioactivity. Now a days, scientists are focussing on modifying the basic properties of MBGs, which are high specific surface area, porosity etc. and found that upon changing these properties the apatite-formation ability of MBG could be fine-tuned [49, 141–143]. Lei et al. prepared MBG microspheres through the sol-gel process with uniform diameter range of 2-5 μm and a mesoporous shell [144]. Zhao et al. prepared MBG microspheres with high P_2O_5 contents (up to 15%) and studied the apatite formation *in vitro* [145]. Studies indicate that the diameter of the microspheres has a positive effect on the bioactivity. Moreover, MBG microspheres with higher P_2O_5 content were found to be more bioactive due to their different ion diffusion rates from the glass network. MBG can also be prepared as ultrathin fibres by electro-spinning techniques with high matrix homogeneities. By controlling the parameters of electro-spinning, the properties of the fibres such as pore volume, surface area and diameter of the hollow core can be tuned. These fibres were found to be highly bioactive when tested *in vitro* [146, 147].

2.9. Ion-doped bioactive glass with and without mesoporosity

2.9.1. Introduction

The clinical demand of bioactive glass is increasing rapidly day by day due to its versatile properties *viz.* bioactivity, resorbability, ostioproductive, osteoconductive and osteoinductive nature, depending upon its flexible compositional range. With increasing population, the diversity of required implants is also expanding. The wide range of application of bioactive glasses include implants for bone defects, repairing or replacing damaged diseased tissues, scaffolds for bone grafting, preparing bone cement, as novel drug carrier and coating material for implants [26, 37]. When implanted in human body, a hydroxyapatite carbonate layer forms on the implant-bone interface which is chemically and structurally similar to the mineral phase of human bone. In the last two decades, researchers found that the sites of implantation of different parts of our body require different chemical and physical properties, and hence bioactive glass with different or modified compositions. Bioactivity of a glass is mainly dependent on its surface reactivity and composition and by modifying those, improvement of the system can be possible. Sometimes modification also needed in order to overcome the disadvantages of traditional bioactive glasses such as high solubility and low fracture toughness.

Recent trends in literature suggest that ionic dissolution products from inorganic materials are keys to understand and assume the behaviour of bioactive glasses *in vitro* and *in vivo*. Since many trace elements such as Sr, Cu, Zn, Mg or Co present in the human body are known for their anabolic effects in bone metabolism, in order to mimic the natural system new approaches for enhancing bioactivity, beneficial and appropriate ions are being introduced [148–151]. It is believed that more similar system such as the host body will increase the bioactivity of the implant. The release of these ions after exposure to a physiological environment tends to improve the bioactive activities of the implant related to both osteogenesis and angiogenesis. Thus, recent trend is to incorporate different ions into the composition of bioactive glasses to enhance their physical characteristics and therapeutic benefit.

This incorporation of different ions in the composition of glass is called doping and it is very crucial for production of functional materials. By definition, a doping element is an additional incorporation in the main composition at a very low concentration compared to the main constituents ranging from a few ppm to a few percent. In many cases, it was found that the functionality of the material is directly dependent on the doping elements. In some other cases, doping may improve surface structure of the implant or the physical attributes of it. In particular, the points related to doping can be listed as follows [152]:

1. The functionality is directly associated with doping.

2. Doping provides a structural control over the material.

3. Doping provokes unexpected structural modifications.

4. Doping brings new unexpected functionality to the material.

It is hard to identify the particular time when doping was first started, but around late 1985 the trend of incorporating different ions were started. First, a number of different ions such as Al, Ag, Fe, Ni, Cr, Cu, Co, Ta, Sb, La, etc. were doped and then tested *in vitro* and *in vivo* [153]. Initially, the dopants were chosen according to their similarity in valence with the elements already present, but with time and following the literature about the essential trace elements required in our body, the interest about dopants has been focussed on some specific elements and their affects [149, 150].

2.9.2. Role of inorganic ions present in human body

Human bone is a highly vascularised tissue which can remodel throughout the life by regulated activity of osteoblasts (bone-forming cells) and osteoclasts (bone-resorbing cells) [154]. The process of bone remodelling is dependent on a variety of local regulatory agents such as growth factors, hormones, etc. [155]. Inorganic ions such as calcium [156–158], phosphorous [159], silicon [160, 161], strontium [162–164], zinc [165], boron [166] and magnesium [167] are also affect the bone metabolism. The acts of the inorganic ions in this context are given in **Table 3**.

Ion	Biological activity	Reference
Si	• Metabolic processes, formation of bone tissue	[160, 168]
	• Intake of Si increase bone mineral density	[169] [170]
	• HAP precipitation	[161]
	• Help to stimulate collagen I formation and osteoblastic differentiation	
Ca	• Favours osteoblast proliferation, differentiation and mineralisation	[156]
	• Activates Ca-sensing receptors in osteoblast cells	[155]
P	• Matrix gla protein (MGP) stimulation	[159]
Zn	• Shows anti-inflammatory effect	[171]
	• Bone formation *in vitro* by activation of protein synthesis in osteoblasts	[172]
	• Increase ATP's activity	
Mg	• Help to form new bone	[173]
	• Increase bone-cell adhesion and stability	[174]
Sr	• Beneficial effects on bone formation *in vivo*	[155]
	• For treating osteoporosis	[175]
Cu	• Promote synergic stimulating effects on angiogenesis when associated with angiogenic growth factor FGF-2	[176] [177]
	• Stimulates proliferation of human endothelial cells	
B	• Stimulates RNA synthesis in fibroblast cells	[178]
	• Stimulates bone formation	[179]
Li	• treatment of both bipolar and unipolar depressive disorder	[180, 181]
	• effects on blood and brain	[182]
	• enhance immunological activities of monocytes and lymphocytes	

Table 3. Acts of different inorganic ions in human body.

By acting as an enzyme cofactors, metal ions influence signalling pathways and stimulate tissue formation [150, 183]. These effects make metal ions interesting for use as doping materials in the field of hard and soft tissue engineering. Several ions, such as Sr, Zn, Cu, Mg, B, etc. have been considered to be promising in enhancing the bioactivity of implant materials by controlling the release of specific ions during *in vivo* dissolution.

2.9.3. Ion-doped bioactive silicate-based glasses

In order to improve the bioactivity, stimulating effects on osteogenesis, angiogenesis and antibacterial effects of bioactive glasses in a specific physiological environment, many methods have been studied incorporating various metal ions in the silicate network. Different substituted silicate glasses exhibit a certain level of acellular bioactivity when tested *in vitro* by standard SBF test, according to Kokubo et al. [21]. The formation of HCA layer on the surface has been the unit of bioactivity measurement as from these results one can assume the bioactivity *in vivo*.

2.9.3.1. *Zinc-bioactive glass*

Zinc is an essential trace element in our body as it is a cofactor for many enzymes. It also helps to stimulate protein synthesis which is essential for DNA replication and also has an important role in the growth, development and differentiation of bone cell [184–187]. In addition, zinc also has antibacterial properties against *Staphylococcus aureus* [188].

Balamurugan et al. synthesised a bioactive glass in CaO-P_2O_5-SiO_2-ZnO system by the sol-gel method containing 5 mol% ZnO which increased ALP activity and osteoblast proliferation [189]. They also examined that incorporation of zinc does not reduce the bioactivity of the bioactive glass. Higher surface area of Zn-substituted glass can be a better nucleation site when immersed in SBF solution making the calcium phosphate phase more crystalline [190, 191]. Recently, Atkinson et al. found that up to 5 mol% of zinc substitution in a sodium-free bioactive glass composition has the ability to induce apatite formation alongside a calcite phase. Increase in Zn content has a tendency to decrease the calcite phase, however it does not affect the apatite deposition [187]. This calcite phase can also bond with bone without the formation of an appetite layer [192]. Du et al. observed that initially Zn retarded the nucleation of HCA at the early stage of SBF soaking, but did not affect the HCA formation in long-term immersion [193]. Scientists have also reported that more than 10 mol% of Zn has a negative effect on bioactivity and after 20% an excessive drop can be seen [194]. ZnO can act as a network modifier or an intermediate oxide or both in the glass structure. It is found that up to a certain amount ZnO works as a network modifier, but with increasing ZnO content it switched from network modifier to an intermediate oxide [191]. Shahrabi et al. found that 5 mol% ZnO may reduce the number of non-bridging oxygen atoms, resulting in a decrease in glass bioactivity [195]. Zinc has the ability to remove cations from silica network and the new bond formed (Si-O-Zn) have considerably lower bond strength than Si-O-Si bond, which leads to decline in glass transition temperature. As observed, zinc can show very good antibacterial activity for the *Bacillus subtilis* and *Pseudomonas aeruginosa* strains [187].

2.9.3.2. *Strontium-bioactive glass*

Strontium (Sr) is a naturally occurring mineral found in water and food. It is also an essential trace element of human body. The total amount of Sr in human body of a 70 kg standard man is around 0.32 g. Recently, researchers have found that Sr positively affects bone metabolism to promote bone formation and osteoblast replication while inhibiting bone resorption by osteoclasts [196]. Evidence also showed that strontium not only enhances osteogenic differentiation, but also helps to stabilise the bone structure [197]. However, too much Sr may increase the number of osteoclast cells which can inhibit bone regeneration and remodelling, leading to osteonecrosis. Thus, strontium has very good effects up to an optimum level. Among the trace elements human body have, only Sr was correlated with bone compression strength [198]. *In vitro* and *in vivo* studies showed that strontium ions upregulate osteoblasts and downregulate osteoclasts [175, 199]. The presence of Sr on the surface of a biomaterial decreases the rate of ion-release at the defect site, which is therapeutically beneficial [200]. Sr-substituted boron glasses show a good adhesion with osteoblast-like cells, Saos-2, thus enhances the cyto-compatibility of borate glass. Lao et al. confirmed that Sr-doped bioactive glasses are more bioactive *in vitro* than their original counterparts. Sr-doped glasses are also able to increase the rate of bone-like apatite layer formation on their surface. Moreover, it also decreases the Ca/P ratio very rapidly, which leads to faster stability of apatite layer, and hence greater bioactivity [201]. Substitution of 5 wt% strontium in place of calcium shows advantageous effect on foetal mouse calvarial bone cells [202].

Strontium-based bioactive glasses has a tendency to increase metabolic activity in osteoblasts and to decrease osteoclast activity. The decrease of osteoclasts is may be caused by decreasing tartrate resistant acid phosphate activity and inhibiting resorption of calcium phosphate films [203]. In some cases, it was found that substitution of Sr in place of Ca is more effective strategy for building materials suitable for bone regeneration therapies [203]. The substitution of Ca by Sr (in mol%) sometimes increases silica content as Sr is heavier than Ca, which results in reduced solubility and hence bioactivity. Though replacing by wt% sometimes increases the rate of HCA formation [201, 204]. In comparison, Sr is slightly larger than Ca, which expands the silica network and increases ion dissolution rates, leading to significantly increased *in vitro* and *in vivo* reactivity. The *in vivo* bioactivity is greater in the case of Sr-doped bioactive glasses due to the biological effects of Sr on bone-forming cells [205].

In corporation of mesoporosity in bioactive glass was found to enhance bone-forming ability, degradation and drug delivery properties compared with traditional bioactive glasses. Therefore, there has been a growing interest on ion-doped mesoporous bioactive glasses and their properties. Zhang et al. found that Sr-MBG shows very good mechanical stability from the viewpoint of its original counterpart, which is required for bone repair [206]. They also observed good apatite forming ability of the Sr-doped MBG. Further study of Sr-MBG scaffolds showed that substitution of Sr for Ca stimulated the proliferation, ALP activity, osteogenic-related gene expression and ECM mineralisation of MC3T3-E1 cells [206].

Zhao et al. tested Sr-MBG scaffold in restoration of the rat critical-sized calvarial defects model and found that Sr-MBG scaffolds have superior osteoconductive property in course to normal MBG scaffolds. Moreover, it was found that Sr-MBG scaffolds has a tendency to stimulate new blood vessel formation in bone defect areas [207]. Very recently, Sriranganathan et al. reported that with increase of the Sr substitution for Ca in high phosphate bioactive glasses decreases the formation of apatite layer directly. They proposed that the apatite formation proceeds via the formation of an octacalcium phosphate ($Ca_8(PO_4)_6H_2{\cdot}5H_2O$) phase, which then transforms into hydroxyl-carbonate apatite. Above a certain concentration of strontium, the octacalcium phosphate phase is unable to form, which ultimately delays the HCA formation [208].

2.9.3.3. *Lithium-bioactive glass*

Lithium has a prolonged medical history as it has been used for over 100 years to treat manic depression [180]. Lithium also marked its importance in the treatment of both bipolar and unipolar depressive disorders. Along with that lithium also has several other effects on blood and brain [181]. Clinicians also observed that lithium often increases the white blood cell counts (granulocytosis) and reduces blood lymphosite counts (lymphomenia). Lithium also has a tendency to enhance immunological activities of monocytes and lymphocytes. Researchers have also found evidence of lithium in bone mineral metabolism [182, 209, 210].

In vitro bioactivity test indicates a decrease in bioactivity with increase in lithium-ion concentration. The theory behind it is that lithium forms lithium oxide groups by reacting with the hydroxyl groups present in the pure sol-gel, which limits crystal formation. Recently, Khorami et al. observed the *in vitro* bioactivity of lithium substituted 45S5 glasses and found no certain advantage of lithium in the reactivity of the bioactive glass composition. A theory based on observations state that *in vitro* reactivity increases with increasing glass solubility. In this study, lithium was replaced for sodium (in wt%) and hence a little decrease in the molar concentration of glass network formers (SiO_2 and P_2O_5) takes place, which may result in an increase in glass solubility. However, the ionic radius of Li^+ is lower than Na^+. Thus, lithium has a strong affinity for bonding to oxygen and tends to contract the free spaces in the silicate network. This phenomenon reduces the rate of glass dissolution and improves chemical durability [211].

The release of lithium ions in SBF is higher for sample with higher lithium content, with an initial burst in the first 24 h followed by more sustained release. Lithium also shows ALP activity and mineralisation in a dose-dependent manner from 0.2 to 0.85 ppm when exposed to murine osteoblast cells [212].

2.9.3.4. *Magnesium-bioactive glass*

Magnesium naturally exists in human body and it is amongst the most important elements in the bone matrix. Enamel, dentin and bone contain 0.44, 1.23 and 0.72 wt% magnesium, respectively [213]. Magnesium is involved in over 300 chemical reactions inside human body. It is also known to activate phagocytosis and regulate active calcium transport. Magnesium also has positive effect in wound healing, bone metabolism, fracture prevention and bone density [214, 215].

When doped, Mg can act as a network former or network modifier. This indicates that an increase in Mg content may lead to more Mg^{2+} ions participating in the silica network by making weaker Si-O-Mg bond rather than stronger Si-O-Si bonds, leading to weakening of overall glass network [216]. With increasing MgO content glass degradation gradually decreases, and the formation of apatite layer is hampered [213, 217].

MgO can affect the surface reactivity of Mg-doped bioactive glasses by indirectly influencing the early stage of mineralisation by favouring the silica atom with non-bridging oxygen speciation [116]. Surface reactivity of Mg-BG increases with increasing MgO/CaO ratio, which can play an important role in glass bioactivity. Based on another study, it was found that the role of Mg^{2+} in the formation of HCA apatite layer in SiO_2-CaO-Na_2O-P_2O_5 system was insignificant. These contradictory observations created a variety of theories based on ionic potential [218], structural parameter [66] or network connectivity [219]. However, all these theories failed to explain glass bioactivity properly. Varanasi et al. observed significant effect of MgO on the osteoblast differentiation [220]. Other studies also support the increased osteoblast proliferation and differentiation. These findings proved the positive effect of magnesium doping in the bioactivity of bioactive glass.

2.9.3.5. *Silver-bioactive glass*

In bone reconstruction surgeries, there are two main factors that should be considered: (1) chemical bond with living bone; (2) prevents bacterial infection. As we know that bioactive glasses show well bioactivity and bond with living bone, but a colonisation of bacteria on the surface of the implant can lead to failure of the treatment. The consequences of implant infections are serious and sometimes it leads to second surgery with a lot of suffering [221].

Due to the antimicrobial properties of silver, the recent focus on development of silver-doped implants is increasing. The antibacterial properties of bioactive glasses containing silver have been investigated by several researchers [222, 223]. The main advantage of incorporating silver ions in a gel-glass system is that the porous glass matrix enables a controlled, sustained delivery of antibacterial agent. Some researchers found that high concentration (2 wt%) of silver ions show cytotoxicity, but in the range of 0.75-1 wt% silver has no toxic influence [224]. Due to the higher efficacy of silver, it has gained the interest of scientists, and after extensive research different mechanisms have been proposed for its antimicrobial activities:

1. Interface with electron transport.
2. Binding to DNA.
3. Interaction with the cell components [225, 226].

Silver incorporation has no significant effect over the bioactivity of the glass [222]. However, silver has a tendency to reduce the dissolution of silica when replaced in place of calcium. As silver is monovalent in comparison with bivalent calcium ion, it takes two silver ions to make two non-bridging oxygen groups in place of one calcium ion. Thus, replacement of calcium by silver lessens the number of non-bridging oxygen groups, and reduces the glass dissolution [191]. Due to its highly promising antibacterial and anti-inflammatory properties, silver-doped bioactive glasses are considered to be very useful for wound healing applications alongside tissue engineering.

3. Clinical relevance of doped bioactive glass

Bioactive glasses are that bone substitutes which posses3. Clinical relevance of doped bioactive glasss the unique property of osteoconduction as well as osteoproduction by stimulating proliferation and differentiation of osteoprogenitor cells through a direct genetic control [24,

227]. The discovery of these new materials led Hench and Wilson to propose the concept of osteostimulation or osteopromotion to define this class of bioactive materials and their effects on the genetic activation of bone cells [228]. Bioactive glasses are surface reactive biomaterials that, when in contact with physiological fluids, release soluble ionic products that have been suggested to stimulate *in vitro* osteogenesis [227, 229]. On critical analysis, Young's modulus of bioactive glass being between 30 and 50 GPa, nearly that of natural bone, is a great advantage. One disadvantage is the low mechanical strength and decreased fracture resistance [230]. This can be easily overcome by altering the composition, using it in low load-bearing areas, and using it for the bioactive stage. Furthermore, bioactive glass manufactured via the sol-gel technique permits the synthesis of material with higher purity and homogeneity at low temperatures [52]. Additives can be easily introduced during the sol-gel process to improve the bioactivity of such glasses. Indeed, improvement of the biological properties of bioactive materials can be achieved by the incorporation of ions (doping) that positively affect osteoblast behaviour and consequently enhance new bone formation [202].

In addition, *in vivo* studies have demonstrated beneficial results from their use in various clinical situations [231–234]. After implantation, interaction with surrounding tissues results in a time-dependent alteration of the material's surface and the formation of a hydroxyl carbonate apatite layer that is very similar to the mineral phase of bone [235]. More recently, a new category of sol-gel glasses has been manufactured with enhanced bioactivity and open pores enclosed in a mesoporous matrix [134, 236]. Furthermore, bioactive glass manufactured via the sol-gel technique permits the synthesis of materials with higher purity and homogeneity at low temperatures [52]. Additives can be easily introduced during the sol-gel process to improve the bioactivity of such glasses. Indeed, improvement of the biological properties of bioactive materials can be achieved by the incorporation of ions that positively affect osteoblast behaviour and consequently enhance *de novo* bone formation.

Metallic ions in body play a crucial role as cofactors of enzymes and excite a chain of reactions related to cell signalling pathways [176]. A number of literatures have been cited on the interaction of metallic ions in various diseases and metabolic disorders such as cancer, CNS disorders, infectious diseases and hormonal disorders [237, 238]. Hence, the effectiveness and selectivity of the beneficial effect of metallic ions can be enhanced by controlling the exact level in the body. Additionally, due to unstable ionic states of certain metallic ions, toxic effects may follow while directly ingested. Hence, wide spread research is underway to develop matrices to control the local release of metallic ions with less systemic toxicity as well as availability of relatively high concentrations of metallic-ion-based drugs to target tissues. The degree of metallic ion loading into matrices for local delivery as well as their controlled and sustained release is of paramount importance for optimal therapeutic use. Common strategy is to load metallic ions into matrices such as hydroxyapatite, bioactive glass, silica and carbon fibres to improve ionic stability and to release for a prolong period of time [148, 239–248]. Due to these superior characteristics, metallic ion doping in biomaterials is an alternative, cost-effective, safe strategy than use of recombinant proteins or genetic engineering approaches [249].

3.1. Doped bioactive glass in bone regeneration

In bone tissue engineering, bioceramics or bioactive glasses and biodegradable polymers [15], often comprise metallic ions as part of the bioceramic or bioactive glass structural composition. The metal ion is generally released during their degradation *in vitro* or *in vivo* [148, 250]. For instance, when bioactive glass (e.g., 45S5 Bioglass) [26, 251] is used as scaffolds to fill a bone defect, critical concentrations of soluble Si, Ca, P and Na ions are released, with the capacity to generate both intracellular and extracellular effects at the interface between the glass and the cellular environment [124, 133, 148, 227, 252–261]. It has also been observed that released ions from bioactive glasses can induce gene expression which in turn helps in bone metabolism by signal transduction as well as enhance cell differentiation and osteogenesis [27, 124, 227, 254]. Furthermore, the ionic dissolution products of bioactive glasses can also encourage angiogenesis [262]. Other metallic ions which may have significant role in bone tissue engineering include copper, magnesium, strontium, manganese, iron, zinc and silver owing to their imminent role as cofactors in metabolic processes in bone, articular tissues and immune system functions [149, 263].

The application of chitosan-doped bioactive glass (BG-CH) was assessed in the guided bone regeneration in ovariectomised rats. The histomorphometric analysis showed increased bone/tissue volume, osteoblast number and osteoblast surface/bone surface and trace elements such as Sr and Fe were detected in the newly formed bone may be responsible for enhanced bone healing and found clinically useful as a therapeutic and implantable material [264].

Zinc being a trace mineral in human body performs a variety of functions in relation to the immune system, cell division, fertility and the body growth and maintenance. Moreover, zinc is also a necessary element for the formation, mineralisation, development and maintenance of healthy bones. These unique properties of zinc evoked the interest of researchers to use it along with silicate-based bioactive glasses for bone tissue engineering and found to have significant ability to enhance antibacterial effects, bioactivity and distinct physical, structural and mechanical properties of bioactive glasses [265]. Zinc also stimulates bone formation and mineralisation by activating aminoacyl-tRNA synthetase in osteoblastic cells, and it stimulates cellular protein synthesis. Zinc plays a role in the preservation of bone mass by inhibiting osteoclast-like cell formation from marrow cells [171]. It also promotes attachment, proliferation of osteoblast and increase ALP expression that is responsible for laying down the bone callus. The doping of Zn into bioactive glasses produces higher chemical stability and densification of glasses matrices. Zinc doping in bioglass for repair of diaphyseal defect creates a good link of interface between bone and Zn-BG during the first speeds, whereas during the last speeds osseoingration, resorption and degradation of bioactive glass and their replacement by bone cells occurs [266].

Strontium (Sr) is a naturally occurring trace element often acts similarly to Ca in the human body; both have strong bone-seeking properties, and Sr can be substituted with Ca in the apatitic phase of bone mineral [267]. Administration of Sr in moderate doses prevented caries in rats [268]. Among the trace metals present in human bone, Sr was the only that was correlated with bone compression strength [198]. Furthermore, over the past few years, Sr has attracted attention through its beneficial effects on bone healing. Indeed, both *in vitro* and *in vivo* studies have demonstrated stimulatory effects of Sr on osteoblasts and an inhibitory effect on osteoclasts, associated with an increase in bone density and resistance [199, 269–271]. Nowadays, strontium ranelate is used as a commercial antiosteoporotic oral drug that has been proven to reduce the incidence of fractures in osteoporotic patients [196, 272]. Addition of strontium-substituted bioactive glass (SrBG) into PCL and fabricating into 3D bioactive composite scaffolds utilising additive manufacturing technology yield higher compressive Young's modulus [273]. Oxidative stress, a pivotal pathological factor inducing bone osteoporosis, can also be reduced by Zn doping of bioglass in overiectomised Wistar rats as Zn significantly enhances superoxide dismutase (SOD), catalase (CAT) and glutathione peroxidase (GPx) and the Ca/P ratio whereas decreases thiobarbituric acid-reactive substances and thus improves bone mineralisation [274]. The study on effects of the substitution of calcium oxide with Sr on bioactive glass also shows promotion of osteogenesis in a differentiating bone cell culture model using mesenchymal stromal cells obtained from rat bone marrow and proved to be potential for bone tissue regeneration [275]. Sr-doped bioglass implant enhances bone regeneration in patients suffering from osteoporosis [276]. The growing evidence of the beneficial effects of strontium on bone justifies the increasing interest in Sr incorporation into biomaterials for hard tissue repair. Thus, strontium-doped bioactive glasses have been recently developed via a sol-gel method that enables a better control of the reaction kinetics [201, 277].

A multifunctional bioactive scaffold should combine angiogenesis capacity, and osteostimulation, for regenerating lost bone tissues. To achieve these objectives when copper (Cu)-containing mesoporous bioactive glass (Cu-MBG) scaffolds with interconnective large pores are used *in vitro* both Cu-MBG scaffolds and their ionic extracts stimulates hypoxia-inducible factor (HIF)-1α and vascular endothelial growth factor (VEGF) expression in human bone marrow stromal cells (hBMSCs). Thus, incorporation of Cu^{2+} ions into MBG scaffolds increase hypoxia-like tissue reaction which enhance angiogenesis and osteogenesis and has promising scope for the treatment of large bone defect [278]. Controlled delivery of 3 wt% CuO from borate bioactive glass scaffolds implanted in rat calverial defect shows significantly better capacity to stimulate angiogenesis and regenerate bone when compared to the undoped glass scaffolds [279]. It is also evident that copper-doped bioglass scaffold *in vivo* acts on BMSCs ((bone-marrow derived mesenchymal stem cells) to stimulate secretion of VEGF which in turn enhances the angiogenic growth into the scaffolds [280]. Copper (Cu) has the property to stimulate vascularisation/angiogenesis and silicate bioceramics have also stimulatory effects on vascularisation *in vitro* due to the release of silicon (Si) ions. Hence, when combined in bioceramic implant Cu and Si have synergistic effects [281].

Biomaterial-centred bacterial infection, one of the major reasons for revision surgery [282], led the researchers to explore such material that could control infection as well as promote bone healing. Incorporation of silver oxide (Ag_2O) proved its promising future to combat against microbial infection on biomedical materials and devices [241, 242, 283–285]. The introduction of Ag_2O into the bioactive glass shows promising bactericidal efficacy against *Escherichia coli, P. aeruginosa* and *S. aureus in vitro* by leaching of Ag^+ ions from bioglass matrix [223, 286–288]. Doping of Ag^+ ions in 45S5 bioglass based scaffolds even proves to be effective against MRSA (methicillin-resistant *S. aureus*) *in vitro* [289]. Silver-doped bioactive gel-glass Ag-S70C30 has beneficial role as antimicrobial wound healing agent in inflammatory response in a local body compartment such as in acne lesions and in non-healing dermal wounds as it has no cytotoxicity against human epidermal keratinocytes [290]. Mesoporous bioactive glasses doped with Ti/Ag have improved hydroxyapatite- (HAP) induced growth and antimicrobial properties and more potency than pure MBGs in bone-tissue regeneration and surgery [291]. Very recently, scaffolds of a borosilicate bioactive glass (composition: $6Na_2O$, $8K_2O$, 8MgO, 22CaO, $36B_2O_3$, $18SiO_2$, $2P_2O_5$; mol%) doped with varying amounts of Ag_2O (0.05, 0.5 and 1.0 wt%) is being used for bone defect repair and as well as to control infection caused by *E. coli* and *S. aureus*. Better adhesion, proliferation and alkaline phosphatase activity of murine osteoblastic MC3T3-E1 cells on the Ag_2O-doped bioactive glass scaffolds is found than on the undoped scaffolds *in vitro* [292].

Wnt pathway has been found to play a central role in controlling embryonic bone development and bone mass [293] during the past decade. In the developing skeletogenesis, Wnt signalling is required for limb bud initiation, early limb patterning, and, finally, late limb morphogenesis events. It has been reported that Wnt-3a and Wnt-7a are expressed in the limb bud and have roles in skeletal pattern determination [294], and that Wnt-14 is involved in joint formation [295]. In addition, Wnt-3a, Wnt-4, Wnt-5a and Wnt-7a all influence cartilage development [295]. Wnt are 39-46 kDa cysteine-rich, secreted glycoproteins that have been identified in organisms ranging from hydra to humans [296]. Recently, it has been suggested that canonical Wnt signalling plays an important role in fracture healing [297]. Lithium (Li) is an element known to mimic the Wnt signalling pathway, which plays a central role in osteoblast proliferation and differentiation [298]. Expression of various Wnts has been reported to be upregulated during fracture repair, and increased β-catenin signalling by lithium administration has been shown to improve fracture healing [299]. Edgington et al. reported that lithium-based dopants to β-TCP induced an effect on the cell-material interaction of osteoblast cells as well as the study exhibited increased proliferative activity at the lower concentration of Li-doping, while the higher concentration showed a decrease in activity, indicating a toxic effect of Li at elevated doses *in vitro* [300]. Lithium activates β-catenin signalling by inhibiting GSK3β [301–303]. It is also reported that lithium enhances bone formation and improves bone mass in mice [304]. Bioactive glasses with Li-containing composition (55% SiO_2-36% CaO-4% P_2O_5-5% Li_2O) synthesised through a quick alkali sol-gel process stimulate apatite formation after immersion in SBF. Furthermore, addition of Li enhances chemical durability and antibacterial activity against *Enterococcus faecalis*. Li-doped bioglass has excellent antibacterial property against tooth infections for the treatment of root canal, other dental applications [305]. Researches reveal that different concentrations of Li_2O (0-12 wt%) substitution for Na_2O in 45S5 bioglass causes *in vitro* more apatite formation and osteoblastic cell responses than non-substituted 45S5 bioglass thus prove its efficacy for bone defect filler [211]. Another study shows that Li doping in therapeutic range (<8.3 ppm) in 45S5 Bioglass causes more HA deposition than non-doped bioglass *in vitro* [306].

There are even some more ions or materials, doping of which positively improve the quality, bioactivity or bone regeneration. Study with boron modified bioactive glass particle shows significantly more thickness of osseointegrated tissue and more area of neoformed bone tissue than non-doped 45S5 glass along with increase in the Ca:P ratio. Boron modification enhances bone formation more than 45S5 glass when implanted into the intramedullary canal of rat tibiae [307]. Modification of bioactive glass by substitution of Na_2O with doping of fluorides, such as CaF_2 and MgF_2 or B_2O_3 increases its mechanical property [308]. Nickel and cobalt both stimulate the hypoxia-inducible factor-1 (HIF-1a), which significantly improving blood vessel formation in tissue engineering applications. No significant structural differences or dissolution rate occur when nickel and cobalt are doped in bioactive glasses [309]. Magnesium-doped melt-derived glasses in the system SiO_2-CaO-Na_2O-P_2O_5 influences the formation and the evolution of the newly formed layers, promotes the dissolution of the silica network, increases the thickness of the silica gel layer as well as slows down the crystallisation of the apatite layer [310]. Silica- and phosphate-based bioactive glass nanoparticles (58SiO_2-33CaO-9P_2O_5) doped with neem (*Azadirachta indica*) leaf powder and silver nanoparticles show good antimicrobial activity against *S. aureus* and *E. coli* and less bioactivity compared with silver-doped glass particles [311].

3.2. Doped bioactive glass as coating of orthopaedic implants

Since the discovery of bioglass it had mainly been used for coating of metallic implant which are bioinert in nature, i.e. bonding ability to bone tissue is poor [312]. On the other hand, bioglass being an excellent osteogenic agent it has also some inherent disadvantages such as poor mechanical properties leading to its limited application in load-bearing implants where metallic alloys are still the materials of choice. Hence, coatings have drawn attention of researchers as a method to improve adherence of bone tissue to metallic alloy to be used as load-bearing implant in orthopaedic surgery. For this purpose, coating material should have thermal coefficient similar to that have bioglass, as well as, has some other properties such as firing cycle during preparation of coating should not degrade the quality of metal and optimum adherence should be achieved with hydroxyapatite formation in contact with body fluid.

To achieve the goal researchers embedded bioglass or hydroxyapatite particles on coating of Ti6Al4V by a simple enamelling technique to enhance their bioactivity and found excellent glass/metal adhesion with well-attached bioactive particles on the surface that can withstand substantial chemical and mechanical stresses [313]. Another family of glasses in the SiO_2-Na_2O-K_2O-CaO-MgO-P_2O_5 system has been synthesised for coatings on Ti-based and Co-Cr alloys by the scientists, where desired achievement were observed to alloys by formation of 100–200 nm thick interfacial layers (Ti5Si3 on Ti-based alloys and Cr*Ox* on Co-Cr) and commercially Ti alloy-based dental implants were fabricated with 100 μm thick glass coatings successfully [314]. Surgical suture materials such as absorbable polyglactin 910 and non-resorbable Mersilk when coated with silver-doped bioactive glass powder (AgBG) and tested *in vitro*, after 3 days of immersion in SBF, hydroxyapatite forms on the coated suture surfaces and thus their bioactive behaviour is enhanced as a result their use in body wall repair and wound healing property is also enhanced [243] it also limits bacterial attachment [315]. *In vivo* histologic and histomorphometric study on osteointegration of gradient coatings composed of bioactive glass and nanohydroxyapatite (BG-nHA) on titanium-alloy orthopaedic implants and surrounding bone tissue. Fluorescence micrograph shows better osteointegration of orthopaedic implant in BG-nHA than uncoated implant [316].

Mesoporous bioactive glass coatings immobilised with L-ascorbic acid phosphate magnesium salt *n*-hydrate (AsMg) on stainless steel plate causes osteoblast MC3T3-E1 cells stimulation by the MBG with enhanced cell attachment, proliferation, differentiation and better developed cytoskeleton as well as, enhanced fibroblast NIH3T3 proliferation *in vitro* [317]. To compare the behaviour of hydroxyapatite and the bioactive glass coated titanium dental implants different clinical and radiological parameters were studied for 12 months in 31 patients. The study revealed equal potency of bioglass as hydroxyapatite to achieve osteointegration in dental implants [318]. Similarly, nanoparticulate bioactive glass coating on the porous titanium implants promotes better osteointegration and stimulates the formation of bone within the pores than non-coated implants [319]. Incorporation of nanosized HAP into ZnO containing bioglass coating on Ti-6Al-4V substrate improves mechanical properties of the coating but do not hamper *in vitro* bioactivity [320]. Composite orthopaedic coatings with antibacterial capability containing chitosan, Bioglass particles (9.8 μm) and silver nanoparticles (Ag-np) were coated in stainless steel 316 substrate and studied *in vitro* in SBF. Result showed low released concentration of Ag ions (<2.5 ppm) was efficiently antibacterial against *S. aureus* up to 10 days and coating enhanced proliferation of MG-63 osteoblast-like cells up to 7 days in culture and it was also found that high concentration of Ag-np (342 μg) have cytotoxic effect [321]. 45S5 bioglass-silica coatings on 316L stainless steel also causes good osteointegration as well as prevents the metallic implant from corrosion in presence of body fluid [322].

3.3. Doped bioactive glass for delivery of growth factors in bone healing

Growth factors are proteins secreted by cells, act on the appropriate target cell or cells to carry out specific action and thereby there over expression have also been shown in different stages of fracture healing. This phenomenon has led the researchers to study their role as well as the potential to be used as therapeutic agent to accelerate fracture healing. Hence, growth factors are also incorporated into bioactive glass implant, scaffold or coating materials to enhance osteogenic property. Incorporation of bioactive glass and fibroblasts into alginate beads stimulates VEGF as a result potentially it can be used for therapeutic angiogenesis [323]. Combination of prolonged localised VEGF presentation from a matrix coated with a bioactive glass enhances bone regeneration as VEGF has beneficial role in osteogenesis [324]. The combination of novel MBG/silk fibrin scaffold and BMP7 and/or PDGF-B adenovirus synergistically promotes wound healing in acute buccal periodontal defects and osteoporosis related fracture by recruitment of recruitment of mesenchymal progenitor cells [325, 326]. Borate bioactive glass microfibres doped with 0-3.0 wt% CuO has remarkable ability to stimulate angiogenesis which help to heal full-thickness skin defects in rodents and promotes human umbilical vein endothelial cells (HUVEC) migration, tubule formation and secretion of vascular endothelial growth factor, as well as the expression of angiogenic-related genes of the fibroblasts *in vitro* [327].

4. Conclusion and final remarks

Innovative research on bone tissue engineering has made considerable strides over the few decades in the development of new materials, processing techniques and their evaluation and applications. Bioresorbable scaffolds with controlled porosity and tailored properties are of paramount necessity in the successful outcome of bone healing. Silicate bioactive glasses have been extensively investigated over last 40 years. Borate and borosilicate bioactive glass compositions are promising and currently being used in tissue engineering. Although the ability of bioactive glass to support osteogenesis has been proved, recent work has shown the angiogenic potential which may be utilised for the benefits of bioactive glass to soft tissue repair. Due to its biodegradable properties, it may release ions during the degradation process. Apart from doping the bioactive glass with several metallic ions, the degrading ions of its own are known to have a beneficial effect on osteogenesis and on angiogenesis. Current findings show that they may also have a favourable effect on chondrogenesis. Metallic ion doping with the presently available bioactive glass may further improve the biological performance of the material that may open a new vista in bone tissue engineering. Future research will take benefit of the advantageous properties of doped bioactive glass in bone healing as well as coating of several metallic implants.

Author details

Samit Kumar Nandi[1*], Arnab Mahato[2], Biswanath Kundu[2] and Prasenjit Mukherjee[3]

*Address all correspondence to: samitnandi1967@gmail.com

1 Department of Veterinary Surgery and Radiology, West Bengal University of Animal and Fishery Sciences, Kolkata, India

2 Bioceramics and Coating Division, CSIR-Central Glass and Ceramic Research Institute, Kolkata, India

3 Teaching Veterinary Clinical complex, West Bengal University of Animal and Fishery Sciences, Kolkata, India

References

[1] Marastoni S, Ligresti G, Lorenzon E, Colombatti A, Mongiat M. Extracellular matrix: a matter of life and death. Connective Tissue Research. 2008;49(3–4):203–6.

[2] Cancedda R. Cartilage and bone extracellular matrix. Current Pharmaceutical Design. 2009;15(12):1334–48.

[3] Brightman AO, Rajwa BP, Sturgis JE, McCallister ME, Robinson JP, Voytik-Harbin SL. Time-lapse confocal reflection microscopy of collagen fibrillogenesis and extracellular matrix assembly in vitro. Biopolymers. 2000;54(3):222–34.

[4] Xiao G, Gopalakrishnan R, Jiang D, Reith E, Benson MD, Franceschi RT. Bone morphogenetic proteins, extracellular matrix and mitogen-activated protein kinase signaling pathways are required for osteoblast-Specific gene expression and differentiation in MC3T3-E1 Cells. Journal of Bone and Mineral Research. 2002;17(1):101–10.

[5] Benders KEM, van Weeren PR, Badylak SF, Saris DBF, Dhert WJA, Malda J. Extracellular matrix scaffolds for cartilage and bone regeneration. Trends in Biotechnology. 2013;31(3):169–76.

[6] Jones JR, Lee PD, Hench LL. Hierarchical porous materials for tissue engineering. Philosophical Transactions of the Royal Society of London A: Mathematical, Physical and Engineering Sciences. 2006;364(1838):263–81.

[7] Goff T, Kanakaris NK, Giannoudis PV. Use of bone graft substitutes in the management of tibial plateau fractures. Injury. 2013;44:S86–S94.

[8] Ricciardi BF, Bostrom MP, editors. Bone graft substitutes: Claims and credibility. Seminars in Arthroplasty; 2013. Elsevier.

[9] Chaikof EL, Matthew H, Kohn J, Mikos AG, Prestwich GD, Yip CM. Biomaterials and scaffolds in reparative medicine. Annals of the New York Academy of Sciences. 2002;961(1):96–105.

[10] Griffith LG. Emerging design principles in biomaterials and scaffolds for tissue engineering. Annals of the New York Academy of Sciences. 2002;961(1):83–95.

[11] Karageorgiou V, Kaplan D. Porosity of 3D biomaterial scaffolds and osteogenesis. Biomaterials. 2005;26(27):5474–91.

[12] Levenberg S, Langer R. Advances in tissue engineering. Current Topics in Developmental Biology. 2004;61:113–34.

[13] Hutmacher DW. Scaffolds in tissue engineering bone and cartilage. Biomaterials. 2000;21(24):2529–43.

[14] Kellomaki M, Niiranen H, Puumanen K, Ashammakhi N, Waris T, Tormala P. Bioabsorbable scaffolds for guided bone regeneration and generation. Biomaterials. 2000;21(24):2495–505.

[15] Rezwan K, Chen QZ, Blaker JJ, Boccaccini AR. Biodegradable and bioactive porous polymer/inorganic composite scaffolds for bone tissue engineering. Biomaterials. 2006;27(18):3413–31.

[16] Torres AL, Gaspar VM, Serra IR, Diogo GS, Fradique R, Silva AP, et al. Bioactive polymeric-ceramic hybrid 3D scaffold for application in bone tissue regeneration. Materials Science and Engineering: C. 2013;33(7):4460–9.

[17] Hench LL, Wilson J. An introduction to bioceramics. World Scientific; Singapore, 1993.

[18] Kokubo T. Bioceramics and their clinical applications. Elsevier; England, 2008.

[19] Hench LL. The future of bioactive ceramics. Journal of Materials Science: Materials in Medicine. 2015;26(2):1–4.

[20] Salinas AJ, Vallet-Regi M. Bioactive ceramics: from bone grafts to tissue engineering. RSC Advances. 2013;3(28):11116–31.

[21] Kokubo T, Takadama H. How useful is SBF in predicting in vivo bone bioactivity? Biomaterials. 2006;27(15):2907–15.

[22] Williams D. Consensus and definitions in biomaterials. Advances in Biomaterials. 1988;8:11–6.

[23] Jones JR. Review of bioactive glass: from Hench to hybrids. Acta Biomaterialia. 2013;9(1):4457–86.

[24] Hench LL, Splinter RJ, Allen WC, Greenlee TK. Bonding mechanisms at the interface of ceramic prosthetic materials. Journal of Biomedical Materials Research. 1971;5(6): 117–41.

[25] Hench LL. Bioceramics: from concept to clinic. Journal of the American Ceramic Society. 1991;74(7):1487–510.

[26] Hench LL. Biomaterials: a forecast for the future. Biomaterials. 1998;19(16):1419–23.

[27] Hench LL, Polak JM. Third-generation biomedical materials. Science. 2002;295(5557): 1014–7.

[28] Hench LL, Hench JW, Greenspan DC. Bioglass: a short history and bibliography. Journal of the Australasian Ceramic Society. 2004;40(1):1–42.

[29] Guarino V, Causa F, Ambrosio L. Bioactive scaffolds for bone and ligament tissue. Expert Review of Medical Devices. 2007;4(3):405–18.

[30] Hutmacher DW, Schantz JT, Lam CXF, Tan KC, Lim TC. State of the art and future directions of scaffold-based bone engineering from a biomaterials perspective. Journal of Tissue Engineering and Regenerative Medicine. 2007;1(4):245–60.

[31] Jones JR. New trends in bioactive scaffolds: the importance of nanostructure. Journal of the European Ceramic Society. 2009;29(7):1275–81.

[32] Jones JR. Bioactive ceramics and glasses. In Tissue engineering using ceramics and polymers. Cambridge, UK: Woodhead Publishing Limited; 2007.

[33] Chen X, Meng Y, Li Y, Zhao N. Investigation on bio-mineralization of melt and sol–gel derived bioactive glasses. Applied Surface Science. 2008;255(2):562–4.

[34] Gupta R, Kumar A. Bioactive materials for biomedical applications using sol–gel technology. Biomedical Materials. 2008;3(3):034005.

[35] Hench LL. The story of Bioglass®. Journal of Materials Science: Materials in Medicine. 2006;17(11):967–78.

[36] Lacefleld W, Hench L. The bonding of Bioglass® to a cobalt–chromium surgical implant alloy. Biomaterials. 1986;7(2):104–8.

[37] Hench LL, Andersson O. Bioactive glass coatings. Advanced Series in Ceramics. 1993;1:239–60.

[38] Bloyer DR, Gomez-Vega JM, Saiz E, McNaney JM, Cannon RM, Tomsia AP. Fabrication and characterization of a bioactive glass coating on titanium implant alloys. Acta Materialia. 1999;47(15):4221–4.

[39] Moritz N, Vedel E, Ylänen H, Jokinen M, Hupa M, Yli-Urpo A. Characterisation of bioactive glass coatings on titanium substrates produced using a CO_2 laser. Journal of Materials Science: Materials in Medicine. 2004;15(7):787–94.

[40] Borrajo JP, Serra J, González P, León B, Munoz FM, Lopez M. In vivo evaluation of titanium implants coated with bioactive glass by pulsed laser deposition. Journal of Materials Science: Materials in Medicine. 2007;18(12):2371–6.

[41] Lopez-Esteban S, Gutierrez-Gonzalez CF, Gremillard L, Saiz E, Tomsia AP. Interfaces in graded coatings on titanium-based implants. Journal of Biomedical Materials Research Part A. 2009;88(4):1010–21.

[42] James P. Glass ceramics: new compositions and uses. Journal of Non-Crystalline Solids. 1995;181(1):1–15.

[43] Lockyer MWG, Holland D, Dupree R. NMR investigation of the structure of some bioactive and related glasses. Journal of Non-Crystalline Solids. 1995;188(3):207–19.

[44] Aboud T, Stoch L. Crystallization behavior in the glass system SiO_2–P_2O_5–Al_2O_3–MgO–Na_2O. Journal of Non-Crystalline Solids. 1997;219:149–54.

[45] Szabo I, Nagy B, Völksch G, Höland W. Structure, chemical durability and microhardness of glass–ceramics containing apatite and leucite crystals. Journal of Non-Crystalline Solids. 2000;272(2):191–9.

[46] Begum AN, Rajendran V, Ylänen H. Effect of thermal treatment on physical properties of bioactive glass. Materials Chemistry and Physics. 2006;96(2):409–17.

[47] Liu J, Miao X. Sol–gel derived bioglass as a coating material for porous alumina scaffolds. Ceramics International. 2004;30(7):1781–5.

[48] Li N, Jie Q, Zhu S, Wang R. Preparation and characterization of macroporous sol–gel bioglass. Ceramics International. 2005;31(5):641–6.

[49] Xia W, Chang J. Well-ordered mesoporous bioactive glasses (MBG): a promising bioactive drug delivery system. Journal of Controlled Release. 2006;110(3):522–30.

[50] Balamurugan A, Sockalingum G, Michel J, Fauré J, Banchet V, Wortham L, et al. Synthesis and characterisation of sol gel derived bioactive glass for biomedical applications. Materials Letters. 2006;60(29):3752–7.

[51] Balamurugan A, Balossier G, Michel J, Kannan S, Benhayoune H, Rebelo A, et al. Sol–gel derived SiO_2–CaO–MgO–P_2O_s bioglass system—preparation and in vitro characterization. Journal of Biomedical Materials Research Part B: Applied Biomaterials. 2007;83(2):546–53.

[52] Li R, Clark A, Hench L. An investigation of bioactive glass powders by sol-gel processing. Journal of Applied Biomaterials. 1991;2(4):231–9.

[53] Hench LL, West JK. The sol-gel process. Chemical Reviews. 1990;90(1):33–72.

[54] Rideal E, Davies J. Interfacial phenomena. New York: Academic Press; 1963.

[55] Kaur G, Pandey OP, Singh K, Homa D, Scott B, Pickrell G. A review of bioactive glasses: their structure, properties, fabrication and apatite formation. Journal of Biomedical Materials Research Part A. 2014;102(1):254–74.

[56] Vallet-Regí M. Ceramics for medical applications. Journal of the Chemical Society, Dalton Transactions. 2001(2):97–108.

[57] R.K. Iler, The colloid chemistry of silica and silicates, Soil Science, 80 (1955) 86.

[58] Brinker CJ, Scherer GW, Roth E. Sol→ gel→ glass. II. Physical and structural evolution during constant heating rate experiments. Journal of Non-Crystalline Solids. 1985;72(2):345–68.

[59] Hench LL, Ulrich DR. Science of ceramic chemical processing. Wiley-Interscience; 1986.

[60] Colby MW, Osaka A, Mackenzie JD. Temperature dependence of the gelation of silicon alkoxides. Journal of Non-Crystalline Solids. 1988;99(1):129–39.

[61] Falcone JS. Soluble silicates. American Chemical Society; 1982.

[62] Iler RK. The chemistry of silica. New York: Wiley; 1979.

[63] Liu S. Aging of gels. University of Florida, Internal report; 1989.

[64] Sepulveda P, Jones JR, Hench LL. Characterization of melt-derived 45S5 and sol–gel–derived 58S bioactive glasses. Journal of Biomedical Materials Research. 2001;58(6): 734–40.

[65] Brinker CJ, Scherer GW. Sol-gel science: the physics and chemistry of sol-gel processing. Academic Press; London, 2013.

[66] Strnad Z. Role of the glass phase in bioactive glass–ceramics. Biomaterials. 1992;13(5): 317–21.

[67] Shelby JE. Introduction to glass science and technology. UK: Royal Society of Chemistry; 2005.

[68] Cormack AN, Tilocca A. Structure and biological activity of glasses and ceramics. Philosophical Transactions of the Royal Society of London A: Mathematical, Physical and Engineering Sciences. 2012;370(1963):1271–80.

[69] Elgayar I, Aliev AE, Boccaccini AR, Hill RG. Structural analysis of bioactive glasses. Journal of Non-Crystalline Solids. 2005;351(2):173–83.

[70] Ylänen H. Bone ingrowth into porous bodies made by sintering bioactive glass microspheres. Åbo Akademi Process Chemistry Group, Combustion and Materials Chemistry; 2000.

[71] Andersson Ö, Liu G, Karlsson K, Niemi L, Miettinen J, Juhanoja J. In vivo behaviour of glasses in the SiO_2–Na_2O–CaO–P_2O_5–Al_2O_3–B_2O_3 system. Journal of Materials Science: Materials in Medicine. 1990;1(4):219–27.

[72] Hench LL, Andersson Ä. An introduction to bioceramics. Singapore: World Scientific; 1993.

[73] Osaka A, Hayakawa S, Tsuru K, Ohtsuki C. Bioactivity of alkali and alkaline earth borosilicate glasses. Borate Glasses, Crystals and Melts. 1997:490–7.

[74] Saranti A, Koutselas I, Karakassides MA. Bioactive glasses in the system CaO–B_2O_3–P_2O: preparation, structural study and in vitro evaluation. Journal of Non-Crystalline Solids. 2006;352(5):390–8.

[75] Yao A, Wang D, Huang W, Fu Q, Rahaman MN, Day DE. In vitro bioactive characteristics of borate-based glasses with controllable degradation behavior. Journal of the American Ceramic Society. 2007;90(1):303–6.

[76] Barrios de Arenas I, Schattner C, Vásquez M. Bioactivity and mechanical properties of Na_2O–CaO–SiO_2–P_2O_5 modified glasses. Ceramics International. 2005;32(5):515–20.

[77] Rude RK, Gruber HE. Magnesium deficiency and osteoporosis: animal and human observations. The Journal of Nutritional Biochemistry. 2004;15(12):710–6.

[78] Okuma T. Magnesium and bone strength. Nutrition. 2001;17(7–8):679–80.

[79] Cowan JA. Structural and catalytic chemistry of magnesium-dependent enzymes. Biometals: An International Journal on the Role of Metal Ions in Biology, Biochemistry, and Medicine. 2002;15(3):225–35.

[80] Gomez S, Rizzo R, Pozzi-Mucelli M, Bonucci E, Vittur F. Zinc mapping in bone tissues by histochemistry and synchrotron radiation-induced X-ray emission: correlation with the distribution of alkaline phosphatase. Bone. 1999;25(1):33–8.

[81] Peretz A, Papadopoulos T, Willems D, Hotimsky A, Michiels N, Siderova V, et al. Zinc supplementation increases bone alkaline phosphatase in healthy men. Journal of Trace Elements in Medicine and Biology. 2001;15(2–3):175–8.

[82] Nishi Y. Zinc and growth. Journal of the American College of Nutrition. 1996;15(4):340–4.

[83] Tapiero H, Townsend DM, Tew KD. Trace elements in human physiology and pathology. Copper. Biomedicine and Pharmacotherapy. 2003;57(9):386–98.

[84] Li X, Wang X, He D, Shi J. Synthesis and characterization of mesoporous CaO–MO–SiO_2–P_2O_5 (M = Mg, Zn, Cu) bioactive glasses/composites. Journal of Materials Chemistry. 2008;18(34):4103–9.

[85] Sitarz M, Bulat K, Szumera M. Influence of modifiers and glass-forming ions on the crystallization of glasses of the $NaCaPO_4$–SiO_2 system. Journal of Thermal Analysis and Calorimetry. 2012;109(2):577–84.

[86] Brink M. Bioactive glasses with a large working range. Abo Akademi University; 1997.

[87] Hench LL, Andersson OH, LaTorre GP. The kinetics of bioactive ceramics. Part III. Surface reactions for bioactive glasses compared with an inactive glass. Bioceramics. 1991;4:156–62.

[88] Hench LL, Andersson OH, LaTorre GP. The kinetics of bioactive ceramics. Bioceramics, USA. 1991:43.

[89] Hench LL, West JK. Biological applications of bioactive glasses. Life Chemistry Reports. 1996;13:187–241.

[90] Skipper LJ, Sowrey FE, Pickup DM, Drake KO, Smith ME, Saravanapavan P, et al. The structure of a bioactive calcia–silica sol–gel glass. Journal of Materials Chemistry. 2005;15(24):2369–74.

[91] Martin RA, Twyman H, Qiu D, Knowles JC, Newport RJ. A study of the formation of amorphous calcium phosphate and hydroxyapatite on melt quenched Bioglass® using surface sensitive shallow angle X-ray diffraction. Journal of Materials Science: Materials in Medicine. 2009;20(4):883–8.

[92] Li P, Zhang F. The electrochemistry of a glass surface and its application to bioactive glass in solution. Journal of Non-Crystalline Solids. 1990;119(1):112–8.

[93] Doostmohammadi A, Monshi A, Fathi MH, Braissant O. A comparative physico-chemical study of bioactive glass and bone-derived hydroxyapatite. Ceramics International. 2011;37(5):1601–7.

[94] Karlsson KH, Fröberg K, Ringbom T. A structural approach to bone adhering of bioactive glasses. Journal of Non-Crystalline Solids. 1989;112(1):69–72.

[95] FitzGerald V, Pickup DM, Greenspan D, Wetherall KM, Moss RM, Jones JR, et al. An atomic scale comparison of the reaction of Bioglass® in two types of simulated body fluid. Physics and Chemistry of Glasses-European Journal of Glass Science and Technology Part B. 2009;50(3):137–43.

[96] Hench LL. Bioactive ceramics: theory and clinical applications. Bioceramics. 1994;7:3–14.

[97] Andersson ÖH, Karlsson KH, Kangasniemi K. Calcium phosphate formation at the surface of bioactive glass in vivo. Journal of Non-Crystalline Solids. 1990;119(3):290–6.

[98] Aitasalo K, Peltola M, Suonpää J, Yli-Urpo A, editors. Bioactive glass S53P4 in frontal sinus obliteration. In A 9-year experience. 13th International Symposium on Ceramics in Medicine; 2000; Bologna, Italy.

[99] Peltola M. Experimental follow-up model for clinical frontal sinus obliteration with bioactive glass (S53P4). Acta Oto-Laryngologica. 2000;120(543):167–9.

[100] Brink M, Turunen T, Happonen RP, Yli-Urpo A. Compositional dependence of bioactivity of glasses in the system Na_2O–K_2O–MgO–CaO–B_2O_3–P_2O_5–SiO_2. Journal of Biomedical Materials Research. 1997;37(1):114–21.

[101] Ylänen H, Karlsson KH, Itälä A, Aro HT. Effect of immersion in SBF on porous bioactive bodies made by sintering bioactive glass microspheres. Journal of Non-Crystalline Solids. 2000;275(1):107–15.

[102] Itälä A, Nordström EG, Ylänen H, Aro HT, Hupa M. Creation of microrough surface on sintered bioactive glass microspheres. Journal of Biomedical Materials Research. 2001;56(2):282–8.

[103] Bovo N. Structure-properties relationships in bioactive glasses for PAA-based polyalkenoate cements. Enginyeria Metallurgica: Universitat Politecnica de catalunya, Barcelona, Spain; 2007.

[104] Hench LL, Pantano CG, Buscemi PJ, Greenspan DC. Analysis of bioglass fixation of hip prostheses. Journal of Biomedical Materials Research. 1977;11(2):267–82.

[105] Oonishi H, Hench LL, Wilson J, Sugihara F, Tsuji E, Matsuura M, et al. Quantitative comparison of bone growth behavior in granules of Bioglass, A-W glass–ceramic, and hydroxyapatite. Journal of Biomedical Materials Research. 2000;51(1):37–46.

[106] Oonishi H, Kushitani S, Yasukawa E, Iwaki H, Hench LL, Wilson J, et al. Particulate bioglass compared with hydroxyapatite as a bone graft substitute. Clinical Orthopaedics and Related Research. 1997;334:316–25.

[107] Oonishi H, Hench LL, Wilson J, Sugihara F, Tsuji E, Kushitani S, et al. Comparative bone growth behavior in granules of bioceramic materials of various sizes. Journal of biomedical materials research. 1999;44(1):31–43.

[108] Schepers EJG, Ducheyne P. Bioactive glass particles of narrow size range for the treatment of oral bone defects: a 1–24 month experiment with several materials and particle sizes and size ranges. Journal of Oral Rehabilitation. 1997;24(3):171–81.

[109] Wang Z, Lu B, Chen L, Chang J. Evaluation of an osteostimulative putty in the sheep spine. Journal of Materials Science: Materials in Medicine. 2011;22(1):185–91.

[110] Fujibayashi S, Neo M, Kim H-M, Kokubo T, Nakamura T. A comparative study between in vivo bone ingrowth and in vitro apatite formation on Na_2O–CaO–SiO_2 glasses. Biomaterials. 2003;24(8):1349–56.

[111] Wheeler DL, Eschbach EJ, Hoellrich RG, Montfort MJ, Chamberland DL. Assessment of resorbable bioactive material for grafting of critical-size cancellous defects. Journal of Orthopaedic Research. 2000;18(1):140–8.

[112] Kokubo T, Kushitani H, Ohtsuki C, Sakka S, Yamamuro T. Chemical reaction of bioactive glass and glass-ceramics with a simulated body fluid. Journal of Materials science: Materials in Medicine. 1992;3(2):79–83.

[113] Oyane A, Kim HM, Furuya T, Kokubo T, Miyazaki T, Nakamura T. Preparation and assessment of revised simulated body fluids. Journal of Biomedical Materials Research Part A. 2003;65(2):188–95.

[114] Takadama H, Hashimoto M, Mizuno M, Kokubo T. Round-robin test of SBF for in vitro measurement of apatite-forming ability of synthetic materials. Phosphorus Research Bulletin. 2004;17(0):119–25.

[115] Clément J, Ekeberg L, Martinez S, Ginebra M, Gil F, Planell J, editors. Influence of the Chemical Composition on the Mechanical Properties and In Vitro Solubility of Phosphate Glasses in the System P_2O_5–CaO–Na_2O. Bioceramics; 1998.

[116] Oliveira JM, Correia RN, Fernandes MH. Effects of Si speciation on the in vitro bioactivity of glasses. Biomaterials. 2002;23(2):371–9.

[117] Lukito D, Xue JM, Wang J. In vitro bioactivity assessment of 70 (wt.)% SiO_2–30 (wt.)% CaO bioactive glasses in simulated body fluid. Materials Letters. 2005;59(26):3267–71.

[118] Agathopoulos S, Tulyaganov DU, Ventura JMG, Kannan S, Karakassides MA, Ferreira JMF. Formation of hydroxyapatite onto glasses of the CaO–MgO–SiO_2 system with B_2O_3, Na_2O, CaF_2 and P_2O_5 additives. Biomaterials. 2006;27(9):1832–40.

[119] Jones JR, Sepulveda P, Hench LL. Dose-dependent behavior of bioactive glass dissolution. Journal of Biomedical Materials Research. 2001;58(6):720–6.

[120] Greenspan DC, Zhong JP, LaTorre GP. Effect of surface area to volume ratio on in vitro surface reactions of bioactive glass particulates. Bioceramics. 1994;7:55–60.

[121] Greenspan DC, Zhong JP, LaTorre GP. Evaluation of surface structure of bioactive glasses *in-vitro*. Bioceramics. 1995;8:477–82.

[122] Balas F, Pérez-Pariente J, Vallet-Regí M, editors. Relationship between bioactivity and textural parameters in glasses. Bioceramics; 1998.

[123] Andrade ÂL, Valério P, Goes AM, de Fátima Leite M, Domingues RZ. Influence of morphology on in vitro compatibility of bioactive glasses. Journal of Non-Crystalline Solids. 2006;352(32):3508–11.

[124] Hench LL, Thompson I. Twenty-first century challenges for biomaterials. Journal of the Royal Society Interface. 2010;7(Suppl 4):S379–91.

[125] Wang C, Xue Y, Lin K, Lu J, Chang J, Sun J. The enhancement of bone regeneration by a combination of osteoconductivity and osteostimulation using β-$CaSiO_3$/β-$Ca_3(PO_4)_2$ composite bioceramics. Acta Biomaterialia. 2012;8(1):350–60.

[126] Yong Cheng H, Zhong Jp. Osteostimulation of bioglass. Chinese Medical Journal (England). 2009;122(19):2386–9.

[127] Vallet-Regí M, Ragel C, Salinas AJ. Glasses with medical applications. European Journal of Inorganic Chemistry. 2003;2003(6):1029–42.

[128] Zhao L, Yan X, Zhou X, Zhou L, Wang H, Tang J, et al. Mesoporous bioactive glasses for controlled drug release. Microporous and Mesoporous Materials. 2008;109(1):210–5.

[129] Xue JM, Shi M. PLGA/mesoporous silica hybrid structure for controlled drug release. Journal of Controlled Release. 2004;98(2):209–17.

[130] Li J, Song Y, Zhang S, Zhao C, Zhang F, Zhang X, et al. In vitro responses of human bone marrow stromal cells to a fluoridated hydroxyapatite coated biodegradable Mg–Zn alloy. Biomaterials. 2010;31(22):5782–8.

[131] Zhu Y, Ikoma T, Hanagata N, Kaskel S. Rattle-type Fe_3O_4@ SiO_2 hollow mesoporous spheres as carriers for drug delivery. Small. 2010;6(3):471–8.

[132] Chen QZ, Thompson ID, Boccaccini AR. 45S5 Bioglass®-derived glass–ceramic scaffolds for bone tissue engineering. Biomaterials. 2006;27(11):2414–25.

[133] Jones JR, Ehrenfried LM, Hench LL. Optimising bioactive glass scaffolds for bone tissue engineering. Biomaterials. 2006;27(7):964–73.

[134] Yan X, Yu C, Zhou X, Tang J, Zhao D. Highly ordered mesoporous bioactive glasses with superior in vitro bone-forming bioactivities. Angewandte Chemie International Edition. 2004;43(44):5980–4.

[135] Kim TG, Shin H, Lim DW. Biomimetic scaffolds for tissue engineering. Advanced Functional Materials. 2012;22(12):2446–68.

[136] Wu C, Chang J. Mesoporous bioactive glasses: structure characteristics, drug/growth factor delivery and bone regeneration application. Interface Focus. 2012;2:292–306.

[137] Yan X, Huang X, Yu C, Deng H, Wang Y, Zhang Z, et al. The in-vitro bioactivity of mesoporous bioactive glasses. Biomaterials. 2006;27(18):3396–403.

[138] Brinker CJ, Lu Y, Sellinger A, Fan H. Evaporation-induced self-assembly: nanostructures made easy. Advanced Materials. 1999;11(7):579–85.

[139] Vallet-Regí M, Garcia MM, Colilla M. Biomedical applications of mesoporous ceramics: drug delivery, smart materials and bone tissue engineering. CRC Press; USA, 2012.

[140] Zhu Y, Kaskel S. Comparison of the in vitro bioactivity and drug release property of mesoporous bioactive glasses (MBGs) and bioactive glasses (BGs) scaffolds. Microporous and Mesoporous Materials. 2009;118(1):176–82.

[141] Lei B, Chen X, Wang Y, Zhao N, Du C, Zhang L. Acetic acid derived mesoporous bioactive glasses with an enhanced in vitro bioactivity. Journal of Non-Crystalline Solids. 2009;355(52):2583–7.

[142] Xia W, Chang J. Preparation, in vitro bioactivity and drug release property of well-ordered mesoporous 58S bioactive glass. Journal of Non-Crystalline Solids. 2008;354(12):1338–41.

[143] Li X, Wang X, He D, Shi J. Synthesis and characterization of mesoporous CaO–MO–SiO_2–P_2O_5 (M = Mg, Zn, Cu) bioactive glasses/composites. Journal of Materials Chemistry. 2008;18(34):4103–9.

[144] Lei B, Chen X, Wang Y, Zhao N. Synthesis and in vitro bioactivity of novel mesoporous hollow bioactive glass microspheres. Materials Letters. 2009;63(20):1719–21.

[145] Zhao S, Li Y, Li D. Synthesis and in vitro bioactivity of CaO–SiO_2–P_2O_5 mesoporous microspheres. Microporous and Mesoporous Materials. 2010;135(1):67–73.

[146] Hong Y, Chen X, Jing X, Fan H, Guo B, Gu Z, et al. Preparation, bioactivity, and drug release of hierarchical nanoporous bioactive glass ultrathin fibers. Advanced Materials. 2010;22(6):754–8.

[147] Hong Y, Chen X, Jing X, Fan H, Gu Z, Zhang X. Fabrication and drug delivery of ultrathin mesoporous bioactive glass hollow fibers. Advanced Functional Materials. 2010;20(9):1503–10.

[148] Hoppe A, Güldal NS, Boccaccini AR. A review of the biological response to ionic dissolution products from bioactive glasses and glass–ceramics. Biomaterials. 2011;32(11):2757–74.

[149] Saltman PD, Strause LG. The role of trace minerals in osteoporosis. Journal of the American College of Nutrition. 1993;12(4):384–9.

[150] Beattie JH, Avenell A. Trace element nutrition and bone metabolism. Nutrition Research Reviews. 1992;5(01):167–88.

[151] Nielsen FH. New essential trace elements for the life sciences. Biological Trace Element Research. 1990;26(1):599–611.

[152] Nedelec JM, Courthéoux L, Jallot E, Kinowski C, Lao J, Laquerriere P, et al. Materials doping through sol–gel chemistry: a little something can make a big difference. Journal of Sol-Gel Science and Technology. 2008;46(3):259–71.

[153] Krajewski A, Ravaglioli A, Fabbri B, Azzoni CB. Doping influence on the interaction between a bioactive glass and a simulated physiological solution: chemical and EPR tests. Journal of Materials Science. 1987;22(4):1228–34.

[154] Cortizo AM, Molinuevo MS, Barrio DA, Bruzzone L. Osteogenic activity of vanadyl (IV)–ascorbate complex: evaluation of its mechanism of action. The International Journal of Biochemistry & Cell Biology. 2006;38(7):1171–80.

[155] Marie PJ, Ammann P, Boivin G, Rey C. Mechanisms of action and therapeutic potential of strontium in bone. Calcified Tissue International. 2001;69(3):121–9.

[156] Maeno S, Niki Y, Matsumoto H, Morioka H, Yatabe T, Funayama A, et al. The effect of calcium ion concentration on osteoblast viability, proliferation and differentiation in monolayer and 3D culture. Biomaterials. 2005;26(23):4847–55.

[157] Marie PJ. The calcium-sensing receptor in bone cells: a potential therapeutic target in osteoporosis. Bone. 2010;46(3):571–6.

[158] Valerio P, Pereira MM, Goes AM, Leite MF. Effects of extracellular calcium concentration on the glutamate release by bioactive glass (BG60S) preincubated osteoblasts. Biomedical Materials. 2009;4(4):045011.

[159] Julien M, Khoshniat S, Lacreusette A, Gatius M, Bozec A, Wagner EF, et al. Phosphate-dependent regulation of MGP in osteoblasts: Role of ERK1/2 and Fra-1. Journal of Bone and Mineral Research. 2009;24(11):1856–68.

[160] Carlisle EM. Silicon: a requirement in bone formation independent of vitamin D1. Calcified Tissue International. 1981;33(1):27–34.

[161] Reffitt DM, Ogston N, Jugdaohsingh R, Cheung HFJ, Evans BAJ, Thompson RPH, et al. Orthosilicic acid stimulates collagen type 1 synthesis and osteoblastic differentiation in human osteoblast-like cells in vitro. Bone. 2003;32(2):127–35.

[162] Delannoy PH, Bazot D, Marie PJ. Long-term treatment with strontium ranelate increases vertebral bone mass without deleterious effect in mice. Metabolism. 2002;51(7):906–11.

[163] Shahnazari M, Sharkey NA, Fosmire GJ, Leach RM. Effects of strontium on bone strength, density, volume, and microarchitecture in laying hens. Journal of Bone and Mineral Research. 2006;21(11):1696–703.

[164] Grynpas MD, Marie PJ. Effects of low doses of strontium on bone quality and quantity in rats. Bone. 1990;11(5):313–9.

[165] Brandão-Neto J, Stefan V, Mendonça BB, Bloise W, Castro AVB. The essential role of zinc in growth. Nutrition Research. 1995;15(3):335–58.

[166] Choi MK, Kim MH, Kang MH. The effect of boron supplementation on bone strength in ovariectomized rats fed with diets containing different calcium levels. Food Science and Biotechnology. 2005;14(2):242–8.

[167] Hartwig A. Role of magnesium in genomic stability. Mutation Research Fundamental and Molecular Mechanisms of Mutagenesis. 2001;475(1):113–21.

[168] Carlisle EM. Silicon: a possible factor in bone calcification. Science. 1970;167(3916):279–80.

[169] Jugdaohsingh R, Tucker KL, Qiao N, Cupples LA, Kiel DP, Powell JJ. Dietary silicon intake is positively associated with bone mineral density in men and premenopausal women of the Framingham offspring cohort. Journal of Bone and Mineral Research. 2004;19(2):297–307.

[170] Damen JJM, Ten Cate JM. Silica-induced precipitation of calcium phosphate in the presence of inhibitors of hydroxyapatite formation. Journal of dental Research. 1992;71(3):453–7.

[171] Yamaguchi M. Role of zinc in bone formation and bone resorption. The Journal of Trace Elements in Experimental Medicine. 1998;11(2–3):119–35.

[172] Kwun IS, Cho YE, Lomeda RAR, Shin HI, Choi JY, Kang YH, et al. Zinc deficiency suppresses matrix mineralization and retards osteogenesis transiently with catch-up possibly through Runx 2 modulation. Bone. 2010;46(3):732–41.

[173] Zreiqat H, Howlett CR, Zannettino A, Evans P, Schulze-Tanzil G, Knabe C, et al. Mechanisms of magnesium-stimulated adhesion of osteoblastic cells to commonly used orthopaedic implants. Journal of Biomedical Materials Research. 2002;62(2):175–84.

[174] Yamasaki Y, Yoshida Y, Okazaki M, Shimazu A, Uchida T, Kubo T, et al. Synthesis of functionally graded $MgCO_3$ apatite accelerating osteoblast adhesion. Journal of Biomedical Materials Research. 2002;62(1):99–105.

[175] Marie PJ. Strontium ranelate: a physiological approach for optimizing bone formation and resorption. Bone. 2006;38(2):10–4.

[176] Gérard C, Bordeleau LJ, Barralet J, Doillon CJ. The stimulation of angiogenesis and collagen deposition by copper. Biomaterials. 2010;31(5):824–31.

[177] Hu Gf. Copper stimulates proliferation of human endothelial cells under culture. Journal of Cellular Biochemistry. 1998;69(3):326–35.

[178] Nielsen FH. Is boron nutritionally relevant? Nutrition Reviews. 2008;66(4):183–91.

[179] Uysal T, Ustdal A, Sonmez MF, Ozturk F. Stimulation of bone formation by dietary boron in an orthopedically expanded suture in rabbits. The Angle Orthodontist. 2009;79(5):984–90.

[180] Vacheron Trystram MN, Braitman A, Cheref S, Auffray L. Antipsychotics in bipolar disorders. Encephale. 2003;30(5):417–24.

[181] Young W. Review of lithium effects on brain and blood. Cell Transplantation. 2009;18(9):951–75.

[182] Kallner G, Petterson U. Renal, thyroid and parathyroid function during lithium treatment: laboratory tests in 207 people treated for 1–30 years. Acta Psychiatrica Scandinavica. 1995;91(1):48–51.

[183] Sun ZL, Wataha JC, Hanks CT. Effects of metal ions on osteoblast-like cell metabolism and differentiation. Journal of Biomedical Material Research. 1997;34(1):29–37.

[184] Lázaro GS, Santos SC, Resende CX, dos Santos EA. Individual and combined effects of the elements Zn, Mg and Sr on the surface reactivity of a $SiO_2 \cdot CaO \cdot Na_2O \cdot P_2O_5$ bioglass system. Journal of Non-Crystalline Solids. 2014;386:19–28.

[185] Li HC, Wang DG, Chen CZ. Effect of zinc oxide and zirconia on structure, degradability and in vitro bioactivity of wollastonite. Ceramics International. 2015;41:10160–9.

[186] Popp JR, Love BJ, Goldstein AS. Effect of soluble zinc on differentiation of osteoprogenitor cells. Journal of Biomedical Materials Research Part A. 2007;81(3):766–9.

[187] Atkinson I, Anghel EM, Predoana L, Mocioiu OC, Jecu L, Raut I, et al. Influence of ZnO addition on the structural, in vitro behavior and antimicrobial activity of sol–gel derived $CaO–P_2O_5–SiO_2$ bioactive glasses. Ceramics International. 2016;42(2):3033–45.

[188] Sánchez-Salcedo S, Shruti S, Salinas AJ, Malavasi G, Menabue L, Vallet-Regi M. In vitro antibacterial capacity and cytocompatibility of $SiO_2–CaO–P_2O_5$ meso-macroporous glass scaffolds enriched with ZnO. Journal of Materials Chemistry B. 2014;2(30):4836–47.

[189] Balamurugan A, Balossier G, Kannan S, Michel J, Rebelo AH, Ferreira JM. Development and in vitro characterization of sol–gel derived $CaO–P_2O_5–SiO_2–ZnO$ bioglass. Acta Biomaterialia. 2007;3(2):255–62.

[190] Courthéoux L, Lao J, Nedelec JM, Jallot E. Controlled bioactivity in zinc-doped sol−gel-derived binary bioactive glasses. The Journal of Physical Chemistry C. 2008;112(35): 13663–7.

[191] El-Kady AM, Ali AF. Fabrication and characterization of ZnO modified bioactive glass nanoparticles. Ceramics International. 2012;38(2):1195–204.

[192] Fujita Y, Yamamuro T, Nakamura T, Kotani S, Ohtsuki C, Kokubo T. The bonding behavior of calcite to bone. Journal of Biomedical Materials Research. 1991;25(8):991–1003.

[193] Du RL, Chang J, Ni SY, Zhai WY, Wang JY. Characterization and in vitro bioactivity of zinc-containing bioactive glass and glass-ceramics. Journal of biomaterials applications. 2006;20(4):341–60.

[194] Aina V, Malavasi G, Pla AF, Munaron L, Morterra C. Zinc-containing bioactive glasses: surface reactivity and behaviour towards endothelial cells. Acta Biomaterialia. 2009;5(4):1211–22.

[195] Shahrabi S, Hesaraki S, Moemeni S, Khorami M. Structural discrepancies and in vitro nanoapatite formation ability of sol–gel derived glasses doped with different bone stimulator ions. Ceramics International. 2011;37(7):2737–46.

[196] Meunier PJ, Roux C, Seeman E, Ortolani S, Badurski JE, Spector TD, et al. The effects of strontium ranelate on the risk of vertebral fracture in women with postmenopausal osteoporosis. New England Journal of Medicine. 2004;350(5):459–68.

[197] Sila-asna M, Bunyaratvej A. Kobe University Repository: Kernel. Kobe Journal of Medical Sciences. 2007;53(1):25–35.

[198] Jensen JEB, Stang H, Kringsholm B, Pritzl G, Sorensen OH. Relationship between trace element content and mechanical bone strength. Bone. 1997;20(Suppl 4):104.

[199] Bonnelye E, Chabadel A, Saltel F, Jurdic P. Dual effect of strontium ranelate: stimulation of osteoblast differentiation and inhibition of osteoclast formation and resorption in vitro. Bone. 2008;42(1):129–38.

[200] Usuda K, Kono K, Dote T, Watanabe M, Shimizu H, Tanimoto Y, et al. An overview of boron, lithium, and strontium in human health and profiles of these elements in urine of Japanese. Environmental Health and Preventive Medicine. 2007;12(6):231–7.

[201] Lao J, Jallot E, Nedelec JM. Strontium-delivering glasses with enhanced bioactivity: a new biomaterial for antiosteoporotic applications? Chemistry of Materials. 2008;20(15): 4969–73.

[202] Isaac J, Nohra J, Lao J, Jallot E, Nedelec JM, Berdal A, et al. Effects of strontium-doped bioactive glass on the differentiation of cultured osteogenic cells. European Cells and Materials. 2011;21:130–43.

[203] Gentleman E, Fredholm YC, Jell G, Lotfibakhshaiesh N, O'Donnell MD, Hill RG, et al. The effects of strontium-substituted bioactive glasses on osteoblasts and osteoclasts in vitro. Biomaterials. 2010;31(14):3949–56.

[204] Hesaraki S, Gholami M, Vazehrad S, Shahrabi S. The effect of Sr concentration on bioactivity and biocompatibility of sol-gel derived glasses based on $CaO–SrO–SiO_2–P_2O_5$ quaternary system. Materials Science and Engineering: C. 2010;30(3):383–90.

[205] O'Donnell MD, Hill RG. Influence of strontium and the importance of glass chemistry and structure when designing bioactive glasses for bone regeneration. Acta Biomaterialia. 6(7):2382–5.

[206] Zhang J, Zhao S, Zhu Y, Huang Y, Zhu M, Tao C, et al. Three-dimensional printing of strontium-containing mesoporous bioactive glass scaffolds for bone regeneration. Acta Biomaterialia. 2014;10(5):2269–81.

[207] Zhao S, Zhang J, Zhu M, Zhang Y, Liu Z, Tao C, et al. Three-dimensional printed strontium-containing mesoporous bioactive glass scaffolds for repairing rat critical-sized calvarial defects. Acta Biomaterialia. 2015;12:270–80.

[208] Sriranganathan D, Kanwal N, Hing KA, Hill RG. Strontium substituted bioactive glasses for tissue engineered scaffolds: the importance of octacalcium phosphate. Journal of Materials Science: Materials in Medicine. 2016;27(2):1–10.

[209] Nordenstrom J, Elvius M, Bagedahl-Strindlund M, Zhao B, Torring O. Biochemical hyperparathyroidism and bone mineral status in patients treated long-term with lithium. Metabolism. 1994;43(12):1563–7.

[210] Davis BM, Pfefferbaum A, Krutzik S, Davis KL. Lithium's effect of parathyroid hormone. American Journal of Psychiatry. 1981;138(4):489–92.

[211] Khorami M, Hesaraki S, Behnamghader A, Nazarian H, Shahrabi S. In vitro bioactivity and biocompatibility of lithium substituted 45S5 bioglass. Materials Science and Engineering: C. 2011;31(7):1584–92.

[212] Miguez-Pacheco V, Büttner T, Maçon ALB., Jones JR, T. Fey D. de Ligny, Greil P, Chevalier J, Malchere A, Boccaccini AR. Development and characterization of lithium-releasing silicate bioactive glasses and their scaffolds for bone repair, Journal of Non-Crystalline Solids. 2016;432:65–72

[213] Ma J, Chen CZ, Wang DG, Hu JH. Synthesis, characterization and in vitro bioactivity of magnesium-doped sol-gel glass and glass–ceramics. Ceramics International. 2011;37(5):1637–44.

[214] Spasov AA, Fomichev EV, Guseva TN, Mazanova LS, Shchava SN. Efficiency of magnesium-containing preparation polykatan in therapy of purulent wounds. Bulletin of Experimental Biology and Medicine. 2001;131(2):132–5.

[215] Sojka JE. Magnesium supplementation and osteoporosis. Nutrition Reviews. 1995;53(3):71–4.

[216] Watts SJ, Hill RG, O'Donnell MD, Law RV. Influence of magnesia on the structure and properties of bioactive glasses. Journal of Non-Crystalline Solids. 2010;356(9):517–24.

[217] Ma J, Chen CZ, Wang DG, Shao X, Wang CZ, Zhang HM. Effect of MgO addition on the crystallization and in vitro bioactivity of glass ceramics in the $CaO–MgO–SiO_2–P_2O_5$ system. Ceramics International. 2012;38(8):6677–84.

[218] Rawlings RD. Bioactive glasses and glass–ceramics. Clinical Materials. 1993;14(2):155–79.

[219] Hill R. An alternative view of the degradation of bioglass. Journal of Materials Science Letters. 1996;15(13):1122–5.

[220] Varanasi VG, Saiz E, Loomer PM, Ancheta B, Uritani N, Ho SP, et al. Enhanced osteocalcin expression by osteoblast-like cells (MC3T3-E1) exposed to bioactive coating glass ($SiO_2–CaO–P_2O_5–MgO–K_2O–Na_2O$ system) ions. Acta Biomaterialia. 2009;5(9):3536–47.

[221] Balamurugan A, Balossier G, Laurent-Maquin D, Pina S, Rebelo AHS, Faure J, et al. An in vitro biological and anti-bacterial study on a sol-gel derived silver-incorporated bioglass system. dental materials. 2008;24(10):1343–51.

[222] Bellantone M, Coleman NJ, Hench LL. Bacteriostatic action of a novel four-component bioactive glass. Journal of biomedical Materials Research. 2000;51(3):484–90.

[223] Bellantone M, Williams HD, Hench LL. Broad-spectrum bactericidal activity of Ag_2O-doped bioactive glass. Antimicrobial Agents and Chemotherapy. 2002;46(6):1940–5.

[224] Luo SH, Xiao W, Wei XJ, Jia WT, Zhang CQ, Huang WH, et al. In vitro evaluation of cytotoxicity of silver-containing borate bioactive glass. Journal of Biomedical Materials Research Part B: Applied Biomaterials. 2010;95(2):441–8.

[225] Efrima S, Bronk BV. Silver colloids impregnating or coating bacteria. The Journal of Physical Chemistry B. 1998;102(31):5947–50.

[226] Liau SY, Read DC, Pugh WJ, Furr JR, Russell AD. Interaction of silver nitrate with readily identifiable groups: relationship to the antibacterial action of silver ions. Letters in Applied Microbiology. 1997;25(4):279–83.

[227] Xynos ID, Edgar AJ, Buttery LDK, Hench LL, Polak JM. Ionic products of bioactive glass dissolution increase proliferation of human osteoblasts and induce insulin-like growth factor II mRNA expression and protein synthesis. Biochemical and Biophysical Research Communications. 2000;276(2):461–5.

[228] Hench LL, Wilson J. Surface-active biomaterials. Science. 1984;226(4675):630–6.

[229] Tsigkou O, Jones JR, Polak JM, Stevens MM. Differentiation of fetal osteoblasts and formation of mineralized bone nodules by 45S5 Bioglass® conditioned medium in the absence of osteogenic supplements. Biomaterials. 2009;30(21):3542–50.

[230] Krishnan V, Lakshmi T. Bioglass: a novel biocompatible innovation. Journal of Advanced Pharmaceutical Technology and Research. 2013;4(2):78–83.

[231] Froum SJ, Weinberg MA, Tarnow D. Comparison of bioactive glass synthetic bone graft particles and open debridement in the treatment of human periodontal defects. A clinical study. Journal of Periodontology. 1998;69(6):698–709.

[232] Anderegg CR, Alexander DC, Freidman M. A bioactive glass particulate in the treatment of molar furcation invasions. Journal of Periodontology. 1999;70(4):384–7.

[233] Froum S, Cho S-C, Rosenberg E, Rohrer M, Tarnow D. Histological comparison of healing extraction sockets implanted with bioactive glass or demineralized freeze-dried bone allograft: a pilot study. Journal of Periodontology. 2002;73(1):94–102.

[234] Peltola M, Aitasalo K, Suonpaa J, Varpula M, Yli-Urpo A. Bioactive glass S53P4 in frontal sinus obliteration: A long-term clinical experience. Head and Neck. 2006;28(9): 834–41.

[235] Hench LL, Paschall HA. Histochemical responses at a biomaterial's interface. Journal of Biomedical Materials Research. 1974;8(3):49–64.

[236] Izquierdo-Barba I, Arcos D, Sakamoto Y, Terasaki O, Lopez-Noriega A, Vallet-Regì Ma. High-performance mesoporous bioceramics mimicking bone mineralization. Chemistry of Materials. 2008;20(9):3191–8.

[237] Taylor A. 9 Therapeutic uses of trace elements. Clinics in Endocrinology and Metabolism. 1985;14(3):703–24.

[238] Gielen M, Tiekink ERT. Metallotherapeutic drugs and metal-based diagnostic agents: the use of metals in medicine. Chichester, UK: John Wiley & Sons; 2005.

[239] Dueland R, Spadaro JA, Rahn BA. Silver antibacterial bone cement: comparison with gentamicin in experimental osteomyelitis. Clinical Orthopaedics and Related Research. 1982;169:264–8.

[240] Yamamoto K, Ohashi S, Aono M, Kokubo T, Yamada I, Yamauchi J. Antibacterial activity of silver ions implanted in SiO_2 filler on oral streptococci. Dental Materials. 1996;12(4):227–9.

[241] Kim TN, Feng QL, Kim JO, Wu J, Wang H, Chen GC, et al. Antimicrobial effects of metal ions (Ag^+, Cu^{2+}, Zn^{2+}) in hydroxyapatite. Journal of Materials Science: Materials in Medicine. 1998;9(3):129–34.

[242] Kawashita M, Tsuneyama S, Miyaji F, Kokubo T, Kozuka H, Yamamoto K. Antibacterial silver-containing silica glass prepared by sol-gel method. Biomaterials. 2000;21(4): 393–8.

[243] Blaker JJ, Nazhat SN, Boccaccini AR. Development and characterisation of silver-doped bioactive-glass-coated sutures for tissue engineering and wound healing applications. Biomaterials. 2004;25(7):1319–29.

[244] Rupp ME, Fitzgerald T, Marion N, Helget V, Puumala S, Anderson JR, et al. Effect of silver-coated urinary catheters: efficacy, cost-effectiveness, and antimicrobial resistance. American Journal of Infection Control. 2004;32(8):445–50.

[245] Dubas ST, Kumlangdudsana P, Potiyaraj P. Layer-by-layer deposition of antimicrobial silver nanoparticles on textile fibers. Colloids and Surfaces A: Physicochemical and Engineering Aspects. 2006;289(1):105–9.

[246] Rivera-Garza M, Olguin MT, Garcia-Sosa I, Alcantara D, Rodriguez-Fuentes G. Silver supported on natural Mexican zeolite as an antibacterial material. Microporous and Mesoporous Materials. 2000;39(3):431–44.

[247] Park S-J, Jang Y-S. Preparation and characterization of activated carbon fibers supported with silver metal for antibacterial behavior. Journal of Colloid and Interface Science. 2003;261(2):238–43.

[248] Alt V, Bechert T, Steinrucke P, Wagener M, Seidel P, Dingeldein E, et al. An in vitro assessment of the antibacterial properties and cytotoxicity of nanoparticulate silver bone cement. Biomaterials. 2004;25(18):4383–91.

[249] Barralet J, Gbureck U, Habibovic P, Vorndran E, Gerard C, Doillon CJ. Angiogenesis in calcium phosphate scaffolds by inorganic copper ion release. Tissue Engineering Part A. 2009;15(7):1601–9.

[250] Habibovic P, Barralet JE. Bioinorganics and biomaterials: bone repair. Acta Biomaterialia. 2011;7(8):3013–26.

[251] Hench LL. Bioceramics. Journal of the American Ceramic Society. 1998;81(7):1705–28.

[252] Wilson J, Low SB. Bioactive ceramics for periodontal treatment: comparative studies in the Patus monkey. Journal of Applied Biomaterials. 1992;3(2):123–9.

[253] Hench LL, Polak JM, Xynos ID, Buttery LDK. Bioactive materials to control cell cycle. Material Research Innovations. 2000;3(6):313–23.

[254] Xynos ID, Edgar AJ, Buttery LDK, Hench LL, Polak JM. Gene-expression profiling of human osteoblasts following treatment with the ionic products of Bioglass® 45S5 dissolution. Journal of Biomedical Materials Research. 2001;55(2):151–7.

[255] Bielby RC, Christodoulou IS, Pryce RS, Radford WJP, Hench LL, Polak JM. Time-and concentration-dependent effects of dissolution products of 58S sol-gel bioactive glass on proliferation and differentiation of murine and human osteoblasts. Tissue Engineering. 2004;10(7–8):1018–26.

[256] Gough JE, Jones JR, Hench LL. Nodule formation and mineralisation of human primary osteoblasts cultured on a porous bioactive glass scaffold. Biomaterials. 2004;25(11): 2039–46.

[257] Bielby RC, Pryce RS, Hench LL, Polak JM. Enhanced derivation of osteogenic cells from murine embryonic stem cells after treatment with ionic dissolution products of 58S bioactive sol-gel glass. Tissue Engineering. 2005;11(3–4):479–88.

[258] Christodoulou I, Buttery LDK, Saravanapavan P, Tai G, Hench LL, Polak JM. Dose- and time-dependent effect of bioactive gel–glass ionic-dissolution products on human fetal osteoblast-specific gene expression. Journal of Biomedical Materials Research Part B: Applied Biomaterials. 2005;74(1):529–37.

[259] Christodoulou I, Buttery LDK, Tai G, Hench LL, Polak JM. Characterization of human fetal osteoblasts by microarray analysis following stimulation with 58S bioactive gel–glass ionic dissolution products. Journal of Biomedical Materials Research Part B: Applied Biomaterials. 2006;77(2):431–46.

[260] Day RM, Boccaccini AR, Shurey S, Roether JA, Forbes A, Hench LL, et al. Assessment of polyglycolic acid mesh and bioactive glass for soft-tissue engineering scaffolds. Biomaterials. 2004;25(27):5857–66.

[261] Jones JR, Ehrenfried LM, Saravanapavan P, Hench LL. Controlling ion release from bioactive glass foam scaffolds with antibacterial properties. Journal of Materials Science: Materials in Medicine. 2006;17(11):989–96.

[262] Gorustovich AA, Roether JA, Boccaccini AR. Effect of bioactive glasses on angiogenesis: a review of in vitro and in vivo evidences. Tissue Engineering Part B: Reviews. 2009;16(2):199–207.

[263] Yazar M, Sarban S, Kocyigit A, Isikan UE. Synovial fluid and plasma selenium, copper, zinc, and iron concentrations in patients with rheumatoid arthritis and osteoarthritis. Biological Trace Element Research. 2005;106(2):123–32.

[264] Jebahi S, Oudadesse H, Saleh GB, Saoudi M, Mesadhi S, Rebai T, et al. Chitosan-based bioglass composite for bone tissue healing: oxidative stress status and antiosteoporotic performance in a ovariectomized rat model. Korean Journal of Chemical Engineering. 2014;31(9):1616–23.

[265] Balasubramanian P, Strobel LA, Kneser U, Boccaccini AR. Zinc-containing bioactive glasses for bone regeneration, dental and orthopedic applications. Biomedical Glasses. 2015;1(1):51–69.

[266] Mosbahi S, Oudadesse H, Wers E, Trigui M, Lefeuvre B, Roiland C, et al. Study of bioactive glass ceramic for use as bone biomaterial in vivo: investigation by nuclear magnetic resonance and histology. Ceramics International. 2016;42(4):4827–36.

[267] Vaughan J. The physiology of bone. 3rd ed. Oxford: Clarendon Press; 1981.

[268] Curzon MEJ. The relation between caries prevalence and strontium concentrations in drinking water, plaque, and surface enamel. Journal of Dental Research. 1985;64(12): 1386–8.

[269] Marie PJ, Hott M, Modrowski D, De Pollak C, Guillemain J, Deloffre P, et al. An uncoupling agent containing strontium prevents bone loss by depressing bone resorption and maintaining bone formation in estrogen-deficient rats. Journal of Bone and Mineral Research. 2005;20(6):1065–74.

[270] Canalis E, Hott M, Deloffre P, Tsouderos Y, Marie PJ. The divalent strontium salt S12911 enhances bone cell replication and bone formation in vitro. Bone. 1996;18(6):517–23.

[271] Baron R, Tsouderos Y. In vitro effects of S12911-2 on osteoclast function and bone marrow macrophage differentiation. European Journal of Pharmacology. 2002;450(1): 11–7.

[272] Reginster J-Y, Felsenberg D, Boonen S, Diez-Perez A, Rizzoli R, Brandi M-L, et al. Effects of long-term strontium ranelate treatment on the risk of nonvertebral and vertebral fractures in postmenopausal osteoporosis: results of a five-year, randomized, placebo-controlled trial. Arthritis and Rheumatism. 2008;58(6):1687–95.

[273] Poh PSP, Hutmacher DW, Stevens MM, Woodruff MA. Fabrication and in vitro characterization of bioactive glass composite scaffolds for bone regeneration. Biofabrication. 2013;5(4):045005.

[274] Jebahi S, Oudadesse H, El Feki H, Rebai T, Keskes H, Pellen P, et al. Antioxidative/oxidative effects of strontium-doped bioactive glass as bone graft. In vivo assays in ovariectomised rats. Journal of Applied Biomedicine. 2012;10(4):195–209.

[275] Santocildes-Romero ME, Crawford A, Hatton PV, Goodchild RL, Reaney IM, Miller CA. The osteogenic response of mesenchymal stromal cells to strontium-substituted bioactive glasses. Journal of Tissue Engineering and Regenerative Medicine. 2015;9(5): 619–31.

[276] Jebahi S, Oudadesse H, Abdessalem N, Keskes H, Rebai T, el Feki H, et al. Comparative study of bone microarchitactural structure after porous bioglass and Strontium doped bioactive glass bone graft in Wistar rat model. Journal of Scientific and Innovative Research. 2014;3(1):16–20.

[277] Lao J, Nedelec J-M, Jallot E. New strontium-based bioactive glasses: physicochemical reactivity and delivering capability of biologically active dissolution products. Journal of Materials Chemistry. 2009;19(19):2940–9.

[278] Wu C, Zhou Y, Xu M, Han P, Chen L, Chang J, et al. Copper-containing mesoporous bioactive glass scaffolds with multifunctional properties of angiogenesis capacity, osteostimulation and antibacterial activity. Biomaterials. 2013;34(2):422–33.

[279] Wang H, Zhao S, Zhou J, Shen Y, Huang W, Zhang C, et al. Evaluation of borate bioactive glass scaffolds as a controlled delivery system for copper ions in stimulating osteogenesis and angiogenesis in bone healing. Journal of Materials Chemistry B. 2014;2(48):8547–57.

[280] Rath SN, Brandl A, Hiller D, Hoppe A, Gbureck U, Horch RE, et al. Bioactive copper-doped glass scaffolds can stimulate endothelial cells in co-culture in combination with mesenchymal stem cells. PLoS One. 2014;9(12):e113319.

[281] Kong N, Lin K, Li H, Chang J. Synergy effects of copper and silicon ions on stimulation of vascularization by copper-doped calcium silicate. Journal of Materials Chemistry B. 2014;2(8):1100–10.

[282] Gristina AG. Biomaterial-centered infection: microbial adhesion versus tissue integration. Science. 1987;237(4822):1588–95.

[283] Matsuura T, Abe Y, Sato Y, Okamoto K, Ueshige M, Akagawa Y. Prolonged antimicrobial effect of tissue conditioners containing silver-zeolite. Journal of Dentistry. 1997;25(5):373–7.

[284] Gatter N, Kohnen W, Jansen B. In vitro efficacy of a hydrophilic central venous catheter loaded with silver to prevent microbial colonization. Zentralblatt für Bakteriologie. 1998;287(1):157–69.

[285] Adams AP, Santschi EM, Mellencamp MA. Antibacterial properties of a silver chloride-coated nylon wound dressing. Veterinary Surgery. 1999;28(4):219–25.

[286] George N, Faoagali J, Muller M. Silvazine™ (silver sulfadiazine and chlorhexidine) activity against 200 clinical isolates. Burns. 1997;23(6):493–5.

[287] Gupta A, Silver S. Molecular genetics: silver as a biocide: will resistance become a problem? Nature Biotechnology. 1998;16(10):888.

[288] El-Kady AM, Ali AF, Rizk RA, Ahmed MM. Synthesis, characterization and microbiological response of silver doped bioactive glass nanoparticles. Ceramics International. 2012;38(1):177–88.

[289] Newby PJ, El-Gendy R, Kirkham J, Yang XB, Thompson ID, Boccaccini AR. Ag-doped 45S5 Bioglass®-based bone scaffolds by molten salt ion exchange: processing and characterisation. Journal of Materials Science: Materials in Medicine. 2011;22(3):557–69.

[290] Lohbauer U, Jell G, Saravanapavan P, Jones JR, Hench LL. Indirect cytotoxicity evaluation of silver doped bioglass Ag-S70C30 on human primary keratinocytes. Key Engineering Materials. 2005;284:431–4.

[291] Lin H, Zhang J, Qu F, Jiang J, Jiang P. In vitro hydroxyapatite-forming ability and antimicrobial properties of mesoporous bioactive glasses doped with Ti/Ag. Journal of Nanomaterials. 2013;2013:24.

[292] Wang H, Zhao S, Cui X, Pan Y, Huang W, Ye S, et al. Evaluation of three-dimensional silver-doped borate bioactive glass scaffolds for bone repair: biodegradability, biocompatibility, and antibacterial activity. Journal of Materials Research. 2015;30(18): 2722–35.

[293] Westendorf JJ, Kahler RA, Schroeder TM. Wnt signaling in osteoblasts and bone diseases. Gene. 2004;341:19–39.

[294] Kengaku M, Capdevila J, Rodriguez-Esteban C, De La Pena J, Johnson RL, Belmonte JCI, et al. Distinct WNT pathways regulating AER formation and dorsoventral polarity in the chick limb bud. Science. 1998;280(5367):1274–7.

[295] Hartmann C, Tabin CJ. Dual roles of Wnt signaling during chondrogenesis in the chicken limb. Development. 2000;127(14):3141–59.

[296] Katoh M. WNT and FGF gene clusters (review). International Journal of Oncology. 2002;21(6):1269–73.

[297] Secreto FJ, Hoeppner LH, Westendorf JJ. Wnt signaling during fracture repair. Current Osteoporosis Reports. 2009;7(2):64–9.

[298] Spencer GJ, Utting JC, Etheridge SL, Arnett TR, Genever PG. Wnt signalling in osteoblasts regulates expression of the receptor activator of $NF_{K}B$ ligand and inhibits osteoclastogenesis in vitro. Journal of Cell Science. 2006;119(7):1283–96.

[299] Chen Q-Z, Rezwan K, Francon V, Armitage D, Nazhat SN, Jones FH, et al. Surface functionalization of Bioglass®-derived porous scaffolds. Acta Biomaterialia. 2007;3(4): 551–62.

[300] Edgington JM, Bandyopadhyay A, Bose S. In vitro characterization of lithium-doped tricalcium phosphate for bone graft. Society for Biomaterials. 2011:Abstract #727.

[301] Phiel CJ, Klein PS. Molecular targets of lithium action. Annual Review of Pharmacology and Toxicology. 2001;41(1):789–813.

[302] Zhang F, Phiel CJ, Spece L, Gurvich N, Klein PS. Inhibitory phosphorylation of glycogen synthase kinase-3 (GSK-3) in response to lithium Evidence for autoregulation of GSK-3. Journal of Biological Chemistry. 2003;278(35):33067–77.

[303] Noble W, Planel E, Zehr C, Olm V, Meyerson J, Suleman F, et al. Inhibition of glycogen synthase kinase-3 by lithium correlates with reduced tauopathy and degeneration in vivo. Proceedings of the National Academy of Sciences of the United States of America. 2005;102(19):6990–5.

[304] Clement-Lacroix P, Ai M, Morvan F, Roman-Roman S, Vayssiere B, Belleville C, et al. Lrp5-independent activation of Wnt signaling by lithium chloride increases bone formation and bone mass in mice. Proceedings of the National Academy of Sciences of the United States of America. 2005;102(48):17406–11.

[305] Kavitha RJ, Subha B, Shanmugam S, Ravichandran K. Synthesis and in vitro characterisation of lithium doped bioactive glass through quick alkali sol-gel method. International Journal of Innovative Research in Science and Engineering. 2014;1(2): 2347–3207.

[306] Miguez-Pacheco V, Buttner T, Macon ALB, Jones JR, Fey T, de Ligny D, et al. Development and characterization of lithium-releasing silicate bioactive glasses and their scaffolds for bone repair. Journal of Non-Crystalline Solids. 2016;432:65–72.

[307] Gorustovich AA, Lopez JMP, Guglielmotti MB, Cabrini RL. Biological performance of boron-modified bioactive glass particles implanted in rat tibia bone marrow. Biomedical Materials. 2006;1(3):100.

[308] Floroian L. Biocompatibility and physical properties of doped bioactive glass ceramics. Bulletin of the Transilvania University of Brasov. 2010;3:52.

[309] Smith JM, Martin RA, Cuello GJ, Newport RJ. Structural characterisation of hypoxia-mimicking bioactive glasses. Journal of Materials Chemistry B. 2013;1(9):1296–303.

[310] Dietrich E, Oudadesse H, Lucas-Girot A, Mami M. In vitro bioactivity of melt-derived glass 46S6 doped with magnesium. Journal of Biomedical Materials Research Part A. 2009;88(4):1087–96.

[311] Prabhu M, Ruby Priscilla S, Kavitha K, Manivasakan P, Rajendran V, Kulandaivelu P. In vitro bioactivity and antimicrobial tuning of bioactive glass nanoparticles added

with neem (*Azadirachta indica*) leaf powder. BioMed Research International. 2014;2014:Article ID 950691.

[312] Hench LL, Andersson OG. Bioactive glass coatings. In: Hench LL, Wilson J, editors. An introduction to bioceramics. Singapore: World Scientific; 1993. p. 239–59.

[313] Gomez-Vega JM, Saiz E, Tomsia AP, Marshall GW, Marshall SJ. Bioactive glass coatings with hydroxyapatite and Bioglass® particles on Ti-based implants. 1. Processing. Biomaterials. 2000;21(2):105–11.

[314] Lopez-Esteban S, Saiz E, Fujino S, Oku T, Suganuma K, Tomsia AP. Bioactive glass coatings for orthopedic metallic implants. Journal of the European Ceramic Society. 2003;23(15):2921–30.

[315] Pratten J, Nazhat SN, Blaker JJ, Boccaccini AR. In vitro attachment of Staphylococcus epidermidis to surgical sutures with and without Ag-containing bioactive glass coating. Journal of Biomaterials Applications. 2004;19(1):47–57.

[316] Xie X-H, Yu X-W, Zeng S-X, Du R-L, Hu Y-H, Yuan Z, et al. Enhanced osteointegration of orthopaedic implant gradient coating composed of bioactive glass and nanohydroxyapatite. Journal of Materials Science: Materials in Medicine. 2010;21(7):2165–73.

[317] Wang X, Li X, Onuma K, Ito A, Sogo Y, Kosuge K, et al. Mesoporous bioactive glass coatings on stainless steel for enhanced cell activity, cytoskeletal organization and AsMg immobilization. Journal of Materials Chemistry. 2010;20(31):6437–45.

[318] Mistry S, Kundu D, Datta S, Basu D. Comparison of bioactive glass coated and hydroxyapatite coated titanium dental implants in the human jaw bone. Australian Dental Journal. 2011;56(1):68–75.

[319] Drnovsek N, Novak S, Dragin U, Ceh M, Gorensek M, Gradisar M. Bioactive glass enhances bone ingrowth into the porous titanium coating on orthopaedic implants. International Orthopaedics. 2012;36(8):1739–45.

[320] Soundrapandian C, Bharati S, Basu D, Datta S. Studies on novel bioactive glasses and bioactive glass-nano-HAp composites suitable for coating on metallic implants. Ceramics International. 2011;37(3):759–69.

[321] Pishbin F, Mourino V, Gilchrist JB, McComb DW, Kreppel S, Salih V, et al. Single-step electrochemical deposition of antimicrobial orthopaedic coatings based on a bioactive glass/chitosan/nano-silver composite system. Acta Biomaterialia. 2013;9(7):7469–79.

[322] Pourhashem S, Afshar A. Double layer bioglass-silica coatings on 316L stainless steel by sol-gel method. Ceramics International. 2014;40(1):993–1000.

[323] Keshaw H, Forbes A, Day RM. Release of angiogenic growth factors from cells encapsulated in alginate beads with bioactive glass. Biomaterials. 2005;26(19):4171–9.

[324] Leach JK, Kaigler D, Wang Z, Krebsbach PH, Mooney DJ. Coating of VEGF-releasing scaffolds with bioactive glass for angiogenesis and bone regeneration. Biomaterials. 2006;27(17):3249–55.

[325] Zhang Y, Cheng N, Miron R, Shi B, Cheng X. Delivery of PDGF-B and BMP-7 by mesoporous bioglass/silk fibrin scaffolds for the repair of osteoporotic defects. Biomaterials. 2012;33(28):6698–708.

[326] Zhang Y, Miron RJ, Li S, Shi B, Sculean A, Cheng X. Novel mesoporous bioGlass/silk scaffold containing adPDGF-B and adBMP7 for the repair of periodontal defects in beagle dogs. Journal of Clinical Periodontology. 2015;42(3):262–71.

[327] Zhao S, Li L, Wang H, Zhang Y, Cheng X, Zhou N, et al. Wound dressings composed of copper-doped borate bioactive glass microfibers stimulate angiogenesis and heal full-thickness skin defects in a rodent model. Biomaterials. 2015;53:379–91.

Chapter 14

Aptamer-Mediated Selective Protein Affinity to Improve Scaffold Biocompatibility

Ludovica Parisi, Carlo Galli, Lisa Elviri, Annalisa Bianchera, Paola Lagonegro, Simone Lumetti, Edoardo Manfredi and Guido Maria Macaluso

Additional information is available at the end of the chapter

http://dx.doi.org/10.5772/63265

Abstract

Protein adsorption on surfaces occurs shortly after scaffold insertion. This process is of pivotal importance to achieve therapeutic success in tissue engineering (TE), and favorable proteins should be adsorbed at the interface without unfolding to preserve their structure and function. Protein misfolding at the interface is a common phenomenon, which can impair cell adhesion and scaffold colonization. Many efforts have been done to improve scaffold biocompatibility by ameliorating protein adsorption, but with poor results. In the present chapter, we propose the use of a novel class of molecules, aptamers, to improve scaffold biocompatibility. Aptamers are small, single stranded oligonucleotides, which specifically bind to a target molecule: they work as antibodies, but without many of the drawbacks associated to the use of antibodies. We propose to immobilize aptamers on scaffolds to retain specific proteins, acting as docking points to guide cell activity. In particular, we show the results obtained by enriching different polymeric scaffolds with aptamers against human fibronectin, a naturally abundant protein in tissues, which plays a pivotal role in cell adhesion. We demonstrate that scaffold enrichment with aptamers lead to a better colonization of the substrate from cells. The results we obtained pave the way to the possibility of further investigating the role of aptamers as useful molecules to improve scaffold biocompatibility in the contest of tissue engineering.

Keywords: aptamers, biocompatibility, fibronectin, scaffold, SELEX, tissue engineering

1. Introduction

Regenerative medicine (RM) is a therapeutic approach that aims to restore structure and function of damaged tissues and organs, in particular to find a solution for those that become permanently damaged and untreatable [1].

RM can be potentially applied to different tissues [2], and one of the most promising fields is that related to bone [3, 4].

Tissue regeneration is a complex task that encompasses completely restoring the lost structure, including its micro-architecture and consequently its functionality. As for bone regeneration, optimal healing is achieved when certain prerequisites are met, namely, osteoinduction, osteoconduction, osteogenesis, and mechanical stability [5].

Osteoinduction is the process that allows the recruitment and stimulation of immature pre-osteoblastic cells to mature osteoblasts and to produce new bone [6]. This phenomenon is regulated by a class of molecules known as inductive agents, mainly represented by bone morphogenetic proteins (BMPs) [3]. As a consequence of osteoinduction, osteogenesis can be achieved. Osteogenesis is carried out by osteoblasts, and consists in the formation of new bone. To improve the outcome of bone regeneration, biomaterials are often used to fill the gaps created by lost tissue. Such biomaterials must be osteoconductive, i.e., capable of supporting bone deposition on their surface [6]. Finally, mechanical stability of the healing site is the fourth factor to consider in order to reach regeneration of sound bone and avoid formation of fibrous tissue [5].

RM for bone tissue currently includes four approaches: molecular, cellular, use of bone substitutes, and tissue engineering (TE).

Progresses in molecular biology and a deeper knowledge of the mechanisms of fracture healing at a molecular level have allowed for the identification of a large number of key molecules that can be used locally or systematically to enhance bone repair [7]. Autologous cells can be an alternative or complementary choice for healing bone fracture. Mesenchymal stem cells (MSCs) have been proposed as a useful in regenerative interventions. MSCs can be collected from bone marrow [8], from peripheral blood [9], or from adipose tissue [10, 11]. Further possibilities to harvest MSCs in dental applications could be other types of stem cells directly isolated from oral tissues such as the dental pulp (DPSCs) or the periodontal ligament (PDLSCs) [12–14]. As mentioned before, biomaterials have also been proposed as a tool to provide a substrate for new bone cells to deposit new bone, acting as gap fillers and osteoconductive scaffold. A wide number of synthetic bone substitutes are now available including hydroxyapatite (HA), β-tricalcium phosphate (β-TCP), and calcium-phosphate cements, glass ceramics, and biocompatible metals [15, 16].

These different approaches are often combined and the investigation of the optimal conditions and tools to regenerate a tissue created a field called tissue engineering.

http://dx.doi.org/10.5772/63265

1.1. Tissue engineering

Tissue engineering (TE) was first defined in 1988 at the first *TE symposium* in California, as *"an interdisciplinary field of research that applies the principles of engineering and the life sciences towards the development of biological substitutes that restore, maintain and improve tissue function"*. It has been demonstrated that TE offers great potential in clinical applications [17, 18], and, in particular, bone tissue engineering seems to harbor a great potential. At present, bioabsorbable scaffolds combined with bone-marrow aspirate and osteoinductive factors (BMPs) have yielded promising results [16], and, more recently, the applicability of a β-TCP scaffold seeded with autogenous bone-marrow cells for bone reconstruction has been shown in a sheep model [19]. Moreover, TE has been used to improve fracture healing and to augment the bone-prosthesis interface in arthroplasty, with promising results and safety [20, 21].

1.1.1. Scaffold

Scaffolds are a central concept in TE. They are 3D porous structures designed to promote cell adhesion, proliferation, and extracellular matrix deposition in order to allow for the restoration of damaged tissue [22].

Scaffolds can be divided into biological and synthetic materials. Biological scaffolds are derived from human and animal tissues, whereas synthetic ones are made of artificial biomaterials [23]. As materials of biological origin, although often possessing favorable characteristics, suffer from scarce availability, safety concerns and sometimes possibility of inflammatory or even immune responses, synthetic biomaterials have been the center of increasing attention. The state of art on scaffolds has evolved over the last years and involves the employment of natural or synthetic polymers. Collagen is the most abundant polymer in tissues and, as a consequence, among the most investigated material for the production of natural-derived scaffolds [24–26]. Together with collagen, chitosan, alginate, and cellulose are promising biomaterial for bone tissue engineering applications [27–30]. Among the synthetic polymers used for scaffold fabrication, polylactic-co-glycolic acid (PLGA) and polycaprolactone (PCL) are probably the most studied [31]. However, their characteristics for TE applications are still suboptimal compared with those of natural polymers [4]. Alternatively to the use of polymers, calcium phosphate, apatite forms, and bioglasses find wide application in bone engineering [32]. Regardless of their chemistry, the main feature scaffolds should possess is biocompatibility.

2. Biocompatibility

The concept of biocompatibility is widely used within biomaterial science, but it is still uncertain what it really means. When it was first used in the early 1940s, a material was considered biocompatible if it could be placed in contact with tissues without altering them: a biocompatible material was conceived to be ideally inert. However, as research progressively revealed that a true biological inertia is not possible, because any thing that enters in contact with a tissue induces a non-self response from the host immune system, the concept of biocompatibility had to be necessarily reviewed. For years materials were considered biocompatible if they were non-toxic, non-immunogenic, non-carcinogenic, non-irritant, and so on against human body. During the 1980s, new evidences brought about another change of view and lead to a more modern definition of biocompatibility. First, it was clear that materials always react with tissues and that they are not inert. Second, it was shown that biological responses to biomaterial are different across tissues, and that the tissue itself affects material biocompatibility. Third, the scientific community realized that some clinical situation require that materials get degraded and removed from the host after accomplishing their function [33]. Accordingly to these concepts, a widely accepted definition of biocompatibility was outlined at the Consensus Conference in Boston in 1987 as follows: "Biocompatibility refers to the ability of a material to perform with an appropriate host response in a specific situation" [34].

In conclusion, focusing on this definition, a material is inserted into a tissue to perform a function, not simply lie inertly, and tissue responses to the material have to be adequate to the specific desired applications [35].

Biocompatibility as defined above is a pivotal concept for TE and scaffolds fabrication. A scaffold can be considered for *in vivo* application if it has been proven to be biocompatible *in vitro*, i.e., if it can support cell adhesion and proliferation. Cellular responses, in turn, heavily depend on protein adsorption on the scaffold surface. Protein adsorption on materials is a spontaneous phenomenon that can be accompanied by protein denaturation, i.e., alteration of protein conformation and function [36]. Protein denaturation on to surfaces may occur for different reasons, mainly due to the chemical and physical characteristics of the material, and for that, a series of methods to enhance the biocompatibility of the surfaces have been developed.

2.1. Modern approaches to enhance scaffold biocompatibility

It has been solidly established that shortly after implantation biomaterials are covered with a thin layer of host proteins, and it is believed that the state of adsorbed proteins play a key role in scaffold colonization from cells [37]. Therefore, controlling the amount, composition and conformation of adsorbed proteins is a viable approach to obtain a highly biocompatible surface [38]. In recent years, several strategies have been developed to guide protein adsorption and thus to improve cell adhesion, including immobilizing short fragment or proteins on scaffolds, or chemically and physically modifying scaffold surfaces.

2.1.1. Chemical and physical treatments

It has been demonstrated that some proteins bind preferentially certain chemical groups. For example it has been shown that fibrinogen binds methyl (–CH3) functionalized surfaces, but not carboxy (–COOH) ones, whereas the hydroxy (–OH) groups enhance the affinity for albumin over fibrinogen [39–41]. Therefore, the first strategy developed to control protein adsorption on scaffolds was enriching surfaces with functional groups, by combining chemical and physical treatments.

http://dx.doi.org/10.5772/63265

Chemical graft modification entails surface activation through different methods, such as chemical reactions or UV, plasma, and ozone exposure [42], followed by covalent grafting of the desired functional groups. Chemical grafting has been used to improve hemocompatibility of vascular grafts by enriching them with heparin and polyethylene glycol (PEG or PEO). The drawbacks of this approach include the loss of protein mobility at the material surface, because they are covalently bound and the possible release of toxic monomers [38].

To overcome issues associated to chemical graft deposition, self-assembled monolayers (SAMs) were developed. SAMs was widely used to study *in vivo* responses of implanted biomaterials in the past, although nowadays is limited to gold- and silver-coated surfaces [38, 43, 44].

An increasingly popular method to graft surfaces with functional groups is plasma modification. Plasma is considered the fourth state of matter and it is obtained when gases are excited by specific electromagnetic frequencies. Plasma modification is cheap and seems to be very effective, but it is still being currently investigated for the development of biomedical devices, including metals, polymers, and ceramics [38, 45].

2.1.2. *Immobilization of RGD and other recognition sequences for integrins*

One of the most recent approaches developed to enhance scaffold biocompatibility is the surface immobilization of small peptides able to mimic proteins involved in cell adhesion, to enrich scaffolds with docking points for cells (Ruoslahti, 1996). The best investigated peptide is the arginine-glycine-aspartic acid (RGD) motif, an ubiquitous adhesive sequence found in many ECM proteins responsible for their interaction with cellular integrin receptors [46]. Several groups have studied the *in vitro* ability of RGD and related motifs to improve osteoblast adhesion, migration, and gene expression [47–49]. Moreover, coating titanium implants with the RGD peptide has been shown to induce a direct activation of macrophages, osteoblasts, and osteoclasts in rat tibia and femur and in dog femur [50–52].

However, Hennessy et al. enriched hyaluronic acid disks with RGD and observed poor cell adhesion and inhibitory effects of the RGD binding domain, probably due to the fast adsorption of fibronectin, vitronectin and fibrinogen within 30 min, which competed with RGD motifs to bind integrins [53].

2.1.3. *Surface coatings*

The application of coatings that mimic the ECM could be an alternative method to improving scaffold biocompatibility. In particular, coatings for bone biomaterials should promote the creation of a suitable environment for osteoblast, osteoclasts, and progenitor cells, that promote implant integration, by improving bone/implant contact (BIC) [46]. Coating titanium implants with collagen, which is the most abundant protein in bone tissue, supports *in vitro* adhesion, migration, and differentiation of osteoblasts [54, 55]. Similarly, coatings of hydroxyapatite-based scaffold with chondroitin sulfate (CS), wide spread in cancellous and cortical bone, Hyaluronic acid (HA) or heparin have demonstrated to increase BMPs secretion and consequently osteoblasts differentiation [56, 57].

All the issues connected to the strategy described, prompted us to develop a new method to enhance scaffold biocompatibility by using a novel class of molecules, called aptamers, to improve protein adsorption and cell adhesion.

3. Aptamers

In the 1980s molecular virology revealed that small structured oligonucleotides could bind proteins with high affinity and specificity. That evidence supported the use of oligonucleotides as specific receptors, which 10 years later lead to the discovery of aptamers [58]. The word “aptamer” was first used in 1990 by Ellington and Szostak to describe small RNAs molecules able to bind small organic dyes. It derives from the fusion of the Latin expression “aptus”, which means “to fit”, and the Greek word “meros”, which means “part” [59]. Since then, aptamers have been defined as short oligonucleotides that by adopting specific 3D conformations are able to bind specific and selected targets [60].

Aptamers are mostly short single-stranded or double-stranded DNA or RNA oligonucleotides, usually 20–80 bp long and 6–30 kDa heavy. Aptamers are constituted of a random sequence region at center, flanked by constant designed primer binding sites and the 3′ and 5′ ends. The sequence region in the center is necessary for target recognition (**Figure 1**), which occurs after aptamer 3D adaptation. In this phenomenon intermolecular interactions, such as Van der Waals forces, hydrogen and electrostatic interactions, stabilize the bond between aptamers and their ligands [61, 62]. The aptamers-ligands interactions are highly specific and capable to discriminate among analogues, i.e., enantioselective aptamers have 12.000-fold higher affinity for L-arginine than for D-arginine [63].

Aptamers are thought to be an excellent alternative to the use of monoclonal antibodies (mAB). Compared with antibodies, aptamers overcome their issues and improve their clinical applicability and suitability for industrialization. First of all, aptamers are low-immunogenic and low-toxic molecules, and they are not directly recognized by the human immune system as foreign agents [64–66]. Unlike antibodies, aptamers have a wider target range, they are smaller so that they can easily penetrate into tissue barriers and cells [67]; moreover they can also bind small ligands, such as ions and small molecules, which cannot be recognized by antibodies [68]. Furthermore, aptamers are thermally stable, and can undergo repeated cycles of denaturation/renaturation without damaging their binding efficiency. Finally, aptamer production and eventually modification is cheaper, easier and faster than that of mAB [68].

The interest of research on aptamers is increasing, as shown by the publication rate on this topic, which has exponentially grown in 25 years [61], leading to more than 5500 published articles in the PubMed database including the term “aptamer” in January 2016. In spite of their popularity, their clinical applications are still limited [62], and as of today only one aptamer-based drug has been approved by the US Food and Drug Administration (FDA). Pfizer/Eyetech launched Macugen, a RNA aptamer against VEGF (vascular endothelial growth factor) for the treatment of wet age-related macular degeneration in 2004 [69]. Barriers to the commercialization of aptamers are essentially two. The former is that some *in vitro* generated aptamers do

http://dx.doi.org/10.5772/63265

not elicit a comparable *in vivo* comparable, whereas the latter is that the SELEX process is time-consuming and not very efficient [62]. In spite of these issues, a recent market report projected the global aptamer market to $5.4 billion by 2019 [70].

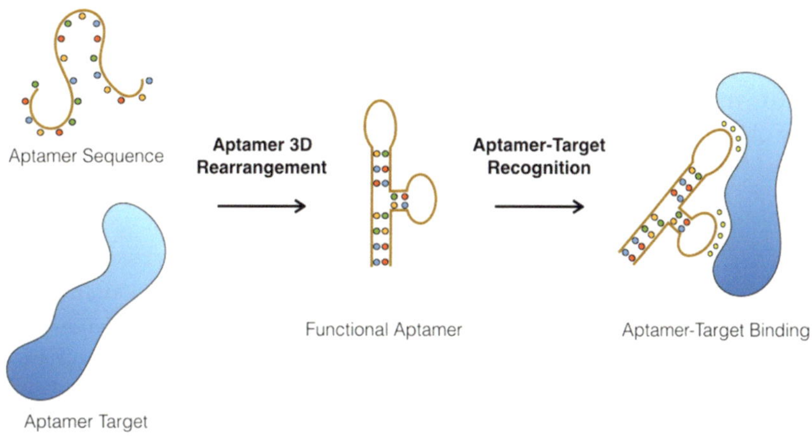

Figure 1. Diagram representing aptamer 3D conformational rearrangement in the presence of the target to form aptamer-target specific complex.

3.1. Aptamers generation

Aptamer selection requires two steps: upstream screening and downstream screening. The upstream screening step identifies full-length aptamers through SELEX (Systematic Evolution of Ligands by EXponential Enrichment), whereas the downstream step aims to isolate the shortest oligonucleotide sequence required for target binding [61].

3.1.1. Upstream screening

In vitro selection or SELEX (Systematic Evolutions of Ligands by EXponential enrichment) is the technique used to isolate aptamers, which was first described by Ellington and Gold in 1990 [59, 71].

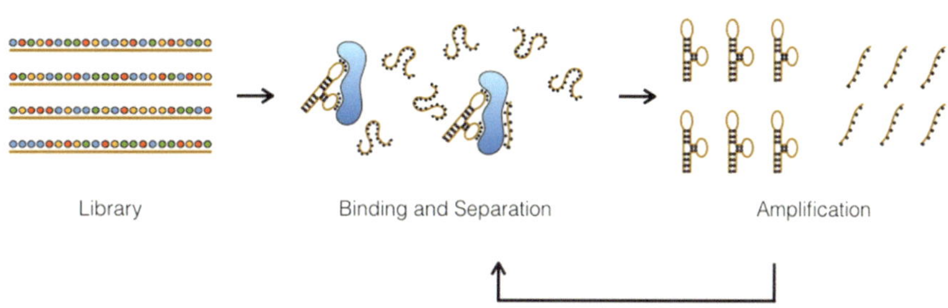

Figure 2. Schematic representation of the SELEX process steps.

The SELEX process consists of three steps, which are then repeated to screen for sequences with higher affinity (**Figure 2**) [58]: (a) the preparation of an initial oligonucleotides pool (library) is followed by (b) the selection of aptamer candidates and by (c) their amplification.

3.1.1.1. Library generation

The whole SELEX process starts with the generation of a synthetic oligonucleotides library, which consists of a pool of ~10^{12} –10^{15} different nucleic acid (ssDNA or RNA) sequences, theoretically able to bind any target molecule. Each sequence represents a possible aptamer candidate and it possesses a central random region, ~25–30 bp long, flanked by two standard primers at the 3′ and 5′ ends [61, 62].

Both ssDNA and RNA libraries can be created and divided in five types, on the basis of the collected sequences. Standard libraries are the most common ones and contain random 20–60 bp long oligonucleotides. Structurally constrained libraries contain oligonucleotides with stable regions, which help aptamers to fold according to a certain secondary structure. Libraries based on a known sequence are constructed by inserting known sequences in the central part of the oligonucleotide. Finally, libraries based on genomic sequences (genomic SELEX) are created by digesting genomic DNA, to find proteins capable to bind it [72].

3.1.1.2. Binding and separation

Once the library is generated, it is incubated with the target. Some of the oligonucleotides in the pool recognize the target and are then considered aptamers (partitioning), whereas unbound sequences are filtered out from the solution (elution) [61].

Several methods are used to discriminate aptamers from other oligonucleotides. The SELEX approach initially employed by Gold and co-workers was based on a nitrocellulose membrane where the T4 DNA polymerase was immobilized [71]. Nowadays, the use of a nitrocellulose membrane is quite out of order because it has some limitations, such as the inability to bind any molecules but proteins and the need to perform at least 12 selection rounds [73, 74]. Alternative strategies have then been developed based on common biochemistry techniques. Chromatographic affinity or magnetic columns are often used for aptamer selection. In the case of chromatographic affinity column, the immobile phase is composed of agarose beads and the targets are immobilized through tags with proteins, such as glutathione *S*-transferase (GST) or His-tag, or through chemical reaction with other molecules. Several aptamers have been selected through this method, however it cannot be applied if the target lacks the tags or the functional group requested for the coupling with the column [75–77]. On the other hand, targets can be immobilized on the surface of magnetic beads and used in magnetic columns, a strategy that is becoming more and more powerful due to the ease of separating aptamers from other nucleotides only by a magnet [78–80]. Furthermore, capillary electrophoresis has been proposed, because of its speed and high resolution. In fact a successful selection of aptamers can be obtained in a few rounds, i.e., Bowser and co-workers selected aptamer against neuropeptide Y and against human IgE in only four rounds [81, 82]. In addition to the methods described above, aptamers against whole cells have been recently selected through the Cell-SELEX method. This technique is complex, because cells cannot be immobilized, unlike target molecules; however, several research groups have been successful. Kobatake's group identified the SBC3, a cell lung cancer cell line with a ssDNA aptamers [83]. Previously, Tan's group selected a series of aptamers able to bind two types of ovarian cancer cells [84], whereas Gold et al. isolated an aptamer for the U251 cell line derived from glioblastomas just in 2003 [85].

Further strategies have been implemented to improve SELEX performance, although their efficiency in selecting aptamers is not still clear.

3.1.1.3. Amplification

After the separation of aptamers from a specific nucleotides, they are amplified by PCR, in the case of ssDNA aptamers, or by RT-PCR in the case of RNA aptamers. Consequently, products of amplification are used as a new sub-library for the following selection round [62].

3.1.2. Downstream screening

After the upstream screening or SELEX, selected aptamers are generally ~80 bp long, but the binding region is actually usually 10–15 nucleotides long [68, 86]. As a consequence, redundant and useless nucleotides can be deleted through a process called "aptamer truncation". Many strategies have been tested to minimize aptamer sequences without damaging its binding ability. Most of these strategies are predictive and based on computational biology. Giangrande et al. were able to truncate an RNA aptamer against PSMA (prostate-specific membrane antigen) while preserving its binding activity and functionality, using structure simulations and target docking algorithms. Partial fragmentation was used by Green et al. to select the shortest sequence of DNA aptamers to bind PDGF (platelet-derived growth factor) [87]. Wang and co-workers detected the non-essential region of the hPTK7 (anti-human protein tyrosine kinase 7), hybridized them with complementary oligonucleotides probes [88]; the same approach was used by Duan and co-workers to select the basic region of anti-CD133 aptamer as marker for cancer stem cells [89].

All the methods described for aptamer truncation are effective; however, their application is hindered by their complexity, length, and cost [61].

3.2. Biomedical applications of aptamers

The similarities between aptamers and mABs lead to their applications in various field, including research tools [90], bioassays [91, 92], food safety [93], and environment monitoring [94], as demonstrated by a plethora of reviews recently published on this topic. However, a major field of interest for aptamers is biomedicine, where aptamers can be used as sensors for biomarker discovery, molecular imaging probes, drug delivery systems and drugs, especially in cancer nanomedicine and therapy [58, 61].

3.2.1. Aptamers as potential drugs

Although the most studied aptamers are against thrombin, VEGF and PDGF, aptamer applications range from cancer to infectious pathogens.

3.2.1.1. Therapeutic aptamers in eye disease

The first therapeutic aptamer approved by the FDA was the Pegaptanib, which today is commercially available as Macugen® (Pfizer and Eyetech) [64, 65]. The Pegaptanib is a 27 ribonucleotide pegylated RNA aptamer antagonist of VEGF165 [95]. Since its approval in 2004, the Macugen® has always been used for the treatment of AMD, a degenerative ocular disease that causes vision loss in older adults due to retinal damage. However, the efficacy of this aptamer was then discovered to be important also for the treatment of diabetic macular edema (DME) and proliferative diabetic retinopathy (PDR) with promising results in clinical trials [96, 97]. At present, the spectrum of use of Pegaptanib is being broadened to other pathologies such as ischemic diabetic macular edema (MIDME), uveitis, choroidal neovascularization secondary to pathologic myopia, and iris neovascularization [98–100].

The limits of anti-VEGF agents to treat AMD are their inability to promote the regression of new blood vessels, which are the cause for the loss of vision. To bypass this limitation, the E10030 aptamer (Fovista™) was developed by Ophthotech Corp in 2012: the E10030 is a 29 pegylated RNA aptamer able to bind PDGF (platelet-derived growth factor), which regulates pericytes maturation. The combined administration of E10030 with Pegaptanib showed successful neovascular regression in preclinical models [101].

3.2.1.2. Therapeutic aptamers for hemostasis

Thrombin is a wide-studied target for anticoagulation, and its *in vivo* inhibition is a major solution to prevent and treat blood clotting abnormalities [61, 102]. Anti-thrombin aptamer (TBA), a 15 bp oligonucleotide, was first selected in 1992 by Toole et al. and it was the most studied aptamer for clinical applications in 2012 [60, 103]. After the evaluation of TBA efficiency *in vivo* [104], the Nu172 aptamer (ARCA Bipharma) was develop as a potential thrombin inhibitor candidate. Nu172 is a 26 bp aptamer able to prevent fibrinogen cleavage of a-thrombin by interacting with the exosite I. Nu172 is currently in phase II clinical trials to be certified for anticoagulation in invasive medical procedures, coronary artery bypass graft and percutaneous interventions [105].

3.2.1.3. Therapeutic aptamers for cancer

The goal of new therapeutic approaches in Oncology is often to block the neoplastic progression through the inhibition of specific cell-pathways, which lead to cell abnormal proliferation. Several clinical trials have proposed the use of aptamers to specifically bind tumor cells and stop cancer development. The specific cell membrane receptors that can be blocked in tumors are numerous, but only few have been investigated with aptamers. A pivot role is played by nucleolin, a protein which is often over-expressed on the surface of cancer cells and that is firstly involved in cell survival, growth and proliferation, as well as in nuclear transport and transcription [106]. In particular, nucleolin seems to manage the internalization of the tumor-homing F3 peptide and its inhibition affects several signaling pathways responsible for abnormal cell proliferation during cancer progression, such as NF-kB and Bcl-2 pathways [107, 108].

AS1411 (Antisoma, PLC) is a 26 bp long aptamer rich in guanosine and screened for against nucleolin [66, 106]. When AS1411 interacts with surface nucleolin, the complex is internalized and prevents its binding with Bcl-2, thus inducing cell apoptosis. AS1411 has shown good growth-inhibitory properties *in vitro* (**Table 1**) and the ability to be accumulated in tumor tissue [66, 109].

Cell Line	Description	Dose of AS1411 administered	Time of exposure to AS1411
A549	Human epithelial lung carcinoma	1 μmol/l	6 days
DU145	Human epithelial prostate carcinoma	2 μmol/l 15 μmol/l	6 days 5 days
MDA-MB-231	Human breast adenocarcinoma	15 μmol/l	5 days
MCF-7	Human breast adenocarcinoma	15 μmol/l	5 days
HeLa	Human cervix adenocarcinoma	15 μmol/l	5 days
Primary cells from leukemia	Human leukemia	10 μmol/l	7 days
Primary cells from lymphoma	Human lymphoma	10 μmol/l	7 days

Table 1. Dose administered and time of exposure of different cell lines to AS1411 aptamer, in order to observe growth ihnibition [66, 109].

3.2.1.4. *Therapeutic aptamers in microbiology*

When aptamers were first described by Ellington and Gold in 1990, their ability to bind viral proteins was clear, and, consequently, their use to treat viral and bacterial diseases has always been investigated [110, 111].

Ebola epidemic of 2014 and other emerging viruses have prompted several research groups to use specific aptamers in the treatment of these diseases by blocking sites essential for virus infectious progression [112–115]. For example, it has been shown that specific aptamers against influenza major targets are able to inhibit or block virus fusion, penetration, and replication [116–120]. Aptamers are also thought to be useful to kill multidrug-resistant (MDR) bacteria *in vivo*, possibly by blocking resistance enzymes such as NMD-1 (New Delhi metallo-β-lactamase) or by inducing the classic pathway of the complement in lieu of antibodies [121–124].

3.2.2. *Aptamers as sensors for biomarker discovery*

Biomarkers are molecules that change their expression level when physiological conditions are altered, and can thus be used to indicate the progression state of a disease or the risk of developing it. Biomarkers are therefore a tool with high potentiality for disease screening and early diagnosis. However, a very limited number of biomarkers have been thus far discovered. The use of mABs to identify disease specific targets is often unfeasible, because these targets are frequently cell epitopes and it is impossible to design and select a mAB against an unknown receptor, and aptamer research is moving to fill the gap. Normally, target cells are amplified, collected, and lysed. The lysate is then incubated with aptamers and target proteins go through a comparative proteomic analysis: briefly, they are separated through the SDS-PAGE and analyzed with mass spectrometry [61].

In recent years, many research groups have worked to find aptamers that specifically bind biomarkers. In particular, the tyrosine kinase 7 has been discovered as a potent marker of T-cell acute lymphoblastic leukemia [125], tenascin-C as biomarker for glioblastoma cells [85], the Igμ heavy chain for Burkitt's lymphoma [126], whereas the stress-induced phosphoprotein I for ovarian cancer [127].

3.2.3. Aptamers as molecular imaging probes for diagnostic

Aptamers have also been proposed as detecting agents in diagnostics, both as molecular beacons or as sensors for bio-imaging [58, 61].

In 2001, Hamaguchi et al. developed an aptamer beacon for thrombin. A thrombin aptamer was modified with complementary sequences at 3′ and 5′ ends to form a stem-loop structure. Furthermore, the 5′-end was labeled with a fluorescent moiety, whereas the 3′ with a quencher. In the absence of thrombin, the complementary 3′ and 5′ ends lie in close proximity and this results in fluorescence quenching, whereas in the presence of thrombin, aptamer acquires its 3D specific conformation, moving the fluorophore and the quencher apart, setting off a fluorescence signal in a dose-depends manner [128]. One year later the same approach was proved by Tan and co-workers [129] and then by several research groups [79, 130–132].

The idea of labeling aptamers with fluorophores was pursued also to develop new probes for computerize tomography (CT) and for magnetic resonance imaging (MRI). In addition, this idea seemed appealing in combination with nanomaterials for CT and MRI analysis (i.e., liposomes, quantum dots (QDs), carbon nanotubes, gold and magnetic nanoparticles), to improve *in vivo* imaging and phototermal therapy, thanks to aptamers' accurate targeting and the rapid diffusion through blood circulation of nanomaterials [58]. This approach was used to image C6 cancer cells using a Cy3-labeled aptamer against nucleolin transmembrane protein in 2010 [133]. The same year Min et al. proposed the use of a QDs-aptamer complex specific for PSMA(+) and PSMA(−) (prostate specific membrane antigen) to detect prostate cancer cells. The complex was able to discriminate between prostate cancer cells and normal or other cancer cells [134]. In 2013, Kim et al. immobilized a VEGFR2 (vascular endothelial growth factor receptor 2) aptamer on a magnetic nanocrystal surface for the detection of the angiogenic vasculature in glioblastoma by MRI with high sensitivity and efficiency [135].

3.2.4. *Aptamers as drug delivery systems*

The ability of aptamers selected through the cell-SELEX to recognize cell antigens have been exploited to deliver a variety of molecules, mainly drugs, into cells [58]. For this purpose, aptamers can be used alone or in combination with other delivery systems, such as polymers or liposomes, in order to enhance their specificity [61].

Building on their previous work on a QDs-aptamer complex specific for PSMA(+) and PSMA(–) (see Section 3.2.3), Min et al. were able to load the construct with doxorubicin, an anticancer drug, and to effectively introduce it inside prostate cancer cells [136]. Levy's group relied on an aptamer against PSMA to introduce a siRNA in prostate cancer cells, which inhibited gene expression within 30 min [137].

To enhance polymers specificity as drug delivery system, they can be funtionalized with aptamers; this strategy has shown to be promising for clinical applications. Farokhzad et al. encapsulated rhodamine-labeled dextran within a nanoparticle of poly (lactic acid)-block-polyethylene glycol copolymer with a terminal carboxylic acid functional group (PLA-PEG-COOH) conjugated to an aptamer against the PSMA antigen of prostate cancer cells. The system was able to enter PSMA over-expressing cells in less than 2 h [138]. The same group further generated a nanoparticle with poly (D,L-lactic-*co*-glycolic acid)-block-poly (ethylene glycol) (PLGA-*b*-PEG) copolymer conjugated with the A10 aptamer against PSMA to deliver docetaxel inside cancer cells. This system was tested *in vivo*, and induced the complete regression of the tumor in five out of seven mice [139]. Following these promising results, several others similar constructs based on the conjugation of polymers and aptamers were efficiently tested [140], and even aptamers conjugated to dendrimers were tested, as reported in a review published in 2011 by Lee et al. [141].

Liposomes were also engineered with aptamers to deliver cisplatin and taxol inside breast cancer cells. The AS1411 aptamer-liposome bioconjugate system efficiently transported cisplatin inside tumorigenic cells, and effectively killed the target cancer cells but not healthy control ones [142]. Moreover, compared with the control liposomes, liposomes conjugated with the AS1411 aptamer and containing taxol, increased the cellular uptake of the construct in the breast cancer cells [143].

Taken together, these results support the use of aptamers as enhancer for drug delivery systems; however, more *in vivo* evaluation is required to allow their use in clinic [61].

4. Aptamers to enhance scaffold biocompatibility

As mentioned earlier in this chapter (see Section 2.1), one of the most investigated topics in TE is developing new methods to improve scaffold biocompatibility. To reach this goal, scaffolds should be highly dynamic and possess surfaces capable to interact with cells, positively modulating protein adsorption [36].

Several research groups have aimed to reach this goal by immobilizing the RGD peptide binding motif on scaffolds (see Section 2.1.2), by modifying chemically or physically scaffold surfaces (see Section 2.1.1) or by coating scaffolds with other highly biocompatible materials (see Section 2.1.3).

In this section we propose a new method to improve natural polymeric scaffold biocompatibility, by using ssDNA aptamers screened for against human fibronectin as docking points, to ameliorate the adsorption of fibronectin, a naturally occurring molecule in damaged tissues, which is mainly involved in cell adhesion and in the regeneration process. The correct adsorption of fibronectin may lead to a faster colonization of the scaffold *in vitro* and to an acceleration of the regeneration process *in vivo*. **Figure 3** summarizes the rationale to use aptamers to enrich biomaterials with specific molecules.

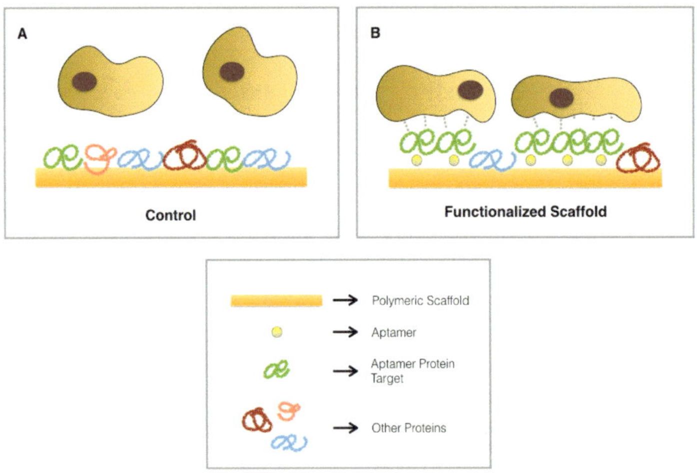

Figure 3. Diagram representing the rationale of functionalizing substrates with aptamers to retain specific proteins. Un-functionalized scaffold adsorbs proteins from the environment based on their availability (A). Aptamer functionalized scaffold specifically binds and retains target protein, by selectively enriching the adsorption for a specific protein (B).

Biomaterial functionalization with aptamers is not new in the literature. Wendel's group pioneered the field in 2007, by coating a vascular prosthesis with aptamers against circulating endothelial progenitor cells (EPCs), to retain specific cells from the bloodstream and quickly create an autologous functional endothelium. Aptamers against EPCs were screened through the Cell-SELEX and covalently grafted on to polydimethylsiloxane (PDMS) and polytetrafluoroethylene (PTFE) substrates. Functionalized scaffolds were incubated with whole porcine blood, washed twice to remove non-specific debris, and stained for CD31 and CD144 by immunofluorescence to identify EPCs. EPCs were observed only on aptamer-grafted prosthesis, whereas no CD31 and CD144 positive cells were retained on control discs [144]. Five years later, Chen et al. designed an artificial ECM using aptamer-grafted polyethylene glycol (PEG) hydrogels: aptamers screened for against cell surface receptors were used as binding sites for cells and they were attached on to the gel through free radical polymerization. It was demonstrated that the amount of cells adhered to hydrogels was proportional to the amount of aptamer incorporated into the hydrogels [145].

Considering those results, we want to show the possibility of enriching natural synthetic scaffolds with aptamers against human Fibronectin to enhance cell adhesion and growth.

For this purpose, we used aptamer screened for against human fibronectin (Base Pair Biotechnologies, Pearland, TX) and modified at their 3′-end with a thiol group and at their 5′-end with biotin.

4.1. Aptamers enhance cell adhesion and proliferation on polymeric scaffolds

Two natural polymer scaffolds were used as substrates: a thiolate hyaluronic acid/polyethylene glycol hydrogel (tHA/PEGDA) and a chitosan modified with D-(+)-raffinose film. tHA/PEGDA gels are 3D matrices normally used for stem cell culture and which offer scant adhesion to cells. For this reason, they are often enriched with adhesion molecules, such as RGD peptides, when firmer adhesion is required. Aptamers were bound to these hydrogels by exploiting the acrylate functional groups of PEGDA, which can easily bind thiol groups on aptamers. Five microliters of aptamer at increasing concentration were mixed to each 50 μl gel.

Chitosan is one of the most investigated natural polymers for TE applications, because it is highly biocompatible [146]. However, some cell types grow slowly on chitosan films, and consequently they were chosen as substrates to be enriched with aptamers. Aptamers were immobilized on 2% chitosan films (r = 3.0 mm; h = 0.25 mm) at increasing concentration by exploiting the spontaneous ability of chitosan to bind sulfur-containing substances [147].

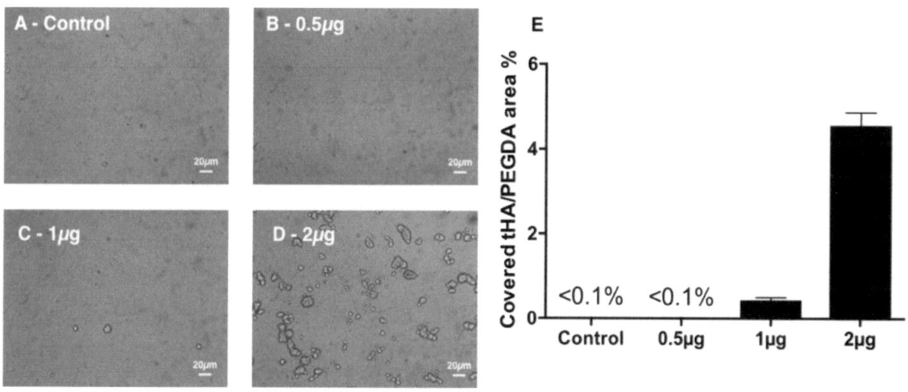

Figure 4. Study of aptamer ability to enhance the proliferation of human osteoblasts (hOB) on tHA/PEGDA hydrogel. Microphotographs, taken with an inverted microscope, showing hOB cells on tHA/PEGDA after 48 h of culture (A–D). The rate of cell growth is proportional to the quantity of aptamer used for the functionalization (E).

Five thousand hOB cells (human osteoblasts) on tHA/PEGDA gels and 5000 MC3T3-E1 cells (murine preosteoblasts from bone/calvaria) on 2% chitosan films were cultured for 7 days. Cells were monitored day by day with an inverted microscope.

Cell proliferation on tHA/PEGDA and chitosan substrates is shown in **Figures 4** and **5**.

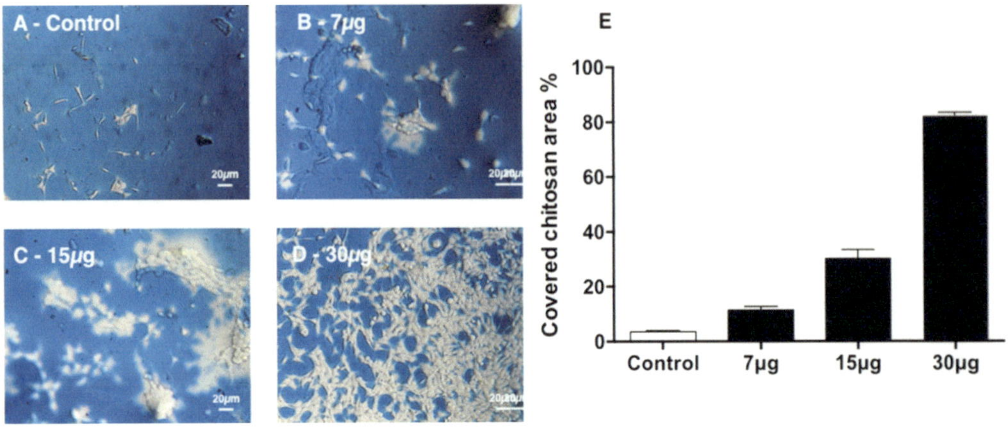

Figure 5. Study of aptamer ability to enhance the proliferation of murine osteoblastic cells (MC3T3-E1) on 2% chitosan films. Microphotographs, taken with an inverted microscope, showing MC3T3-E1 cells on 2% chitosan films after 48 h of culture and stained with the Trypan Blue to discriminate viable and dead cells. The rate of cell growth is proportional to the quantity of aptamer used for the functionalization (E).

In both the cases, aptamers increase the number of adhering cells and the rate of cell growth is proportional to the amount of aptamer used. Cell morphology appear round both in control groups and in aptamer-rich samples, unlike the flattened spindle shape morphology that is normally observed on tissue culture plastic substrates, and is routinely associated to firm cell adhesion. Although cell adhesion does appear improved in the presence of aptamers, as indicated by a significantly higher number of cells, the culture substrate is mechanically elastic and the normal morphological features of a good adhesion cannot be achieved.

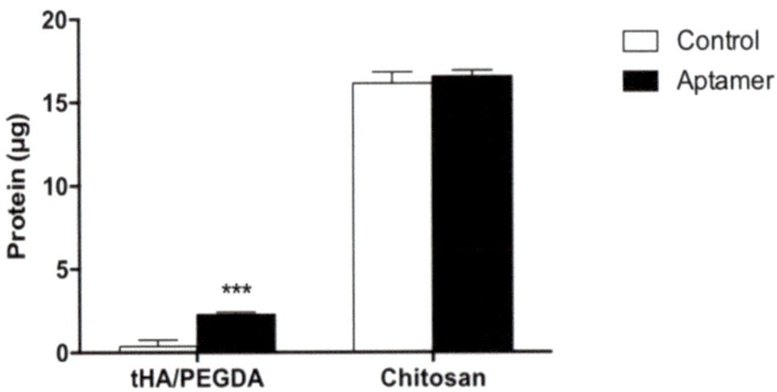

Figure 6. Histograms representing the amount of protein adsorbed on polymeric scaffolds with or without aptamers. Scaffolds were incubated for 2 h with 30 µg of proteins. The amount of protein bind by the scaffold was quantitated through the Bradford.

Although aptamers act on both substrates presumably in comparable ways, by binding fibronectin, the rationale for their use is possibly different, as suggested by results of protein

http://dx.doi.org/10.5772/63265

adsorption assays reported in **Figure 6**, where 30 μg of serum protein were incubated for 2 h on different scaffolds with or without aptamers and quantitated with Bradford.

The presence of aptamers on tHA/PEGDA quantitatively increases the amount of fibronectin on the gel and this may explain the improved cell adhesion and proliferation. Cells on control gels do not get in contact with adsorbed proteins and lack good attachment points for their integrins. Availability of a higher amount of adhesive protein then results in more firmly adhering cells. On the other hand, chitosan is known to bind massive amounts of protein from the supernatant and aptamers do not affect the quantity of adsorbed proteins. A viable hypothesis for the effects of aptamers on chitosan is therefore that aptamers may affect the quality of adsorbed protein. Aptamers may preserve the natural conformation of fibronectin on films, without unfolding it and maintaining a favorable exposure of adhesion sequences for cells.

Evidences reported show that aptamers are a viable approach to improve the biocompatibility of scaffolds, ameliorating the process of adhesive protein adsorption on surfaces both quantitatively and qualitatively, and should further investigated to create tissue-specific scaffold for tissue engineering.

5. Summary

Scaffolds for tissue engineering should support an appropriate cellular activity. In particular, cell adhesion and proliferation depend mainly on the efficiency of protein adsorption at the interface, a process deeply influenced by surface chemistry. Nowadays, a wide number of treatments have been proposed to enhance scaffold biocompatibility, including physical and chemical treatments or biological coatings. In this chapter we reported on the use of aptamers to improve scaffold biocompatibility.

After a general presentation on tissue engineering in Section 1, Section 2 described the rationale to control protein adsorption on biomaterial surfaces. A panoramic view of the methods developed and reported in literature to improve scaffold biocompatibility was reviewed. At the end of the section the possibility of using aptamers for this goal was outlined.

Section 3 contained general information about aptamers. The technique to obtain aptamers (SELEX) was well described and a general view on the use of aptamers in biomedical applications was outlined. Finally, in Section 4 after the explanation of the rationale to use aptamers as enhancers for scaffold biocompatibility, our preliminary results were reported. In particular, we investigated the possibility to immobilize aptamers on different substrates to improve scaffold biocompatibility *in vitro*, with similar results. Aptamers were bound to tHA/PEGDA hydrogels or to chitosan films: in both the cases the adsorption of proteins was ameliorated, as well as the adhesion and proliferation of cells. The results obtained paved the way to further investigation of the use of aptamers in combination with scaffolds for tissue engineering applications.

Acknowledgements

The study was supported by a 2013 grant by the American Academy of Implant Dentistry Foundation. We thank Dr. Bill Jackson and Dr. Lisa Thurston (Base Pair Biotechnologies, Pearland, TX, USA) for their precious advice. We also thank Dr. Gallia Graiani and Dr. Andrea Toffoli (Dentistry Center, University of Parma), Dr. Benedetta Ghezzi, Dr. Anna Lidia Perruccio, Dr. Maria Siciliano, Dr. Alessandra Zecca (Department of Biomedical Biotechnological and Translational Sciences, University of Parma) for their assistance.

Conflict of interest

The authors have no conflict of interest to disclose.

Author details

Ludovica Parisi[1,2], Carlo Galli[1,2,4*], Lisa Elviri[3], Annalisa Bianchera[3], Paola Lagonegro[4], Simone Lumetti[1,2], Edoardo Manfredi[1,2] and Guido Maria Macaluso[1,2,4]

*Address all correspondence to: carlo.galli@unipr.it

1 Department of Biomedical Biotechnological and Translational Sciences, University of Parma, Parma, Italy

2 Dentistry Center, University of Parma, Parma, Italy

3 Department of Pharmacy, University of Parma, Parma, Italy

4 IMEM-CNR, University of Parma, Parma, Italy

References

[1] Mason, C. and P. Dunnill, A brief definition of regenerative medicine. Regen Med, 2008. 3(1): p. 1–5.

[2] Langer, R. and J.P. Vacanti, Tissue engineering. Science, 1993. 260(5110): p. 920–926.

[3] Dimitriou, R., et al., Bone regeneration: current concepts and future directions. BMC Med, 2011. 9: p. 66.

[4] Oryan, A., et al., Bone regenerative medicine: classic options, novel strategies, and future directions. J Orthop Surg Res, 2014. 9(1): p. 18.

[5] Giannoudis, P.V., T.A. Einhorn, and D. Marsh, Fracture healing: the diamond concept. Injury, 2007. 38 Suppl 4: p. S3–S6.

[6] Albrektsson, T. and C. Johansson, Osteoinduction, osteoconduction and osseointegration. Eur Spine J, 2001. 10 Suppl 2: p. S96–S101.

[7] Dimitriou, R., E. Tsiridis, and P.V. Giannoudis, Current concepts of molecular aspects of bone healing. Injury, 2005. 36(12): p. 1392–1404.

[8] Pountos, I., et al., Efficacy of minimally invasive techniques for enhancement of fracture healing: evidence today. Int Orthop, 2010. 34(1): p. 3–12.

[9] Matsumoto, T., et al., Therapeutic potential of vasculogenesis and osteogenesis promoted by peripheral blood CD34-positive cells for functional bone healing. Am J Pathol, 2006. 169(4): p. 1440–1457.

[10] Im, G.I., Y.W. Shin, and K.B. Lee, Do adipose tissue-derived mesenchymal stem cells have the same osteogenic and chondrogenic potential as bone marrow-derived cells? Osteoarthritis Cartilage, 2005. 13(10): p. 845–853.

[11] Niemeyer, P., et al., Comparison of mesenchymal stem cells from bone marrow and adipose tissue for bone regeneration in a critical size defect of the sheep tibia and the influence of platelet-rich plasma. Biomaterials, 2010. 31(13): p. 3572–3579.

[12] Seo, B.M., et al., Investigation of multipotent postnatal stem cells from human periodontal ligament. Lancet, 2004. 364(9429): p. 149–155.

[13] Seo, B.M., et al., Recovery of stem cells from cryopreserved periodontal ligament. J Dent Res, 2005. 84(10): p. 907–912.

[14] Egusa, H., et al., Stem cells in dentistry – part I: stem cell sources. J Prosthodont Res, 2012. 56(3): p. 151–165.

[15] Finkemeier, C.G., Bone-grafting and bone-graft substitutes. J Bone Joint Surg Am, 2002. 84-A(3): p. 454–464.

[16] Giannoudis, P.V., H. Dinopoulos, and E. Tsiridis, Bone substitutes: an update. Injury, 2005. 36 Suppl 3: p. S20–S27.

[17] Rose, F.R. and R.O. Oreffo, Bone tissue engineering: hope vs hype. Biochem Biophys Res Commun, 2002. 292(1): p. 1–7.

[18] Salgado, A.J., O.P. Coutinho, and R.L. Reis, Bone tissue engineering: state of the art and future trends. Macromol Biosci, 2004. 4(8): p. 743–765.

[19] Kokemueller, H., et al., Prefabrication of vascularized bioartificial bone grafts in vivo for segmental mandibular reconstruction: experimental pilot study in sheep and first clinical application. Int J Oral Maxillofac Surg, 2010. 39(4): p. 379–387.

[20] Ohgushi, H., et al., Tissue engineered ceramic artificial joint – ex vivo osteogenic differentiation of patient mesenchymal cells on total ankle joints for treatment of osteoarthritis. Biomaterials, 2005. 26(22): p. 4654–4661.

[21] Kim, S.J., et al., A multi-center, randomized, clinical study to compare the effect and safety of autologous cultured osteoblast (Ossron) injection to treat fractures. BMC Musculoskelet Disord, 2009. 10: p. 20.

[22] Langer, R. and D.A. Tirrell, Designing materials for biology and medicine. Nature, 2004. 428(6982): p. 487–492.

[23] Dhandayuthapani, S., et al., Bromelain-induced apoptosis in GI-101A breast cancer cells. J Med Food, 2012. 15(4): p. 344–349.

[24] Kikuchi, M., Hydroxyapatite/collagen bone-like nanocomposite. Biol Pharm Bull, 2013. 36(11): p. 1666–1669.

[25] Lee, S.S., et al., Bone regeneration with low dose BMP-2 amplified by biomimetic supramolecular nanofibers within collagen scaffolds. Biomaterials, 2013. 34(2): p. 452–459.

[26] Pastorino, L., et al., Oriented collagen nanocoatings for tissue engineering. Colloids Surf B Biointerfaces, 2014. 114: p. 372–378.

[27] Nishiyama, Y., P. Langan, and H. Chanzy, Crystal structure and hydrogen-bonding system in cellulose Ibeta from synchrotron X-ray and neutron fiber diffraction. J Am Chem Soc, 2002. 124(31): p. 9074–9082.

[28] Agnihotri, S.A., N.N. Mallikarjuna, and T.M. Aminabhavi, Recent advances on chitosan-based micro- and nanoparticles in drug delivery. J Control Release, 2004. 100(1): p. 5–28.

[29] Aravamudhan, A., et al., Cellulose and collagen derived micro-nano structured scaffolds for bone tissue engineering. J Biomed Nanotechnol, 2013. 9(4): p. 719–731.

[30] Perez, R.A., et al., Utilizing core-shell fibrous collagen-alginate hydrogel cell delivery system for bone tissue engineering. Tissue Eng Part A, 2014. 20(1–2): p. 103–114.

[31] Mistura, D.V., et al., Development, characterization, and cellular adhesion of poly(L-lactic acid)/poly(caprolactone triol) membranes for potential application in bone tissue regeneration. Artif Organs, 2013. 37(11): p. 978–984.

[32] Perez, R.A. and M.P. Ginebra, Injectable collagen/alpha-tricalcium phosphate cement: collagen-mineral phase interactions and cell response. J Mater Sci Mater Med, 2013. 24(2): p. 381–393.

[33] Williams, D.F., On the mechanisms of biocompatibility. Biomaterials, 2008. 29(20): p. 2941–2953.

[34] Donaruma, L.G., Definitions in biomaterials, D. F. Williams, Ed., Elsevier, Amsterdam, 1987, 72 pp. J Polym Sci Part C: Polym Lett, 1988. 26(9): p. 414.

[35] Williams, D.F., The Williams dictionary of biomaterials, L.U. Press. 1999.

[36] A., M., Dinamiche delle interazioni materiale-ambiente biologico, in Biomateriali – dagli impianti protesici alla medicina rigenerativa, Patròn Editore, editor, Bologna, 2005. p. 27–47.

[37] Tang, L. and W. Hu, Molecular determinants of biocompatibility. Expert Rev Med Devices, 2005. 2(4): p. 493–500.

[38] Thevenot, P., et al., Surface chemistry influences cancer killing effect of TiO_2 nanoparticles. Nanomedicine, 2008. 4(3): p. 226–236.

[39] Tegoulia, V.A., et al., Surface properties, fibrinogen adsorption, and cellular interactions of a novel phosphorylcholine-containing self-assembled monolayer on gold. Langmuir, 2001. 17(14): p. 4396–4404.

[40] Martins, M.C., B.D. Ratner, and M.A. Barbosa, Protein adsorption on mixtures of hydroxyl- and methyl-terminated alkanethiols self-assembled monolayers. J Biomed Mater Res A, 2003. 67(1): p. 158–171.

[41] Agashe, M., et al., Molecular simulation to characterize the adsorption behavior of a fibrinogen gamma-chain fragment. Langmuir, 2005. 21(3): p. 1103–1117.

[42] Ruckenstein, E. and Z.F. Li, Surface modification and functionalization through the self-assembled monolayer and graft polymerization. Adv Colloid Interface Sci, 2005. 113(1): p. 43–63.

[43] Tang, L., L. Liu, and H.B. Elwing, Complement activation and inflammation triggered by model biomaterial surfaces. J Biomed Mater Res, 1998. 41(2): p. 333–340.

[44] Barbosa, J.N., et al., The influence of functional groups of self-assembled monolayers on fibrous capsule formation and cell recruitment. J Biomed Mater Res A, 2006. 76(4): p. 737–743.

[45] Dyshlovenko, S., et al., Pulsed laser modification of plasma-sprayed coatings: experimental processing of hydroxyapatite and numerical simulation. Surface Coat Technol, 2006. 201(6): p. 2248–2255.

[46] Forster, Y., et al., Surface modification of implants in long bone. Biomatter, 2012. 2(3): p. 149–157.

[47] Rezania, A., et al., The detachment strength and morphology of bone cells contacting materials modified with a peptide sequence found within bone sialoprotein. J Biomed Mater Res, 1997. 37(1): p. 9–19.

[48] Dee, K.C., T.T. Anderson, and R. Bizios, Osteoblast population migration characteristics on substrates modified with immobilized adhesive peptides. Biomaterials, 1999. 20(3): p. 221–227.

[49] Zreiqat, H., et al., Differentiation of human bone-derived cells grown on GRGDSP-peptide bound titanium surfaces. J Biomed Mater Res A, 2003. 64(1): p. 105–113.

[50] Ferris, D.M., et al., RGD-coated titanium implants stimulate increased bone formation in vivo. Biomaterials, 1999. 20(23–24): p. 2323–2331.

[51] Elmengaard, B., J.E. Bechtold, and K. Soballe, In vivo effects of RGD-coated titanium implants inserted in two bone-gap models. J Biomed Mater Res A, 2005. 75(2): p. 249–255.

[52] Rammelt, S., et al., Coating of titanium implants with collagen, RGD peptide and chondroitin sulfate. Biomaterials, 2006. 27(32): p. 5561–5571.

[53] Hennessy, K.M., et al., The effect of RGD peptides on osseointegration of hydroxyapatite biomaterials. Biomaterials, 2008. 29(21): p. 3075–3083.

[54] Geissler, U., et al., Collagen type I-coating of Ti6Al4V promotes adhesion of osteoblasts. J Biomed Mater Res, 2000. 51(4): p. 752–760.

[55] Roehlecke, C., et al., Synergistic effect of titanium alloy and collagen type I on cell adhesion, proliferation and differentiation of osteoblast-like cells. Cells Tissues Organs, 2001. 168(3): p. 178–187.

[56] Huang, L., et al., The effect of hyaluronan on osteoblast proliferation and differentiation in rat calvarial-derived cell cultures. J Biomed Mater Res A, 2003. 66(4): p. 880–884.

[57] Takada, T., et al., Sulfated polysaccharides enhance the biological activities of bone morphogenetic proteins. J Biol Chem, 2003. 278(44): p. 43229–43235.

[58] Song, K.M., S. Lee, and C. Ban, Aptamers and their biological applications. Sensors (Basel), 2012. 12(1): p. 612–631.

[59] Ellington, A.D. and J.W. Szostak, In vitro selection of RNA molecules that bind specific ligands. Nature, 1990. 346(6287): p. 818–822.

[60] Mascini, M., I. Palchetti, and S. Tombelli, Nucleic acid and peptide aptamers: fundamentals and bioanalytical aspects. Angew Chem Int Ed Engl, 2012. 51(6): p. 1316–1332.

[61] Ku, T.H., et al., Nucleic acid aptamers: an emerging tool for biotechnology and biomedical sensing. Sensors (Basel), 2015. 15(7): p. 16281–16313.

[62] Sun, H. and Y. Zu, A highlight of recent advances in aptamer technology and its application. Molecules, 2015. 20(7): p. 11959–11980.

[63] Geiger, A., et al., RNA aptamers that bind L-arginine with sub-micromolar dissociation constants and high enantioselectivity. Nucleic Acids Res, 1996. 24(6): p. 1029–1036.

[64] Eyetech Study, G., Preclinical and phase 1A clinical evaluation of an anti-VEGF pegylated aptamer (EYE001) for the treatment of exudative age-related macular degeneration. Retina, 2002. 22(2): p. 143–152.

[65] Eyetech Study, G., Anti-vascular endothelial growth factor therapy for subfoveal choroidal neovascularization secondary to age-related macular degeneration: phase II study results. Ophthalmology, 2003. 110(5): p. 979–986.

[66] Ireson, C.R. and L.R. Kelland, Discovery and development of anticancer aptamers. Mol Cancer Ther, 2006. 5(12): p. 2957–2962.

[67] Xiang, D., et al., Nucleic acid aptamer-guided cancer therapeutics and diagnostics: the next generation of cancer medicine. Theranostics, 2015. 5(1): p. 23–42.

[68] Jayasena, S.D., Aptamers: an emerging class of molecules that rival antibodies in diagnostics. Clin Chem, 1999. 45(9): p. 1628–1650.

[69] Ng, E.W. and A.P. Adamis, Anti-VEGF aptamer (pegaptanib) therapy for ocular vascular diseases. Ann N Y Acad Sci, 2006. 1082: p. 151–171.

[70] Nucleic acid aptamers for diagnostics and therapeutics: global markets. Available from: http://www.marketresearch.com/BCC-Research-v374/Nucleic-Acid-Aptamers-Diagnostics-Therapeutics-8412378/.

[71] Tuerk, C. and L. Gold, Systematic evolution of ligands by exponential enrichment: RNA ligands to bacteriophage T4 DNA polymerase. Science, 1990. 249(4968): p. 505–510.

[72] Kulbachinskiy, A.V., Methods for selection of aptamers to protein targets. Biochemistry (Mosc), 2007. 72(13): p. 1505–1518.

[73] Tombelli, S., M. Minunni, and M. Mascini, Analytical applications of aptamers. Biosens Bioelectron, 2005. 20(12): p. 2424–2434.

[74] Gopinath, S.C., Methods developed for SELEX. Anal Bioanal Chem, 2007. 387(1): p. 171–182.

[75] Vianini, E., M. Palumbo, and B. Gatto, In vitro selection of DNA aptamers that bind L-tyrosinamide. Bioorg Med Chem, 2001. 9(10): p. 2543–2548.

[76] Levesque, D., et al., In vitro selection and characterization of RNA aptamers binding thyroxine hormone. Biochem J, 2007. 403(1): p. 129–138.

[77] Song, K.M., et al., Gold nanoparticle-based colorimetric detection of kanamycin using a DNA aptamer. Anal Biochem, 2011. 415(2): p. 175–181.

[78] Niazi, J.H., S.J. Lee, and M.B. Gu, Single-stranded DNA aptamers specific for antibiotics tetracyclines. Bioorg Med Chem, 2008. 16(15): p. 7245–7253.

[79] Wang, A.Z., et al., Superparamagnetic iron oxide nanoparticle-aptamer bioconjugates for combined prostate cancer imaging and therapy. ChemMedChem, 2008. 3(9): p. 1311–1315.

[80] Joeng, C.B., et al., ssDNA aptamers that recognize diclofenac and 2-anilinophenylacetic acid. Bioorg Med Chem, 2009. 17(15): p. 5380–5387.

[81] Mendonsa, S.D. and M.T. Bowser, In vitro selection of high-affinity DNA ligands for human IgE using capillary electrophoresis. Anal Chem, 2004. 76(18): p. 5387–5392.

[82] Mendonsa, S.D. and M.T. Bowser, In vitro selection of aptamers with affinity for neuropeptide Y using capillary electrophoresis. J Am Chem Soc, 2005. 127(26): p. 9382–9383.

[83] Kunii, T., et al., Selection of DNA aptamers recognizing small cell lung cancer using living cell-SELEX. Analyst, 2011. 136(7): p. 1310–1312.

[84] Van Simaeys, D., et al., Study of the molecular recognition of aptamers selected through ovarian cancer cell-SELEX. PLoS One, 2010. 5(11): p. e13770.

[85] Daniels, D.A., et al., A tenascin-C aptamer identified by tumor cell SELEX: systematic evolution of ligands by exponential enrichment. Proc Natl Acad Sci U S A, 2003. 100(26): p. 15416–15421.

[86] Gold, L., et al., Diversity of oligonucleotide functions. Annu Rev Biochem, 1995. 64: p. 763–797.

[87] Green, L.S., et al., Inhibitory DNA ligands to platelet-derived growth factor B-chain. Biochemistry, 1996. 35(45): p. 14413–14424.

[88] Zhou, J., et al., Structural prediction and binding analysis of hybridized aptamers. J Mol Recognit, 2011. 24(1): p. 119–126.

[89] Shigdar, S., et al., RNA aptamers targeting cancer stem cell marker CD133. Cancer Lett, 2013. 330(1): p. 84–95.

[90] Qiao, L., et al., A new application of aptamer: one-step purification and immobilization of enzyme from cell lysates for biocatalysis. J Biotechnol, 2015. 203: p. 68–76.

[91] Saberian-Borujeni, M., et al., Nanoscaled aptasensors for multi-analyte sensing. Bioimpacts, 2014. 4(4): p. 205–215.

[92] Chen, A. and S. Yang, Replacing antibodies with aptamers in lateral flow immunoassay. Biosens Bioelectron, 2015. 71: p. 230–242.

[93] Wu, J., et al., Recent trends in SELEX technique and its application to food safety monitoring. Mikrochim Acta, 2014. 181(5–6): p. 479–491.

[94] Hayat, A. and J.L. Marty, Aptamer based electrochemical sensors for emerging environmental pollutants. Front Chem, 2014. 2 41 doi: 10.3389/fchem.2014.00041.

[95] Lee, J.H., F. Jucker, and A. Pardi, Imino proton exchange rates imply an induced-fit binding mechanism for the VEGF165-targeting aptamer, Macugen. FEBS Lett, 2008. 582(13): p. 1835–1839.

[96] Inc, E., Phase 3 study presented at world ophthalmology congress evaluates investigational use of macugen in patients with diabetic macular edema. 2010.

[97] Sultan, M.B., et al., A phase 2/3, multicenter, randomized, double-masked, 2-year trial of pegaptanib sodium for the treatment of diabetic macular edema. Ophthalmology, 2011. 118(6): p. 1107–1118.

[98] Hermann Eye Center, WV. A Pilot Study for the Treatment of Iris Neovascularization With Macugen. In: ClinicalTrials.gov [Internet]. Bethesda (MD): National Library of Medicine (US). 2006 . Available from: https://clinicaltrials.gov/ct2/show/NCT00295828 NLM Identifier: NCT00295828.

[99] Rosenbaum JT. Future for biological therapy for uveitis. Curr Opin Ophthalmol. 2010 Nov;21(6):473–7.

[100] Pfizer. Long-Term Use Of Pegaptanib In Patients For Subfoveal Choroidal Neovascularization Secondary To Age-Related Macular Degeneration In: ClinicalTrials.gov [Internet]. Bethesda (MD): National Library of Medicine (US). 2008- . Available from: https://clinicaltrials.gov/ct2/show/NCT00845273 NLM Identifier: NCT00845273.

[101] Jo, N., et al., Inhibition of platelet-derived growth factor B signaling enhances the efficacy of anti-vascular endothelial growth factor therapy in multiple models of ocular neovascularization. Am J Pathol, 2006. 168(6): p. 2036–2053.

[102] Di Cera, E., Thrombin as procoagulant and anticoagulant. J Thromb Haemost, 2007. 5 Suppl 1: p. 196–202.

[103] Bock, L.C., et al., Selection of single-stranded DNA molecules that bind and inhibit human thrombin. Nature, 1992. 355(6360): p. 564–566.

[104] Griffin, L.C., et al., In vivo anticoagulant properties of a novel nucleotide-based thrombin inhibitor and demonstration of regional anticoagulation in extracorporeal circuits. Blood, 1993. 81(12): p. 3271–3276.

[105] ARCA Biopharma. Study of NU172 as Anticoagulation in Patients Undergoing Off-pump CABG Surgery (SNAP-CABG-OFF). In: ClinicalTrials.gov [Internet]. Bethesda (MD): National Library of Medicine (US). 2008- . Available from: https://clinicaltrials.gov/ct2/show/NCT00808964 NLM Identifier: NCT00808964.

[106] Bates, P.J., et al., Discovery and development of the G-rich oligonucleotide AS1411 as a novel treatment for cancer. Exp Mol Pathol, 2009. 86(3): p. 151–164.

[107] Girvan, A.C., et al., AGRO100 inhibits activation of nuclear factor-kappaB (NF-kappaB) by forming a complex with NF-kappaB essential modulator (NEMO) and nucleolin. Mol Cancer Ther, 2006. 5(7): p. 1790–1799.

[108] Soundararajan, S., et al., The nucleolin targeting aptamer AS1411 destabilizes Bcl-2 messenger RNA in human breast cancer cells. Cancer Res, 2008. 68(7): p. 2358–2365.

[109] Bates, P.J., et al., Antiproliferative activity of G-rich oligonucleotides correlates with protein binding. J Biol Chem, 1999. 274(37): p. 26369–26377.

[110] Bruno, J.G., Predicting the uncertain future of aptamer-based diagnostics and therapeutics. Molecules, 2015. 20(4): p. 6866–6887.

[111] Duclair, S., et al., High-affinity RNA aptamers against the HIV-1 protease inhibit both in vitro protease activity and late events of viral replication. Mol Ther Nucl Acids, 2015. 4: p. e228.

[112] Cheng, C., et al., Potent inhibition of human influenza H5N1 virus by oligonucleotides derived by SELEX. Biochem Biophys Res Commun, 2008. 366(3): p. 670–674.

[113] Binning, J.M., et al., Development of RNA aptamers targeting Ebola virus VP35. Biochemistry, 2013. 52(47): p. 8406–8419.

[114] Shum, K.T., J. Zhou, and J.J. Rossi, Aptamer-based therapeutics: new approaches to combat human viral diseases. Pharmaceuticals (Basel), 2013. 6(12): p. 1507–1542.

[115] Wandtke, T., J. Wozniak, and P. Kopinski, Aptamers in diagnostics and treatment of viral infections. Viruses, 2015. 7(2): p. 751–780.

[116] Gopinath, S.C. and P.K. Kumar, Aptamers that bind to the hemagglutinin of the recent pandemic influenza virus H1N1 and efficiently inhibit agglutination. Acta Biomater, 2013. 9(11): p. 8932–8941.

[117] Kwon, H.M., et al., An RNA aptamer that specifically binds to the glycosylated hemagglutinin of avian influenza virus and suppresses viral infection in cells. PLoS One, 2014. 9(5): p. e97574.

[118] Musafia, B., R. Oren-Banaroya, and S. Noiman, Designing anti-influenza aptamers: novel quantitative structure activity relationship approach gives insights into aptamer-virus interaction. PLoS One, 2014. 9(5): p. e97696.

[119] Shiratori, I., et al., Selection of DNA aptamers that bind to influenza A viruses with high affinity and broad subtype specificity. Biochem Biophys Res Commun, 2014. 443(1): p. 37–41.

[120] Suenaga, E. and P.K. Kumar, An aptamer that binds efficiently to the hemagglutinins of highly pathogenic avian influenza viruses (H5N1 and H7N7) and inhibits hemagglutinin-glycan interactions. Acta Biomater, 2014. 10(3): p. 1314–1323.

[121] Bruno, J.G., et al., Development of DNA aptamers for cytochemical detection of acetylcholine. In Vitro Cell Dev Biol Anim, 2008. 44(3–4): p. 63–72.

[122] Bruno, J.G., et al., A novel screening method for competitive FRET-aptamers applied to *E. coli* assay development. J Fluoresc, 2010. 20(6): p. 1211–1223.

[123] Schlesinger, S.R., et al., Metallo-β-lactamases and aptamer-based inhibition. Pharmaceuticals 2011, 4, 419–428 doi: 10.3390/ph4020419

[124] Stecker, J.R., et al., Dynamics and visualization of MCF7 adenocarcinoma cell death by aptamer-C1q-mediated membrane attack. Nucleic Acid Ther, 2012. 22(4): p. 275–282.

[125] Shangguan, D., et al., Cell-specific aptamer probes for membrane protein elucidation in cancer cells. J Proteome Res, 2008. 7(5): p. 2133–2139.

[126] Mallikaratchy, P., et al., Aptamer directly evolved from live cells recognizes membrane bound immunoglobin heavy mu chain in Burkitt's lymphoma cells. Mol Cell Proteomics, 2007. 6(12): p. 2230–2238.

[127] Van Simaeys, D., et al., Identification of cell membrane protein stress-induced phosphoprotein 1 as a potential ovarian cancer biomarker using aptamers selected by cell systematic evolution of ligands by exponential enrichment. Anal Chem, 2014. 86(9): p. 4521–4527.

[128] Hamaguchi, N., A. Ellington, and M. Stanton, Aptamer beacons for the direct detection of proteins. Anal Biochem, 2001. 294(2): p. 126–131.

[129] Li, J.J., X. Fang, and W. Tan, Molecular aptamer beacons for real-time protein recognition. Biochem Biophys Res Commun, 2002. 292(1): p. 31–40.

[130] Levy, M., S.F. Cater, and A.D. Ellington, Quantum-dot aptamer beacons for the detection of proteins. Chembiochem, 2005. 6(12): p. 2163–2166.

[131] Bagalkot, V., et al., Quantum dot-aptamer conjugates for synchronous cancer imaging, therapy, and sensing of drug delivery based on bi-fluorescence resonance energy transfer. Nano Lett, 2007. 7(10): p. 3065–3070.

[132] Zhou, D., Quantum dot-nucleic acid/aptamer bioconjugate-based fluorimetric biosensors. Biochem Soc Trans, 2012. 40(4): p. 635–639.

[133] Lee, K.Y., et al., Bioimaging of nucleolin aptamer-containing 5-(*N*-benzylcarboxyamide)-2′-deoxyuridine more capable of specific binding to targets in cancer cells. J Biomed Biotechnol, 2010. 2010: p. 168306.

[134] Min, K., et al., Simultaneous electrochemical detection of both PSMA (+) and PSMA (–) prostate cancer cells using an RNA/peptide dual-aptamer probe. Chem Commun (Camb), 2010. 46(30): p. 5566–5568.

[135] Kim, G.D., et al., 6″-Debromohamacanthin A, a bis (indole) alkaloid, inhibits angiogenesis by targeting the VEGFR2-mediated PI3K/AKT/mTOR signaling pathways. Mar Drugs, 2013. 11(4): p. 1087–1103.

[136] Min, K., et al., Dual-aptamer-based delivery vehicle of doxorubicin to both PSMA (+) and PSMA (–) prostate cancers. Biomaterials, 2011. 32(8): p. 2124–2132.

[137] Chu, T.C., et al., Aptamer mediated siRNA delivery. Nucl Acids Res, 2006. 34(10): p. e73.

[138] Farokhzad, O.C., et al., Nanoparticle-aptamer bioconjugates: a new approach for targeting prostate cancer cells. Cancer Res, 2004. 64(21): p. 7668–7672.

[139] Farokhzad, O.C., et al., Targeted nanoparticle-aptamer bioconjugates for cancer chemotherapy in vivo. Proc Natl Acad Sci U S A, 2006. 103(16): p. 6315–6320.

[140] Guo, J., et al., Aptamer-functionalized PEG-PLGA nanoparticles for enhanced anti-glioma drug delivery. Biomaterials, 2011. 32(31): p. 8010–8020.

[141] Lee, I.H., et al., Targeted chemoimmunotherapy using drug-loaded aptamer-dendrimer bioconjugates. J Control Release, 2011. 155(3): p. 435–441.

[142] Cao, Z., et al., Reversible cell-specific drug delivery with aptamer-functionalized liposomes. Angew Chem Int Ed Engl, 2009. 48(35): p. 6494–6498.

[143] Wu, J., et al., Nucleolin targeting AS1411 modified protein nanoparticle for antitumor drugs delivery. Mol Pharm, 2013. 10(10): p. 3555–3563.

[144] Hoffmann, J., et al., Immobilized DNA aptamers used as potent attractors for porcine endothelial precursor cells. J Biomed Mater Res A, 2008. 84(3): p. 614–621.

[145] Chen, N., et al., Cell adhesion on an artificial extracellular matrix using aptamer-functionalized PEG hydrogels. Biomaterials, 2012. 33(5): p. 1353–1362.

[146] Gasperini, L., J.F. Mano, and R.L. Reis, Natural polymers for the microencapsulation of cells. J R Soc Interface, 2014. 11(100): p. 20140817.

[147] Elviri, L., et al., Macroporous chitosan hydrogels: effects of sulfur on the loading and release behaviour of amino acid-based compounds. Carbohydr Polym, 2015. 132: p. 50–58.

Chapter 15

Stem Cells for Bone Regeneration: Role of Trophic Factors

Yogambha Ramaswamy, Khoon S Lim,
Hala Zreiqat and Zufu Lu

Additional information is available at the end of the chapter

http://dx.doi.org/10.5772/63357

Abstract

Stem cells play a critical role in tissue regeneration and repair, maintenance and turnover and the control of haematopoiesis in the various tissues. These cells have an incredible ability to differentiate into specific cell types like osteoblasts, chondrocytes or myocytes and to develop bone, cartilage or muscle tissues. Now it is believed that the cells do not differentiate by themselves but rather the secretion of the bioactive (trophic) factors which are responsible for the functional outcome of the tissue. Stem cells reside in complicated and dynamic three-dimensional (3D) microenvironments in vivo known as stem cell niches. The niches are composed of extracellular matrix (ECM), soluble and tethered proteins and supporting cells, which have a profound influence on the functionality of the cells, including differentiation and trophic factor release. In this chapter, we review and emphasize the influence of stem cell microenvironment on the secretion of trophic factors and their perspective application for bone regeneration.

Keywords: bone, stem cells, tissue regeneration, niche, trophic factors

1. Introduction

Bone is a highly vascularized tissue with an intrinsic property to self-repair, regenerate and remodel. It has an excellent ability to heal traumatic injuries (e.g. fractures) without any formation of scars. However, there still exist a number of clinical scenarios where their self-repair and regenerative capabilities fail. Some of the classic examples include large bone defects caused by traumatic injury, infection, tumour resection and skeletal abnormalities due to congenital diseases. Bone-related injuries resulting from these clinical scenarios have significant impacts on the health and lifestyle of individuals. In the USA alone, more than half a million patients experience problems due to bone defects each year, with medical cost associated with these defects being more than $2.5 billion/annum and this figure is expected to double by 2020. It is estimated that about 2.2 million bone graft procedures are performed around the world annually [1–3]. The current strategies used for augmenting bone regeneration include different bone-grafting methods, such as autologous bone grafts and allografts [4]. Autologous bone grafts have relatively successful clinical outcomes; however, donor site morbidity, limited supply and the complicated surgical procedures associated with bone harvests hinder the efficacy of such procedures. On the other hand, allogenic bone grafts are excellent in terms of sourcing large quantities of donor tissue required for treating large bone defects; however, the issues related to immunogenicity, rejection reaction and disease transmission render this treatment less ideal [4, 5]. The shortcomings associated with these treatments have led to exploring tissue engineering approaches and stem cell-based therapies for bone repair.

There is great promise for stem cell-based therapeutics for the treatment of numerous diseases and injuries; as such, substantial investment has been made over the past decade for new therapies. Stem cells play a critical role in tissue regeneration and repair, maintenance, turnover and the control of haematopoiesis in the bone marrow. They are considered as an attractive cell population for bone repair due to their proliferation, osteogenic potential and secretion of potent endogenous trophic factors to enhance local vascularization. These cells have an incredible ability to differentiate into specific cell types like osteoblasts, chondrocytes or myocytes and to develop bone, cartilage or muscle tissues. It is believed that the stem cells can help in repairing the damaged tissue not only by direct differentiation process but also indirectly through the secretion of their bioactive (trophic) factor [6]. In case of any tissue damage, the stem cells can be attracted to the damage site wherein they secrete bioactive factors that can function to trophically assist the repair and regeneration process.

In this chapter, we discuss about the (1) role of the stem cells in bone regeneration and their trophic factors and (2) the influence of stem cell microenvironment on the secretion of trophic factors and their effects on bone regeneration. The stem cell-based therapies using trophic factors may have profound clinical applications.

2. Stem cells and bone regeneration

Bone regenerates through complex and organized biological events of bone induction and conduction. This process involves a number of cell types and molecular signalling pathways in a defined sequence to maximize the repair and regeneration of the skeletal tissue. The organic matrix of the bone tissue is composed of collagen type I fibres (approximately 95%) proteoglycans and numerous non-collagenous proteins (5%) [7]. Non-collagenous proteins participate in the process of matrix maturation, mineralization and may regulate the functional activity of bone cells. Primarily, the functional integrity of bone tissue is maintained by the cell types such as osteoblasts (bone-forming cells) and osteoclasts (bone-resorbing cells).

During the phase of bone formation, the osteoblasts are recruited from mesenchymal stem cells (MSCs) present in bone marrow [8]. On the other hand, osteoclasts are derived from haematopoietic stem cells through committed osteoclast progenitors that fuse to form mature multinucleated cells [9]. The regeneration process occurs through osteogenesis initiated by skeletal stem cell also known as mesenchymal stem cells. During embryogenesis, the development of the skeletal tissue occurs by intramembranous and endochondral ossification. Bone formations begin with aggregation of MSCs to form condensations and within the mesenchymal condensation core; cells differentiate into chondrocytes in endochondral ossification or directly into osteoblasts in the intramembranous bone formation pathway [10]. Therefore, stem cells play a key role in bone regeneration and are considered to have the potential to treat bone defects either through cell-based therapies or tissue engineering. Stem cell-mediated bone regeneration provides a number of potential therapeutic advantages as compared to the use of autograft tissues. As such, therapeutic uses of stem cells are being explored extensively for bone tissue regeneration applications. MSCs and adipose-derived stem cells (ADSCs) have received considerable attention in this regard and have been extensively evaluated for bone regeneration.

Numerous studies in animal models clearly demonstrate that stem cells have the potential to treat critical-sized segmental defects, mandibular defects and effective spinal fusion to name a few. More recently, Liu et al. showed that systemic injection of MSCs into mandibular defects of dogs can increase new bone formation as compared to the defect without any cells [11]. Some clinical reports also suggest that MSCs and ADSCs can be used for treating fractures of the distal tibia, osteonecrosis of the femoral head and maxillary defects [12–16]. Although these results are promising, the efficacy of translating these outcomes into clinical practice at a large scale is still in infancy.

In addition to the cell-based therapies, stem cells are combined with biomaterials and implanted into the defect site and this tissue engineering approach is considered to be a promising strategy to treat bone defects. Numerous small animal studies have shown that treating the bone defects with a combination of biomaterials and MSCs can augment bone regeneration. Human bone marrow MSCs and macroporous calcium phosphate cement were combined and transplanted into critical-sized cranial defects in rats. The constructs generated much more new bone and blood vessels than the control calcium phosphate cement without cells [16]. Porous tantalum rods were implanted with or without autologous bone marrow stromal cells (BMSCs) on hind legs in dogs and the scaffold combined with cells enhanced new bone formation after 12 weeks of implantation [17]. These studies indicate that the combination of scaffolds with stem cells can enhance bone regeneration to greater extent. Likewise, composite scaffolds consisting of polycaprolactone and tricalcium phosphate (TCP) combined with autologous MSCs or recombinant human bone morphogenetic protein 7 was transplanted into critical-sized defects of the long bones of the sheep. The composite scaffold loaded with growth factor and MSCs was able to induce enhanced bone formation, indicating the importance of soluble factor in effective bone regeneration [18]. The osteogenic capability of ADSCs cells in healing critical-size mouse calvarial defects showed that implantation of apatite-coated poly lactic-co-glycolic acid scaffolds seeded with ADSCs can heal critical-size skeletal defects without genetic manipulation or the addition of exogenous growth factors [19, 20]. These animal studies with a combination of scaffolds and stem cells have shown great promise with excellent bone regeneration capabilities; however, translation of these into clinical use is limited. A study by Kawate et al. used a tissue engineering approach and transplanted β-TCP with MSCs and a free vascularized fibula into three young patients with steroid-induced osteonecrosis of the femoral head. Two out of the three patients showed healing of the defect with new bone formation and vascularization within 27 months of implantation. Although these studies with a tissue engineering approach was promising, problems still persist in terms of validating the source of the stem cells, the safety, the cost involved and more importantly understanding the molecular mechanisms involved and these questions has to be addressed before any clinical application can be achieved [21].

3. Stem cell trophic factors

In the recent past, stem cell technology has revolutionized the field of regenerative medicine and has been an attractive platform for the purposes of tissue repairs and cancer treatments. Stem cells are ideal for regenerative purposes due to their multipotentiality and self-renewing capabilities and this concept is fairly well established through many in vitro, in vivo and preclinical studies [22]. These cells play important roles in many biological processes, includ-

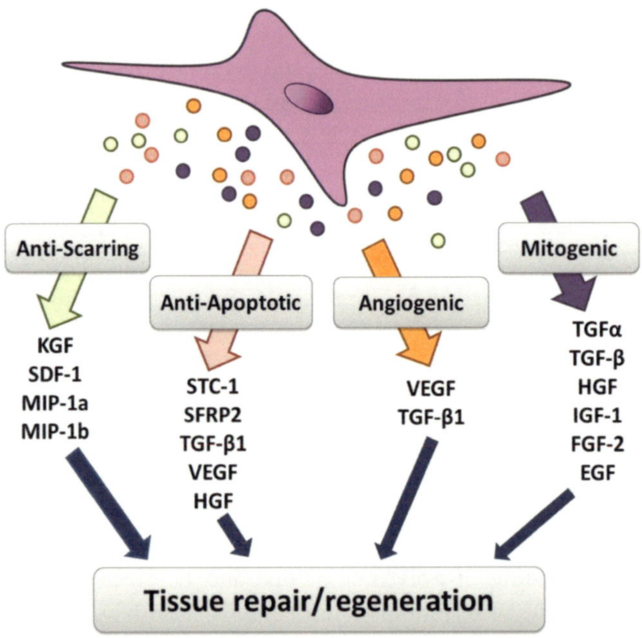

Figure 1. Various paracrine factors released by mesenchymal stem cells which play an important role in mitogenesis, angiogenesis, apoptosis and scarring. Endothelial Growth Factor (EGF), Fibroblast Growth Factor (FGF), Hepatocyte Growth Factor (HGF), Insulin Growth Factor (IGF), Kerotinocyte growth factor (KGF), Macrophage Inflammatory Proteins (MIP), Secreted Frizzled-Related Protein 2, Stanniocalcin-1(STC-1), Stromal cell derived factor (SDF), Transforming Growth Factor (TGF), Vascular Endothelial Growth Factor (VEGF).

ing anti-inflammation, cell migration, proliferation and differentiation, and signal pathway activation or inhibition. There is strong understanding that stem cells (especially MSCs) are able to repair the tissue by modulating the environment they reside, influencing the immune response, supporting angiogenesis, and also through the productive cross talk with the resident cells as illustrated in schematic diagram (**Figure 1**). It is believed that the stem cells may be able to achieve these activities through the secretion of a broad panel of biomolecules called as trophic factors including growth factors, cytokines and chemokines and also the factors released in the extracellular vesicles (exosomes and microvesicles) [23–25]. Therefore, in recent years, researchers have a notion that the secret to the stem cell-based therapy may lie in the stem cell-secreted biomolecules rather than the cell itself as a therapeutic tool. Hence, there is a curious enthusiasm to explore and understand more about these secretion factors in order to enable a switch from use of stem cells to the use of stem cell secretion factors in regenerative medicine [22, 26]. MSCs are reported to secrete a variety of trophic factors such as transforming growth factors (TGF-α and β), hepatocyte growth factor (HGF), epithelial growth factor (EGF), basic fibroblast growth factor (FGF-2), insulin-like growth factor-1 (IGF-1), and vascular endothelial growth factor (VEGF) which induces mitogenesis and angiogenesis and are also anti-apoptotic. Other trophic factors like interleukins, stromal cell-derived factor-1 and prostaglandin 2 are the key immunomodulatory cytokines [6, 25, 27, 28] as illustrated in **Figure 2**. Some fundamental studies have demonstrated that administration of stem cell condition medium containing bioactive factors released by the cells in culture medium can exert regenerative properties. Stem cell-derived secretory molecules has shown some promising tissue-repairing properties in cardiovascular [29], renal [6, 30], liver [31], lung injury [32], and neurodegenerative disease models [22, 33]. Trophic factors secreted by MSCs have induced proliferation of endogenous cardiac progenitor cells in vitro. Nakanishi et al. highlighted that conditioned media from rat MSCs can promote proliferation and migration of isolated cardiac progenitor cells and prevent their apoptosis when subjected to hypoxia and serum starvation [34]. Furthermore, human MSC secretions harvested in conditioned medium, reduced infarct size and preserved cardiac function in a large animal model of myocardial infarction [35]. MSC-conditioned media harvested after 24 h enhanced the paracrine effect and prevented oxygen-induced neonatal lung injury in a rat model [36]. An interesting study by Du et al. showed that MSC-conditioned media could even protect hepatocytes and sinusoidal endothelial cells and stimulate their regeneration in reduced-size rat liver transplantation [37]. The outcomes of this work was well complemented by another study undertaken by Van Poll et al., who provided clear evidence that introduction of MSC-conditioned media in a D-galactosamine-induced rat model of acute liver injury could enhance proliferation of hepatocytes and reduce apoptotic hepatocellular death, thereby increasing the survival rates and preventing hepatic failures [38]. The role of trophic factors in the treatment of chronic kidney disease is well demonstrated by Koppen et al. in a rat model. This study showed that administration of human embryonic MSC-conditioned media decreases the progression of chronic kidney disease with reduced hypertension and glomerular injury indicating the therapeutic benefits of trophic factors for kidney-related injuries and disease [39]. Most of the investigators have shown the beneficial effects of trophic factors from MSCs; however, it is not just confined to these cells alone. Adipose-derived stem cells which are also gaining popularity as an attractive source of cells for regenerative purposes is showing similar properties. Sowa et al. showed that growth factors from ADSCs can promote peripheral nerve regeneration through paracrine secretion of trophic factors regardless of donor age or anatomic site of origin. The effects of mouse ADSCs-conditioned medium were tested on Schwann cells and dorsal root ganglion neurons in vitro. The results showed that ADSCs produced factors which were capable of promoting survival and proliferation of Schwann cells and enhancing the neurite outgrowth in dorsal root ganglion neurons in vitro [40]. Yamada et al. showed that ADSC-secreted molecules could induce a trophic effect in pancreatic islet culture conditions in vitro. These results suggested that trophic factors, particularly VEGF, secreted by human ADSCs enhanced the survival and function of porcine islet cells [41]. These studies suggest that the stem cell trophic factors alone have the potential for therapeutic use and can enhance effects in regeneration. The concept of utilizing the stem cell secretome for tissue repair is undoubtedly a step forward towards cell-free regenerative medicine and the effect of trophic factors in many other types of tissues like bone, ligament and for wound healing purposes is being explored.

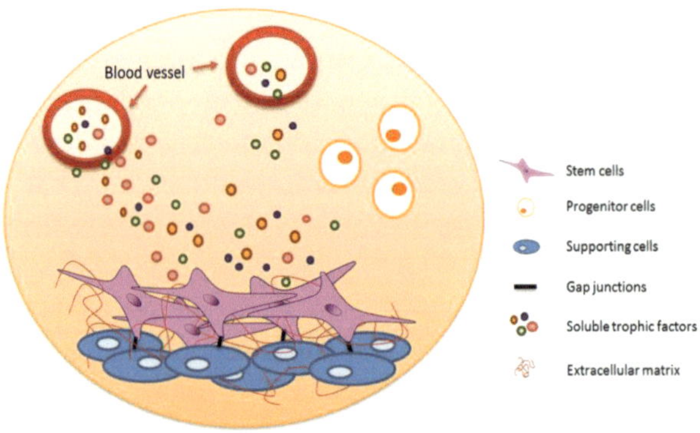

Figure 2. Architecture of the stem cell niche consisting of extracellular matrix, support cells, soluble trophic factors, transmembrane cell adhesion molecules and progenitor cells.

4. Stem cell trophic factors for bone regeneration

So far the use of stem cells in bone regeneration has largely been focussed on either transplanting the stem cells directly to the defect site or through the tissue engineering approaches. However, in recent years, the paracrine effects of stem cells in bone regeneration are being extensively explored and this can have positive implications in the field of bone regeneration. The secretion factors of the stem cells (e.g. MSCs) may have potential therapeutic applications in rheumatoid arthritis, osteoarthritis, genetic bone and cartilage disorders as well as bone metastasis [42]. The secretion factors released from the MSCs during their, osteogenic differentiation process induce recruitment and differentiation of endogenous progenitors. Murine MSCs was cultured in osteogenic medium and the condition media was collected and assessed for its effects on differentiation and migration of exogenous MSCs. The results showed that MSCs maintained in osteogenic medium, secreted factors at specific time points that induced alkaline phosphatase activity in exogenous MSCs as well as their migration thus showing the important contribution of trophic factors in the process of bone repair [43]. A study by Ando et al. showed that MSC-derived trophic factors can accelerate the healing process in distraction osteogenesis. In this study, serum-free conditioned medium derived from human MSCs was locally administered into the distraction gap in a high-speed distraction osteogenesis mouse model. The introduction of the MSC condition media supported the recruitment of murine bone marrow stromal cells and endothelial promoting osteoblast proliferation, differentiation and angiogenesis [44]. The role of trophic factors in treating rheumatoid arthritis is well demonstrated by Ishikawa et al. using dental pulp stem cells (DPSCs). This study showed that delivery of serum-free conditioned media from DPSCs into a collagen type II antibody-induced arthritis mouse model of the rheumatoid arthritis can inhibit inflammation-induced M2-type conditions I and suppress osteoclastogenesis and bone destruction in collagen type II antibody-induced arthritis [45]. An excellent study by Doorn et al. showed that trophic factors from human MSCs can contribute immensely to bone formation. In this study, human MSCs (hMSCs) were treated with small molecule dibutyryl cyclic adenosine monophosphate (db-cAMP) and the condition media was collected. This was used to culture a variety of cells including human umbilical vein endothelial cells, osteosarcoma, breast cancer and mouse myoblast cell line. The treatment of the condition media from cAMP-treated hMSCs to various cells could improve their proliferation and induce osteogenic differentiation with differential effects on migration. This study indicated that the trophic factors secreted by hMSCs can be tuned for a specific application [26, 46]. An in vitro study to investigate the role of brain-derived neurotrophic factor (BDNF) in spinal cord repair has shown that the condition media with the increased levels of BDNF was able to protect the motoneurons and enhance its survival rate, thus indicating the therapeutic benefits the trophic factors can have in the treatments of spinal cord injuries [47].

Furthermore, Cantinieaux et al. also showed the paracrine-mediated actions of bone marrow stromal cells for treating spinal cord injuries. An in vitro and in vivo study was conducted to evaluate the effects of factors released by the bone marrow stromal cells in a spinal cord injury in a rat model. The in vitro studies showed that bone marrow stromal cell-conditioned medium protected the neurons from apoptosis, activated macrophages and also exhibited some proangiogenic properties. Similar beneficial effects of trophic factors from the bone marrow stromal cells condition was also observed in the in vivo studies with histological analysis showing the proangiogenic action and tissue protection effect [48].

In addition, the effect of secretion factors from human umbilical cord-derived mesenchymal stem cells on the osteogenesis of human MSCs has shown to initiate osteogenic differentiation with increased amount of calcium deposit, and upregulation of osteogenic gene expression [49]. These outcomes suggests that stem cell trophic factors may have key solutions for bone repair and regenerations and further mechanistic understanding can reveal their potential for further clinical applications.

5. Stem cell microenvironment: biophysical cues and trophic factors

Stem cells reside in complicated and dynamic three-dimensional (3D) microenvironments in vivo known as stem cell niches where they undergo self-renewal and differentiation. Their function is maintained through an array of complex signals derived from this niche [50–52]. Structurally, the niche is composed of extracellular matrix (ECM), soluble proteins like chemokines, cytokines and growth factors, supporting cells and physical factors. [53, 54]. ECM proteins are the influential components of the niche and they primarily help in maintaining stem cell homoeostasis and direct lineage commitment. ECM forms the vital communication network for transferring the cell signals emanated from soluble and matrix-bound factors and from cell-matrix interactions and the composition of the ECM can govern the fate of the cells considerably [55–57]. This concept is very well demonstrated through the preservation of the decellularized matrix which was able to guide stem cell differentiation into the cell types residing in the tissue from which the ECM was derived. On the basis of these properties, decellularized organs have been used in tissue engineering and for developing cell therapy approaches [58, 59]. ECM parameters are extremely dynamic and are spatially and temporarily controlled during development suggesting that they play a morphogenetic role in guiding differentiation and arrangement of cells. Support cells play an important role in restricting the stem cells to their niche through the cell surface adhesion proteins. The interactions between the stem cells and the support cells are largely governed by cadherin proteins that form adherens junctions. As such, stem cells are able to maintain their stemness and self-renewal when they are in the vicinity of the support cells [60]. Once the cell divides, one daughter cell remains in contact with the support cell and the other migrates from the niche and commits itself to a particular lineage [61]. Recent study by Polisetti et al. provided excellent insights into molecular mechanisms of progenitor cell niche anchorage mediated by integrins-, cadherins- and dystrophin-associated proteins that regulates both stable and dynamic cell-matrix and cell-cell interactions within the limbal niche [62]. Additionally, support cells such as perivascular stromal cells including nestin+ mesenchymal stromal cell (MSC) [63], leptin receptor (Lepr) expressing mesenchymal cell and Mx1+ stromal cells [64] have shown to play vital roles in regulating the functions of hematopoietic cells in bone marrow. Support cells such as osteoblasts were believed to play an important role in preserving the HSCs in a quiescent state and help in their maintenance or just form a niche supportive of early lymphoid progenitors [65, 66]. These studies suggest the importance of support cells in the architecture of stem cell niche which eventually affects the functions of stem cells [67]. Soluble molecules are another important component of the niche besides ECM and support cells and are absolutely critical for directing the stem cell fate. Soluble factors can be in the form of growth factors, cytokines, enzymes, transforming growth factors, bone morphogenic factors and vitamin C to name a few [68, 69]. These factors can be either added to the culture conditions or secreted by the stem cells or the supporting cells in the niche. These factors can then bind to the membrane receptors of the cells and trigger the cell signalling pathways altering the gene expression of the stem cells [61, 70, 71]. Soluble molecules that are prevalent in most of the niches include Wnts, hedgehog proteins, FGF and bone morphogenetic proteins (BMP) . Some of these molecules are key factors in regulating the self-renewal of haematopoietic stem cells. It is well established through many studies that Wnts and hedgehog proteins play a key role in osteogenesis especially in bone formation, maintaining cellular differentiation and regulating the formation of bone and cartilage, whereas FGFs and BMPs have profound impact on the osteoprogenitor differentiation and the regulation of the endochondral and intramembranous ossification [60, 72]. Similarly, soluble growth factors and cell membrane-bound factors such as platelet-derived growth factor (PDGF), TGF-β, VEGF, BMP and Notch signalling have been implicated as having multivariable effects on cardiac development [73, 74]. In recent years, it has been established that the stem cell niche is not just confined to the soluble factors and cell-cell interactions but also to the definable physical and mechanical cues, which influences the decision-making capability of the stem cells. A number of investigators have demonstrated that stem cells have the ability to sense and transduce the physical and mechanical cues. The cues such as mechanical strain, stiffness, shear stress and topography can regulate the fate of the cells. It has been shown that application of mechanical strain can increase proliferation and decrease differentiation in human embryonic cells, which affects the cell alignment in the direction of the strain and also directs the MSCs to myogenic phenotype. It has been shown that MSCs can express high levels of ligament-specific markers under the influence of rotational strain [75–78]. Additionally, the fate of the stem cells can also be influenced by the substrate stiffness. The effect of stiffness on stem cell differentiation has been well demonstrated by numerous investigators and an excellent study by Engler et al. showed that variation in the substrate stiffness can modulate the differentiation of stem cells into various specific lineages such as neuronal, muscle and osteogenic lineages. This lineage commitment was found to depend largely on the elasticity of the substrate [53]. A similar result was highlighted by Saha et al., and Banerjee et al., who showed that changes in the substrate stiffness can present a defining influence on the differentiation of neural progenitor cells with stiff substrates modulating the cells to astrocytes while the softer ones towards neuronal differentiation [79, 80]. Stem cells are also sensitive to the shear stress and this can result in the morphological changes which in turn affects the cell behaviour at the molecular level. A study by Illi et al. showed that shear stress can stimulate the molecular pathways leading to histone modifications in mouse embryonic stem cells resulting in epigenomic regulations [81]. In addition, the shear stress has been shown to affect the differentiation of stem cells into vascular cells. Exposure of stem cells to shear stress increased the expression of endothelial cell-specific markers such as von Willebrand factor and vascular endothelial-cadherin [75]. Topographical cues can also influence various behaviours of the stem cells similar to stress, strain and stiffness. Topographical modifications in the substrate can change the morphological features of the cells which can vary the orientation of the cytoskeletal structure of the cells thus affecting the function of the stem cell fate. Dalby et al. showed the influence of ordered and disordered nanoscale pattern on differentiation of MSCs. This study showed that osteogenesis was more predominant with ordered nanoscale pattern with an increase in the expression of genes responsible for osteogenic differentiation as compared to the disordered pattern [82]. A similar outcome was reported by Zouani et al. who showed that substrates with large nanodepths (100 μm) induced higher osteogenic differentiation as compared to the small depths (10 μm) indicating that stem cells can sense and respond to the topographical changes and regulate their function [83–85].

Such studies have convinced that the mechanical cues can influence the fate of the stem cells; however, the mechanistic insights as to how these cues direct the differentiation of stem cells is just beginning to be unravelled. Stem cells can sense the stiff microenvironment and transduce the signals through the Rho kinase [86, 87], TGF-β [88, 89], Src family kinases [90] and phosphor-tyrosine signalling pathways [91, 92]. Other studies by Dupont et al. and Swift et al. have shown that yes-associated protein and transcriptional coactivator with PDZ-binding motif also have a significant role in regulating the stem cell differentiation mechanism in response to mechanical parameters. While more and more mechanistic data begins to emerge, it is only clear that mechanical cues are potent physical parameters in the regulation of stem cell differentiation [93–96]. The release and beneficial effects of trophic factors from the stem cells will also depend on the microenvironment it is residing in. Changes in the microenvironment with respect to the biological and mechanical cues can affect the release of trophic factors which can have profound implications in their functionality. More studies are now beginning to emerge to decipher these concepts using various artificial platforms. For example, Abdeen et al. studied the combined role of stiffness and matrix protein on the secretory profile of MSCs and their effects on human microvascular endothelial cells. In this work, the conditioned media from MSCs adherent to polyacrylamide hydrogel with controlled matrix rigidity and protein composition was collected and applied to a model angiogenesis assay using HMVECs within Matrigel. The result from this study showed that secretion of the trophic factors was related to a combined effect of stiffness and adhesion protein for directing proangiogenic signalling [97]. Jose et al. pretreated the MSCs with glycine-histidine-lysine (GHK), a peptide fragment of osteonectin and a matrix cellular protein with reported proangiogenic potential. The study revealed a dose-dependent increase in VEGF concentration in media conditioned by GHK-treated MSC, which increased endothelial cell proliferation, migration and tubule formation. This study suggested that microenvironment of the stem cells can have significant influence on the trophic factors and their functionality [98]. Furthermore, Silva et al. showed that the secretome of the bone marrow MSCs were affected when the cells were cultured on fibronectin peptide-modified hydrogels as compared to the unmodified gels and this change in the secretome-induced higher metabolic viabilities and neuronal cell densities [99]. Hoch et al. also showed that cell-secreted decellularized extracellular matrices can preserve the bone-forming phenotype of the differentiated MSC. In this study, osteogenically induced MSCs were cultured on the decellularized matrices and the osteogenic and angiogenic potential was measured after the withdrawal of the induction media. It was found that culturing osteogenically induced MSCs on decellularized matrix can enhance calcium deposition and secretion of proangiogenic factor such as VEGF [100].

It has also been noted that the changes in the microenvironment of the stem cells due to biomolecules can also affect the trophic factors secretion by the stem cells and this can in turn affect the functionality of the cells by our group and others. We have shown that short-term exposure of human osteoblasts to tumour necrosis factor (TNF-α) can promote osteogenic differentiation and also stimulate human osteoblasts to secrete soluble factors that can foster a microenvironment favouring osteogenic differentiation of ADSC [101]. A similar study was performed by Czekanska et al., whereby MSCs were stimulated with interleukin-1β (IL1β), granulocyte-colony stimulating factor (GCSF), stromal cell-derived factor 1 (SDF1) and stem cell factor (SCF) for about 2 h. The results showed that a mere 2-h stimulation could affect the expression of multiple cytokine genes and proteins in MSC significantly. IL1β strongly promoted the secretion of a wide range of proteins with chemotactic, proinflammatory and angiogenic properties, whereas SCF regulated the expression of proteins involved in proliferation, chondrogenesis and ECM regulation. This outcome was clear evidence that the changes in secretome can be directed towards a desired final functional outcome through the selection of the most appropriate cytokine [102, 103].

Through numerous studies reported in the literature, it is quite evident that the stem cell function greatly depends on the architecture of the niche; any physical or biochemical disruption can affect the stem cell function profoundly.

6. Conclusions

Stem cells are in a way considered to be the "building blocks" of regenerative medicine and are believed to possess solutions to many types of injuries and diseases. Enormous amount of research is focussed on deciphering and understanding the functionalities of these cells through the cell-based therapy, through tissue engineering or purely through their paracrine activities.

The idea of "stem cell free regenerative" medicine has undoubtedly captured a great deal of attention in the recent few years. Most studies suggest that the use of stem cells secretory molecules such as trophic factors, microvesicles or exosomes can be advantageous and valuable in the treatment of injuries or diseases compared to the cell-based therapies. There are more to be explored in terms of their mechanisms at a molecular level, the effect of microenvironment on their release, and the long-term effects of these kinds of treatments in an in vivo scenario. Answers to these questions can help in validating cell-free regenerative technology as a potential therapeutic tool.

Author details

Yogambha Ramaswamy[1], Khoon S Lim[2], Hala Zreiqat[1] and Zufu Lu[1*]

*Address all correspondence to: zufu.lu@sydney.edu.au

1 Biomaterials and Tissue Engineering Research Unit, School of AMME, The University of Sydney, Sydney, Australia

2 Christchurch Regenerative Medicine and Tissue Engineering (CReaTE) Group, Department of Orthopaedic Surgery and Musculoskeletal Medicine, University of Otago Christchurch, Christchurch, New Zealand

References

[1] Australian Orthopedic Association, 2014. https://www.aoa.org.au/ accessed on 12/11/15

[2] Amini, A.R., C.T. Laurencin, and S.P. Nukavarapu, *Bone tissue engineering: recent advances and challenges*. Critical Reviews in Biomedical Engineering, 2012. 40(5): p. 363–408.

[3] Marino, J.T. and B.H. Ziran, *Use of solid and cancellous autologous bone graft for fractures and nonunions*. Orthopedic Clinics of North America, 2010. 41(1): p. 15–26.

[4] Dimitriou, R., et al., *Bone: regeneration current concepts and future directions*. BioMed Central, 2011. 9(66): p. 1–28.

[5] Walmsley, G., et al., *Osteogenic differentiation of adipose-derived stromal cells: advancements and future directions for bone tissue engineering*. Science Proceedings, 2016. 3: p. 1–6.

[6] Tsuji, K. and S. Kitamura, *Trophic factors from tissue stem cells for renal regeneration*. Stem Cells International, 2015. 2015: p. 7.

[7] Barrère, F., C.A. van Blitterswijk, and K. de Groot, *Bone regeneration: molecular and cellular interactions with calcium phosphate ceramics*. International Journal of Nanomedicine, 2006. 1(3): p. 317–332.

[8] Logar, D., et al., *Expression of bone resorption genes in osteoarthritis and in osteoporosis*. Journal of Bone and Mineral Metabolism, 2007. 24(4): p. 219–225.

[9] Nakamura, I., et al., *Involvement of αvβ3 integrins in osteoclast function*. Journal of Bone and Mineral Metabolism, 2007. 25(6): p. 337–344.

[10] Deschaseaux, F., L. Sensébé, and D. Heymann, *Mechanisms of bone repair and regeneration*. Trends in Molecular Medicine, 2009. 15(9): p. 417–429.

[11] Liu, X., et al., *Mesenchymal stem cells systemically injected into femoral marrow of dogs home to mandibular defects to enhance new bone formation*. Tissue Engineering Part A, 2013. 20(3–4): p. 883–892.

[12] Liebergall, M., et al., *Stem cell-based therapy for prevention of delayed fracture union: a randomized and prospective preliminary study*. Molecular Therapy, 2013. 21(8): p. 1631–1638.

[13] Mesimäki, K., et al., *Novel maxillary reconstruction with ectopic bone formation by GMP adipose stem cells*. International Journal of Oral and Maxillofacial Surgery, 2009. 38(3): p. 201–209.

[14] Gangji, V., V. De Maertelaer, and J.-P. Hauzeur, *Autologous bone marrow cell implantation in the treatment of non-traumatic osteonecrosis of the femoral head: Five year follow-up of a prospective controlled study*. Bone, 2011. 49(5): p. 1005–1009.

[15] Zhao, D., et al., *Treatment of early stage osteonecrosis of the femoral head with autologous implantation of bone marrow-derived and cultured mesenchymal stem cells*. Bone, 2012. 50(1): p. 325–330.

[16] Chen, W., et al., *Umbilical cord and bone marrow mesenchymal stem cell seeding on macroporous calcium phosphate for bone regeneration in rat cranial defects*. Biomaterials, 2013. 34(38): p. 9917–9925.

[17] Wei, X., et al., *Tantalum coating of porous carbon scaffold supplemented with autologous bone marrow stromal stem cells for bone regeneration in vitro and in vivo*. Experimental Biology and Medicine, 2016. 241: p. 592–602.

[18] Reichert, J.C., et al., *A Tissue Engineering Solution for segmental defect regeneration in load-bearing long bones*. Science Translational Medicine, 2012. 4(141): p. 141ra93.

[19] Cowan, C.M., et al., *Adipose-derived adult stromal cells heal critical-size mouse calvarial defects*. Nature Biotechnology, 2004. 22(5): p. 560–567.

[20] Levi, B., et al., *Human adipose derived stromal cells heal critical size mouse calvarial defects*. PLoS One, 2010. 5(6): p. e11177.

[21] Kawate, K., et al., *Tissue-engineered approach for the treatment of steroid-induced osteonecrosis of the femoral head: transplantation of autologous mesenchymal stem cells cultured with beta-tricalcium phosphate ceramics and free vascularized fibula*. Artificial Organs, 2006. 30(12): p. 960–962.

[22] Bollini, S., et al., *The regenerative role of the fetal and adult stem cell secretome*. Journal of Clinical Medicine, 2013. 2(4): p. 302–327.

[23] Baglio, S.R., D.M. Pegtel, and N. Baldini, *Mesenchymal stem cell secreted vesicles provide novel opportunities in (stem) cell-free therapy*. Frontiers in Physiology, 2012. 3(359.10): p. 3389.

[24] Gallina, C., V. Turinetto, and C. Giachino, *A new paradigm in cardiac regeneration: the mesenchymal stem cell secretome*. Stem Cells International, 2015. 2015(765846): p. 765846.

[25] Lavoie, J.R. and M. Rosu-Myles, *Uncovering the secretes of mesenchymal stem cells*. Biochimie, 2013. 95(12): p. 2212–2221.

[26] Doorn, J., et al., *Therapeutic applications of mesenchymal stromal cells: paracrine effects and potential improvements*. Tissue Engineering Part B: Reviews, 2011. 18(2): p. 101–115.

[27] Maumus, M., C. Jorgensen, and D. Noël, *Mesenchymal stem cells in regenerative medicine applied to rheumatic diseases: Role of secretome and exosomes*. Biochimie, 2013. 95(12): p. 2229–2234.

[28] Murphy, M.B., K. Moncivais, and A.I. Caplan, *Mesenchymal stem cells: environmentally responsive therapeutics for regenerative medicine*. Experimental & Molecular Medicine, 2013. 45(11): p. e54.

[29] Mirotsou, M., et al., *Paracrine mechanisms of stem cell reparative and regenerative actions in the heart*. Journal of Molecular and Cellular Cardiology, 2011. 50(2): p. 280–289.

[30] Cantaluppi, V., et al., *Rationale of mesenchymal stem cell therapy in kidney injury*. American Journal of Kidney Diseases, 2013. 61(2): p. 300–309.

[31] Kuo, T.K., et al., *Stem cell therapy for liver disease: parameters governing the success of using bone marrow mesenchymal stem cells*. Gastroenterology, 2008. 134(7): p. 2111–2121. e3.

[32] Gotts, J.E. and M.A. Matthay, *Mesenchymal stem cells and acute lung injury*. Critical Care Clinics, 2011. 27(3): p. 719–733.

[33] Uccelli, A., et al., *Neuroprotective features of mesenchymal stem cells*. Best Practice & Research Clinical Haematology, 2011. 24(1): p. 59–64.

[34] Nakanishi, C., et al., *Activation of cardiac progenitor cells through paracrine effects of mesenchymal stem cells*. Biochemical and Biophysical Research Communications, 2008. 374(1): p. 11–16.

[35] Timmers, L., et al., *Human mesenchymal stem cell-conditioned medium improves cardiac function following myocardial infarction*. Stem Cell Research, 2011. 6(3): p. 206–214.

[36] Waszak, P., et al., *Preconditioning enhances the paracrine effect of mesenchymal stem cells in preventing oxygen-induced neonatal lung injury in rats*. Stem Cells and Development, 2012. 21(15): p. 2789–2797.

[37] Du, Z., et al., *Mesenchymal stem cell–conditioned medium reduces liver injury and enhances regeneration in reduced-size rat liver transplantation*. Journal of Surgical Research, 2013. 183(2): p. 907–915.

[38] van Poll, D., et al., *Mesenchymal stem cell–derived molecules directly modulate hepatocellular death and regeneration in vitro and in vivo*. Hepatology, 2008. 47(5): p. 1634–1643.

[39] van Koppen, A., et al., *Human embryonic mesenchymal stem cell-derived conditioned medium rescues kidney function in rats with established chronic kidney disease*. PLoS One, 2012. 7(6): p. e38746.

[40] Sowa, Y., et al., *Adipose-derived stem cells produce factors enhancing peripheral nerve regeneration: influence of age and anatomic site of origin*. Stem Cells and Development, 2011. 21(11): p. 1852–1862.

[41] Yamada, S., et al., *Trophic effect of adipose tissue–derived stem cells on porcine islet cells*. Journal of Surgical Research, 2014. 187(2): p. 667–672.

[42] Djouad, F., et al., *Mesenchymal stem cells: innovative therapeutic tools for rheumatic diseases*. Nature Reviews Rheumatology, 2009. 5(7): p. 392–399.

[43] Li, F., N. Whyte, and C. Niyibizi, *Differentiating multipotent mesenchymal stromal cells generate factors that exert paracrine activities on exogenous MSCs: Implications for paracrine activities in bone regeneration*. Biochemical and Biophysical Research Communications, 2012. 426(4): p. 475–479.

[44] Ando, Y., et al., *Stem cell-conditioned medium accelerates distraction osteogenesis through multiple regenerative mechanisms*. Bone, 2014. 61: p. 82–90.

[45] Ishikawa, J., et al., *Factors secreted from dental pulp stem cells show multifaceted benefits for treating experimental rheumatoid arthritis*. Bone, 2016. 83: p. 210–219.

[46] Doorn, J., et al., *Pro-osteogenic trophic effects by PKA activation in human mesenchymal stromal cells*. Biomaterials, 2011. 32(26): p. 6089–6098.

[47] Ritfeld, G.J., et al., *The role of brain-derived neurotrophic factor in bone marrow stromal cell-mediated spinal cord repair*. Cell Transplantation, 2015. 24(11): p. 2209–2220.

[48] Cantinieaux, D., et al., *Conditioned medium from bone marrow-derived mesenchymal stem cells improves recovery after spinal cord injury in rats: an original strategy to avoid cell transplantation*. PLoS One, 2013. 8(8): p. e69515.

[49] Wang, K.-X., et al., *The effects of secretion factors from umbilical cord derived mesenchymal stem cells on osteogenic differentiation of mesenchymal stem cells*. PLoS One, 2015. 10(3): p. e0120593.

[50] Thomson, J.A., et al., *Embryonic stem cell lines derived from human blastocysts*. Science, 1998. 282(5391): p. 1145–1147.

[51] Takahashi, K. and S. Yamanaka, *Induction of pluripotent stem cells from mouse embryonic and adult fibroblast cultures by defined factors*. Cell, 2006. 126(4): p. 663–676.

[52] Watt, F.M. and B.L. M. Hogan, *Out of Eden: Stem cells and their niches*. Science, 2000. 287(5457): p. 1427–1430.

[53] Engler, A.J., et al., *Matrix elasticity directs stem cell lineage specification*. Cell, 2006. 126(4): p. 677–689.

[54] Ward Jr., D.F., et al., *Mechanical strain enhances extracellular matrix-induced gene focusing and promotes osteogenic differentiation of human mesenchymal stem cells through an extracellular-related kinase-dependent pathway*. Stem Cells and Development, 2007. 16(3): p. 467–480.

[55] Brizzi, M.F., G. Tarone, and P. Defilippi, *Extracellular matrix, integrins, and growth factors as tailors of the stem cell niche*. Current Opinion in Cell Biology, 2012. 24(5): p. 645–651.

[56] Peerani, R. and P.W. Zandstra, *Enabling stem cell therapies through synthetic stem cell–niche engineering*. The Journal of Clinical Investigation, 2010. 120(1): p. 60–70.

[57] Discher, D.E., D.J. Mooney, and P.W. Zandstra, *Growth factors, matrices, and forces combine and control stem cells*. Science, 2009. 324(5935): p. 1673–1677.

[58] Gattazzo, F., A. Urciuolo, and P. Bonaldo, *Extracellular matrix: a dynamic microenvironment for stem cell niche*. Biochimica et Biophysica Acta (BBA)-General Subjects, 2014. 1840(8): p. 2506–2519.

[59] Nakayama, K.H., et al., *Decellularized rhesus monkey kidney as a three-dimensional scaffold for renal tissue engineering*. Tissue Engineering Part A, 2010. 16(7): p. 2207–2216.

[60] Lutolf, M.P. and H.M. Blau, *Artificial stem cell niches*. Advanced Materials, 2009. 21(32–33): p. 3255–3268.

[61] Nava , M.M., M.T. Raimondi, and R. Pietrabissa, *Controlling self-renewal and differentiation of stem cells via mechanical cues*. BioMedical Research International, 2012. 2012 p. 797410.

[62] Polisetti, N., et al., *Cell adhesion molecules and stem cell-niche-interactions in the limbal stem cell niche*. Stem Cells, 2016. 34(1): p. 203–219.

[63] Méndez-Ferrer, S., et al., *Mesenchymal and haematopoietic stem cells form a unique bone marrow niche*. Nature, 2010. 466(7308): p. 829–834.

[64] Park, D., et al., *Endogenous bone marrow MSCs are dynamic, fate-restricted participants in bone maintenance and regeneration*. Cell Stem Cell, 2012. 10(3): p. 259–272.

[65] Calvi, L., et al., *Osteoblastic cells regulate the haematopoietic stem cell niche*. Nature, 2003. 425(6960): p. 841–846.

[66] Zhang, J., et al., *Identification of the haematopoietic stem cell niche and control of the niche size*. Nature, 2003. 425(6960): p. 836–841.

[67] Kumar, B., et al., *Exosome-mediated microenvironment dysregulation in leukemia*. Biochimica et Biophysica Acta (BBA)-Molecular Cell Research, 2016. 1863(3): p. 464–470.

[68] Kawaguchi, J., P.J. Mee, and A.G. Smith, *Osteogenic and chondrogenic differentiation of embryonic stem cells in response to specific growth factors*. Bone, 2005. 36(5): p. 758–769.

[69] Zhang, H., et al., *Biomimetic three-dimensional microenvironment for controlling stem cell fate*. Interface Focus, 2011. 1: p. rsfs20110035.

[70] Reilly, G.C. and A.J. Engler, *Intrinsic extracellular matrix properties regulate stem cell differentiation*. Journal of Biomechanics, 2010. 43(1): p. 55–62.

[71] Liu, Z.J., Y. Zhuge, and O.C. Velazquez, *Trafficking and differentiation of mesenchymal stem cells*. Journal of Cellular Biochemistry, 2009. 106(6): p. 984–991.

[72] Arvidson, K., et al., *Bone regeneration and stem cells*. Journal of Cellular and Molecular Medicine, 2011. 15(4): p. 718–746.

[73] Arshi, A., et al., *Rigid microenvironments promote cardiac differentiation of mouse and human embryonic stem cells*. Science and Technology of Advanced Materials, 2016.

[74] Yamashita, J., et al., *Flk1-positive cells derived from embryonic stem cells serve as vascular progenitors*. Nature, 2000. 408(6808): p. 92–96.

[75] Shitiz, K., et al., *Control of stem cell fate and function by engineering physical microenvironments*. Integrative Biology, 2012. 4(9): p. 1008–1018.

[76] Altman, G., et al., *Cell differentiation by mechanical stress*. Faseb Journal, 2002. 16(2): p. 270–272.

[77] Saha, S., et al., *Inhibition of human embryonic stem cell differentiation by mechanical strain*. Journal of cellular physiology, 2006. 206(1): p. 126–137.

[78] Park, J.S., et al., *Differential effects of equiaxial and uniaxial strain on mesenchymal stem cells*. Biotechnology and Bioengineering, 2004. 88(3): p. 359–368.

[79] Saha, K., et al., *Substrate modulus directs neural stem cell behavior*. Biophysical Journal, 2008. 95(9): p. 4426–4438.

[80] Banerjee, A., et al., *The influence of hydrogel modulus on the proliferation and differentiation of encapsulated neural stem cells*. Biomaterials, 2009. 30(27): p. 4695–4699.

[81] Illi, B., et al., *Epigenetic histone modification and cardiovascular lineage programming in mouse embryonic stem cells exposed to laminar shear stress*. Circulation Research, 2005. 96(5): p. 501–508.

[82] Dalby, M.J., et al., *The control of human mesenchymal cell differentiation using nanoscale symmetry and disorder*. Nature Materials, 2007. 6(12): p. 997–1003.

[83] Griffin, M.F., et al., *Control of stem cell fate by engineering their micro and nanoenvironment*. World Journal of Stem Cells, 2015. 7(1): p. 37.

[84] Viswanathan, P., et al., *3D surface topology guides stem cell adhesion and differentiation*. Biomaterials, 2015. 52: p. 140–147.

[85] Zouani, O.F., et al., *Altered nanofeature size dictates stem cell differentiation*. Journal of Cell Science, 2012. 125(5): p. 1217–1224.

[86] Provenzano, P.P. and P.J. Keely, *Mechanical signaling through the cytoskeleton regulates cell proliferation by coordinated focal adhesion and Rho GTPase signaling*. Journal of Cell Science, 2011. 124(8): p. 1195–1205.

[87] Chaudhuri, P.K., et al., *Topography induces differential sensitivity on cancer cell proliferation via Rho-ROCK-Myosin contractility*. Scientific Reports, 2016. 6: p. 19672.

[88] Allen, J.L., M.E. Cooke, and T. Alliston, *ECM stiffness primes the TGFβ pathway to promote chondrocyte differentiation*. Molecular Biology of The Cell, 2012. 23(18): p. 3731–3742.

[89] Horiguchi, M., M. Ota, and D.B. Rifkin, *Matrix control of transforming growth factor-β function*. Journal of Biochemistry, 2012. 152(4): p. 321–329.

[90] Jasaitis, A., et al., *E-Cadherin-dependent stimulation of traction force at focal adhesions via the Src and PI3K signaling pathways*. Biophysical Journal, 2012. 103(2): p. 175–184.

[91] Arnsdorf, E.J., et al., *Mechanically induced osteogenic differentiation–the role of RhoA, ROCKII and cytoskeletal dynamics*. Journal of Cell Science, 2009. 122(4): p. 546–553.

[92] Sun, Y., C.S. Chen, and J. Fu, *Forcing stem cells to behave: a biophysical perspective of the cellular microenvironment*. Annual Review of Biophysics, 2012. 41: p. 519.

[93] Shin, J.-W. and D.J. Mooney, *Improving stem cell therapeutics with mechanobiology*. Cell Stem Cell, 2016. 18(1): p. 16–19.

[94] Ivanovska, I.L., et al., *Stem cell mechanobiology: diverse lessons from bone marrow*. Trends in Cell Biology, 2015. 25(9): p. 523–532.

[95] Dupont, S., et al., *Role of YAP/TAZ in mechanotransduction*. Nature, 2011. 474(7350): p. 179–183.

[96] Halder, G., S. Dupont, and S. Piccolo, *Transduction of mechanical and cytoskeletal cues by YAP and TAZ*. Nature Reviews Molecular Cell Biology, 2012. 13(9): p. 591–600.

[97] Abdeen, A.A., et al., *Matrix composition and mechanics direct proangiogenic signaling from mesenchymal stem cells*. Tissue Engineering Part A, 2014. 20(19–20): p. 2737–2745.

[98] Jose, S., et al., *Enhanced trophic factor secretion by mesenchymal stem/stromal cells with glycine-histidine-lysine (GHK)-modified alginate hydrogels*. Acta Biomaterialia, 2014. 10(5): p. 1955–1964.

[99] Silva, N.A., et al., *Modulation of bone marrow mesenchymal stem cell secretome by ECM-like hydrogels*. Biochimie, 2013. 95(12): p. 2314–2319.

[100] Hoch, A.I., et al., *Cell-secreted matrices perpetuate the bone-forming phenotype of differentiated mesenchymal stem cells*. Biomaterials, 2016. 74: p. 178–187.

[101] Lu, Z., et al., *Short-term exposure to tumor necrosis factor-alpha enables human osteoblasts to direct adipose tissue-derived mesenchymal stem cells into osteogenic differentiation*. Stem Cells and Development, 2012. 21(13): p. 2420–2429.

[102] Czekanska, E.M., et al., *Enhancing inflammatory and chemotactic signals to regulate bone regeneration*. European Cells & Materials, 2014. 28: p. 320–334.

[103] Crowder, S.W., et al., *Material cues as potent regulators of epigenetics and stem cell function*. Cell Stem Cell, 2016. 18(1): p. 39–52.